INJURY-FREE RUNNING

YOUR ILLUSTRATED GUIDE TO BIOMECHANICS, GAIT ANALYSIS, AND INJURY PREVENTION

SECOND EDITION

TOM MICHAUD

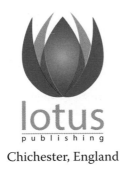

lotus
publishing

Chichester, England

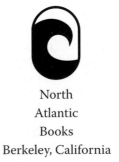

North
Atlantic
Books
Berkeley, California

First published in 2021 by
Lotus Publishing
Apple Tree Cottage, Inlands Road, Nutbourne, Chichester, PO18 8RJ, and
North Atlantic Books
Berkeley, California

Illustrations Tom Michaud
Text Design Medlar Publishing Solutions Pvt Ltd., India
Cover Design Chris Fulcher
Printed and Bound in India by Replika Press

Injury-Free Running: Your Illustrated Guide to Biomechanics, Gait Analysis, and Injury Prevention, Second Edition is sponsored and published by the Society for the Study of Native Arts and Sciences (dba North Atlantic Books), an educational nonprofit based in Berkeley, California, that collaborates with partners to develop cross-cultural perspectives; nurture holistic views of art, science, the humanities, and healing; and seed personal and global transformation by publishing work on the relationship of body, spirit, and nature.

North Atlantic Books' publications are available through most bookstores. For further information, visit our website at www.northatlanticbooks.com or call 800-733-3000.

Medical Disclaimer

The following information is intended for general information purposes only. Individuals should always consult their health care provider before administering any suggestions made in this book. Any application of the material set forth in the following pages is at the reader's discretion and is his or her sole responsibility.

British Library Cataloging-in-Publication Data
A CIP record for this book is available from the British Library
ISBN 978 1 913088 16 3 (Lotus Publishing)
ISBN 978 1 62317 631 0 (North Atlantic Books)

Library of Congress Cataloging-in-Publication Data
Names: Michaud, Thomas C., author.
Title: Injury-free running : your illustrated guide to biomechanics, gait analysis, and injury prevention / Tom Michaud.
Description: Second edition. | Chichester, England : Lotus Publishing ; Berkeley, California : North Atlantic Books, 2021. | Revised edition of: Injury-free running : how to build strength, improve form, and treat/prevent injuries. Newton Biomechanics, 2014. | Includes bibliographical references and index.
Identifiers: LCCN 2020046187 (print) | LCCN 2020046188 (ebook) | ISBN 9781623176310 (trade paperback) | ISBN 9781623176327 (ebook)
Subjects: LCSH: Running--Physiological aspects. | Running injuries--Prevention.
Classification: LCC RC1220.R8 M525 2021 (print) | LCC RC1220.R8 (ebook) | DDC 617.1/027642--dc23
LC record available at https://lccn.loc.gov/2020046187
LC ebook record available at https://lccn.loc.gov/2020046188

CONTENTS

FOREWORD

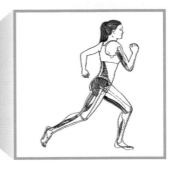

One of the most inspiring scientists and clinicians I know is my good friend running guru Dr. Tom Michaud. He has changed my life, and I share his message in my own book *Run for Your Life*. The first book I read and studied as background was Dr. Michaud's *Human Locomotion*. Evolutionary biology is the foundation of health, and if we understand it, we can better address why one gets ill or injured. We are living in a world mismatched with our genetic code when it comes to how we move, sleep, and eat. Dr. Michaud's approach harks back to our eminent clinicians of the past: Treat every athlete and patient as a puzzle and figure it out. Start with the basics of movement for both running and walking.

Half a century ago, Oregon coach and Nike co-founder Bill Bowerman, in his book *Jogging*, talked about "easy running" as the best way to train the cardiac, respiratory, and circulatory systems. Bowerman also mentioned that for beginners, a walk/run style was ideal. For those who are new to the fitness routine, running is likely to be intense, so walk first; however, as you become more fit, walking will not be strenuous enough. So, in your journey to health, learning the skill of pain-free jogging will pay dividends as you become more fit and can spend more time jogging and less time walking.

The first edition of *Injury-Free Running* is a required text for all my run store employees at

Two Rivers Treads as well as enthusiasts and clinicians of running. In this second edition, Dr. Michaud expands further on the same foundation that Bowerman established and millions of American followed. Bowerman's *Jogging* was a best-seller and sold over a million copies—perhaps that same kind of success awaits Dr. Michaud. In any case, the message for many runners is to slow down, get back to the basics of movement in all facets of your life, and respect your anatomy and physiology.

In the course of my running journey, I have crossed paths with Dr. Michaud many times. At 53 years old, it is never too late for me to learn new things and share them with others. Although slowing now with age and new priorities, I have strung together 30 straight years of sub-three-hour marathons while working full time as a physician and on the side directing races, not to mention owning and managing a small community running retail. Facets of my run store have grown out of what I have learned from Dr. Michaud, including the assessment of foot strength and function as well as strength and movement.

Looking back at these marathons has given me a new perspective on running. In today's culture there is a trend and emphasis on hacks when pursuing the path to success. I agree that for immediate performance enhancement this might be true, but the jury is out if we are talking about long-term health and a lifetime of running. There are also lots of folks who read stuff, write stuff, and make claims as to what is true based on short-term results, but who do not actually run or treat runners, although many are former runners themselves.

The late Dr. George Sheehan often wrote: "We are all an experiment of one." This is true, but I think one must understand the principles of overall health and how to treat the body to keep the experiment going. Since my foot surgeries in 2000, I have read, absorbed, and respected the writings of Dr. Michaud. Most proponents of "pain is gain" cannot produce this type of sustainable performance data with themselves or with any of their clients or athletes. I have not missed a Boston Marathon since 2000 (and have not had any running-related injuries since then either), and despite some years of extreme weather, my times are all consistent with gentle physiological age-related decline. I have finished well over 100 marathons and multiple ultras and haven't "worn my knees out"—a testament to the teachings of Dr. Michaud.

So, what is the "secret sauce" of long-term healthy running?

Since 2015 we have been training the US Air Force Basic Trainees to slow down, get stronger, and move better. "Self-paced runs" used to be efforts where the Airman felt compelled to stay with the lead group or pick a group running faster than they should based on the culture of military fitness, where you must push every day. Runners "stretched" and never learned how to move. The results of this mode of training were off-the-chart musculoskeletal injuries. So, we are reversing this now and teaching the principles of Dr. Michaud, before loading the system with speed and power. After training in this manner, I performed a VO_2 max test on myself at age 50; the result was 65 ml/kg/min, the highest score for any age at the military facility, where they have done over 1,000 tests. When people ask me how I train, I share the principles of Dr. Michaud and thank him for giving me the courage to continue to train this way.

It is everyone's birthright to run. There is something magical about both feet being in the air at the same time. In my community, through our run store, we teach the principles at every "Couch to 5K" and new runner workshop. Smiles go around the room with the release of tension when we dispel the impression that running needs to be painful. So pick up and read this book—it will change your life and the lives of others who wish to live a vigorous life as they age. Thank you, Dr. Michaud.

Mark Cucuzzella MD FAAFP
Professor West Virginia University School of Medicine
LtCol US Air Force (ret.)
Race Director Freedom's Run
DrMarksDesk.com

PREFACE

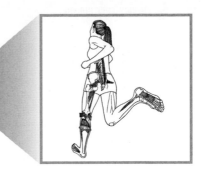

Since the first edition of this book was published in 2013, new techniques for treating and preventing injuries have been developed. More importantly, some amazing new research has proven that there actually is an ideal running form. While previous studies suggested that because runners who are forced to modify their self-selected stride length or cadence become less efficient, it was assumed that runners have an innate ability to choose the ideal running form that is just right for them. The latest research shows that the "runners self-select the best running form" theory just isn't true.

In 2017, scientists from the UK (1) performed a detailed biomechanical and metabolic evaluation on nearly 100 recreational runners and proved that making very specific changes in running alignment can not only make you more efficient but also allow you to run faster. I personally feel that these modifications in running form will also decrease your overall risk of injury. For slower recreational runners trying to remain injury free, a 2019 study showed that switching to a running technique called "ground running" reduces impact intensity by 35% and decreases musculoskeletal loading by 34% (2). Interestingly, switching to ground running from conventional running increases the runners' metabolic rate by 5%, confirming that ground running is an excellent way to both stay fit and avoid injury. Because it takes almost no training to convert from regular running to ground running, you can markedly reduce your risk of injury with little to no effort.

Because parts of this book are moderately technical, Chapter 1 reviews everything you need to know about anatomy, while Chapter 2 explains everything that happens in your body while you walk and run. The importance of storing energy in muscles and tendons, and returning it to them, is always emphasized. Chapter 3 discusses new tests you can do at home to determine your risk of injury, and reviews new techniques for improving tendon resiliency and muscle strength. Not only will the exercise routines outlined in this book help you run faster, but they should also help you avoid injury.

A completely new chapter has been added that explains how to perform an at-home gait analysis. Chapter 4 reviews every aspect of gait analysis, and will walk you through the steps necessary to develop the ideal running style based on your running speed. This is followed by Chapter 5, an updated chapter on running shoes, as over the last five years a range of innovative models have completely changed the industry. Inspired in part by the early minimalist shoes, running shoe manufacturers have developed a wide range of interesting models, from the maximalist Hokas to the ultrafast Nike Alphaflys, which are actually capable of storing and returning energy. You'll learn that unless you're planning on running a marathon in less than two hours, you don't need to spend $250 on a pair of shoes to run fast and/or avoid injury. It turns out that comfort is the key to improving efficiency and remaining injury free.

The last chapter of this book, Chapter 6, has also been modified to reflect the latest research regarding injury prevention, and a few novel treatment protocols have been added. For example, a great study by Sullivan et al. on plantar fasciitis proved that weakness of the toe and peroneal muscles (also known as the "peroneals" or "fibularis muscles") are key in the development of plantar fasciitis (3). Until this paper came out, no one had even considered that weakness in the peroneals played a role in the development of plantar fasciitis. Other interesting studies have demonstrated that runners with retropatellar disorders can get back to running sooner when foot exercises are included in their treatment protocols (4), and that strengthening the soleus may be the key to treating and preventing Achilles injuries. The section on stress fractures details the precise steps you can take to get back to running, and the latest nutritional information is reviewed. A few surprising studies have shown that too much vitamin D can actually weaken your bones (5), and that Keto diets can cause rapid reductions in bone density and should therefore be avoided (6).

It seems like in the last five years more than ever, sports medicine specialists are finally realizing that rather than prescribing nonsteroidal anti-inflammatories and injecting tendons with corticosteroids (which are worse than no treatment at all), the best way to improve performance and avoid injury is by increasing muscle and tendon resiliency, improving neuromotor coordination, finding the ideal running shoe, and developing the precise running form that matches your biomechanical needs. Unlike the elite and recreational runners of the 1980s and 1990s who were treated with medications and ineffective stretches, today's runners have access to state-of-the-art information that, with a little bit of effort, can allow them to run faster and avoid injury for a long time to come.

REFERENCES

1. Folland J, Allen S, Black M, et al. Running technique is an important component of running economy and performance. *Med Sci Sports Exerc.* 2017;49:1412–1423.
2. Bonnaerens S, Fiers P, Galle S, et al. Grounded running reduces musculoskeletal load. *Med Sci Sports Exerc.* 2019;51:708–715.
3. Sullivan J, et al. Musculoskeletal and activity-related factors associated with plantar heel pain. *Foot Ankle Int.* 2015;36:37–45.
4. Molgaard C, Rathleff M, Andreasen J, et al. Foot exercises and foot orthoses are more effective than knee focused exercises in individuals with patellofemoral pain. *J Sci Med Sport.* 2018;21:10–15.
5. Glerup H, Mikkelsen K, Poulsen L, et al. Hypovitaminosis D myopathy without biochemical signs of osteomalacic bone involvement. *Calcif Tissue Int.* 2000;66:419–424.
6. Heikura I, Burke L, Hawley J, et al. A short-term ketogenic diet impairs markers of bone health in response to exercise. *Front Endocrinol.* 2020;10:880.

CHAPTER 1

A REVIEW OF ANATOMY AND THREE-DIMENSIONAL MOTION

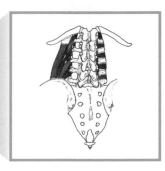

We take it for granted but the process of running around on two legs is an extremely unusual way to get around. Of the more than 4,000 species of mammals on earth today, only one is upright while walking. Even Plato commented on the curious nature of our preferred form of locomotion by referring to humans as the only "featherless bipeds" (there weren't many kangaroos in ancient Greece).

The reason that 99% of animals on this planet prefer using all four limbs while walking and running is that moving around on two legs presents an engineering conundrum: When the foot first hits the ground, the entire limb must be supple in order to absorb shock and accommodate discrepancies in terrain, while shortly thereafter, these same structures become rigid so they can tolerate the accelerative forces associated with propelling the body forward. This is in contrast to quadrupeds, which have the luxury of being able to absorb shock with their forelimbs while their hindlimbs serve to support and to accelerate (picture a cat jumping on and off a ledge).

Shock absorption is particularly important in marathon running, since the feet of long-distance runners contact the ground an average of 10,000 times per hour, absorbing between two and seven times their body weight with each strike. In the course of a marathon, this translates into a force of over 12 million pounds that must be dissipated by the body. Obviously, even a minor glitch in our shock absorption system will result in injury. To make matters worse, the forces associated with accelerating the body forward are even greater than the forces associated with initially contacting the ground.

To understand the complex structural interactions responsible for shock absorption and acceleration, it is important to understand exactly how our joints, muscles, tendons, ligaments, and bones interact while walking and running. Because most runners are not familiar with anatomy and clinical biomechanics, the following section will provide an illustrated review of all the major muscles, tendons, ligaments, and bones associated with running. This review goes down to the cellular level, as understanding how our tissues repair and remodel is the key to preventing injuries and maintaining peak performance (e.g., healthy muscles and tendons store and return energy to enhance efficiency and off load our bones). To make this section easier to understand, the Greek/Latin origins of the names of our muscles and bones are listed. You will see that early anatomists never wanted anatomy to be complicated, as almost all of our muscles and bones are named according to their shape: The piriformis muscle looks like a pear, while the navicular bone resembles a ship.

The anatomy section is followed with a review of the words used to describe three-dimensional motion. At first, terms like "dorsiflexion" and "eversion" may seem complicated, but after hearing them a few times, they will quickly become part of your vocabulary. Last but not least, the final portion of this chapter summarizes what each muscle does while we run and what can go wrong if the muscle is weak and/or tight. All of this information will be covered in greater detail in subsequent chapters.

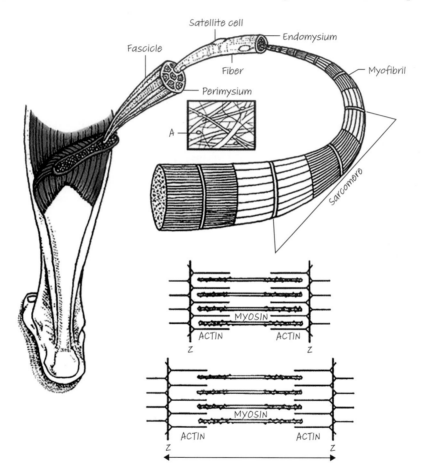

Fig. 1.1. **Muscle anatomy.** *If you take a cross-section of any muscle, you'll see small compartments called "fascicles." Fascicles are visible to the naked eye and can be seen when cutting a piece of steak. Fascicles in turn are subdivided into fibers, which are embedded in connective tissue called the "perimysium." The perimysium is a type of dense connective fascia, which is loaded with a mixture of strong supportive collagen fibers and a stretchable protein called "elastin." The cells inside the perimysium are fibroblasts (**A**), which repair and remodel damaged collagen and elastin fibers. The perimysium is the structure we try to lengthen when getting massages and/or performing foam rolling.*

Attached to the sides of fibers are satellite cells, which rebuild muscle fibers damaged during exercise. As will be discussed briefly, special sensory cells called "spindles" are also attached to the sides of muscle fibers. Spindle cells tell our nervous system exactly how fast and how far each joint is moving, and that information is analyzed to calculate the metabolic cost of each running step and make changes to improve efficiency. Last but not least, fibers are subdivided into myofibrils, which are made of proteins called "actin" and "myosin." These proteins are the motors that drive muscle contraction. New research shows that when muscles are exercised in their lengthened positions (as in the bottom of this illustration), satellite cells kick into gear to accelerate remodeling. This information has been used to design exercises to help improve running performance.

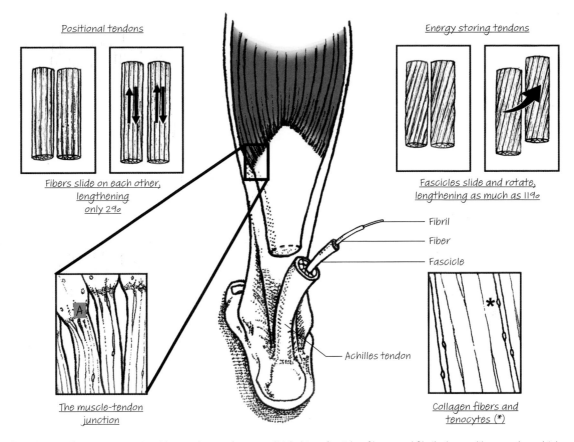

Positional tendons

Fibers slide on each other, lengthening only 2%

The muscle-tendon junction

Energy storing tendons

Fascicles slide and rotate, lengthening as much as 11%

Fibril
Fiber
Fascicle

Achilles tendon

Collagen fibers and tenocytes (*)

Fig. 1.2. Tendon anatomy. *As with muscles, tendons are divided into fascicles, fibers, and fibrils, but unlike muscles, which are almost 80% water, tendons are made of strong parallel collagen fibers, containing very few blood vessels and hardly any water. The limited blood supply and reduced water content allow tendons to function like steel cables: Their parallel fibers of type I collagen can withstand large forces without the slightest damage.*

*When a tendon is injured, small repair cells called tenocytes, located between collagen fibers, rebuild the collagen fibers.

Recent research shows there are two completely different types of tendon: energy-storing tendons and positional tendons. The positional tendons are located where high force output is needed, such as in the muscles of your hips and thighs. When exposed to a stretching force, the small fibers slide back and forth over one another, moving only a small distance. This action allows the force generated by the muscle to then be transferred directly through the tendon to the bone. In contrast, energy-storing tendons, which are located almost exclusively below the knee, are designed with their fascicles angled slightly to one another, allowing them to slide and rotate on one another, and lengthening as much as 11%. This sudden lengthening is extremely important for maintaining running efficiency, as the stretching tendon stores and returns free energy like a bouncing rubber ball.

*The improved storage of energy in, and the return of energy to, the energy-storing tendons explains why the world's fastest marathon runners have the longest Achilles tendons. Elasticity present in energy-storing tendons also prevents injury, as it dampens force that would otherwise go into the muscle. The weak link in the application of force from tendon to muscle is the muscle–tendon junction. This is the most common site of a muscle tear, as the interface between the muscle and the tendon frequently rips (**A** in inset). Just as strengthening muscles in their lengthened positions stimulates muscle repair, strengthening tendons while they are maintained in a stretched position enhances tendon flexibility. Maximizing tendon flexibility is vital for avoiding injury and preventing age-related decreases in running performance because as we age, tendons naturally stiffen, which can be avoided with specific exercises and proper nutrition.*

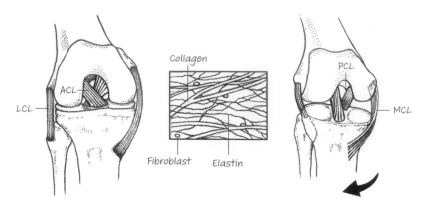

Fig. 1.3. ***Ligament anatomy.*** *While tendons connect muscles to bones, ligaments connect neighboring bones to one another. They are structured similarly to tendons except they contain more elastin fibers, which makes them more flexible (**arrow**). Unfortunately, ligaments are not as strong as tendons and the higher elastin content makes them prone to tearing. (**ACL** = anterior cruciate ligament; **PCL** = posterior cruciate ligament; **LCL** = lateral collateral ligament; **MCL** = medial collateral ligament.)*

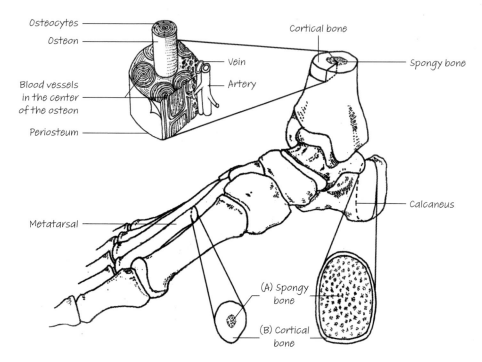

Fig. 1.4. ***Bone anatomy.*** *Bone is comprised of two different types of bony tissue: cortical bone and medullary bone. Cortical bone is also referred to as "compact bone," while medullary bone is also known as "spongy bone." The basic functional unit of cortical bone is the osteon, and it contains small blood vessels running through its core. Sprinkled throughout the osteon are osteocytes, which are important in repairing and remodeling bone. Cortical bone, which is surrounded by the pain-sensitive periosteum, is extremely powerful and resists bending forces like a steel pipe. In contrast, spongy bone is softer and is loaded with small chambers that allow for the production of red blood cells.*

*The ratio of cortical to spongy bone is dependent upon the stresses applied to the bone: Bones that are exposed to high bending forces, such as the metatarsals of your forefoot, are made almost exclusively of cortical bone (**A**). In contrast, bones that absorb shock, such as your calcaneus (**B**), are made primarily of soft spongy bone, which allows them to expand and absorb shock like a cushion.*

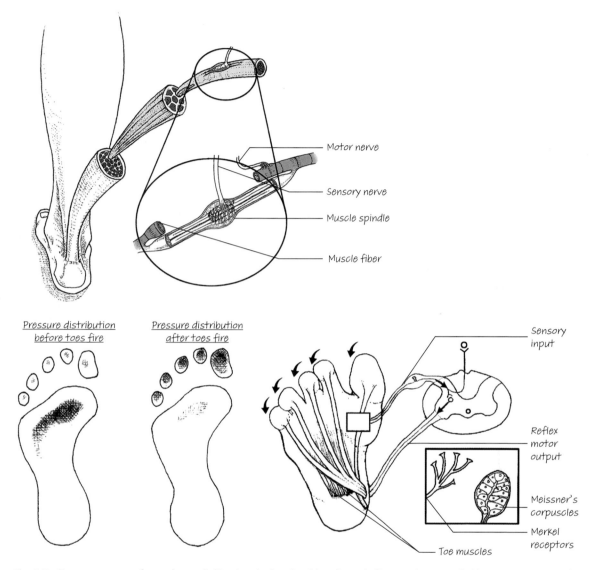

Fig. 1.5. *Sensory nerves of muscles and skin.* *Attached to the sides of muscle fibers and surrounded by epimysium, muscle spindles tell your central nervous system exactly how rapidly your muscles are firing and what they are doing while you are running. Contracture in the perimysium can inhibit information from spindles, increasing the risk of injury. The skin on the bottom of your feet is also important for injury prevention. Special receptors called "Meissner's corpuscles" and "Merkel receptors" provide information regarding the transfer of pressure along bottom of your foot. When too much pressure occurs in one area, the skin receptors fire and produce a reflex contraction of the specific muscles necessary to offload the region receiving excessive pressure. For example, if excessive pressure is centered beneath your forefoot, the skin receptors cause your toe muscles to pull down, thereby redistributing pressure over a broader area (inset). Interestingly, foot massage and mobilization have been shown to increase the sensitivity of sensory receptors in the bottom of your feet, which can improve performance and help prevent injury.*

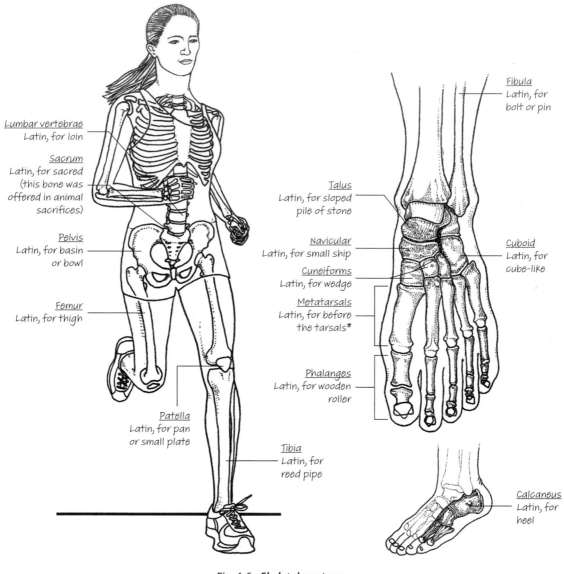

Fig. 1.6. *Skeletal anatomy.*
*The tarsals are all of the foot bones located behind the metatarsals:
the calcaneus, talus, cuboid, navicular, and the cuneiforms. The word tarsals is Latin for flat surface.

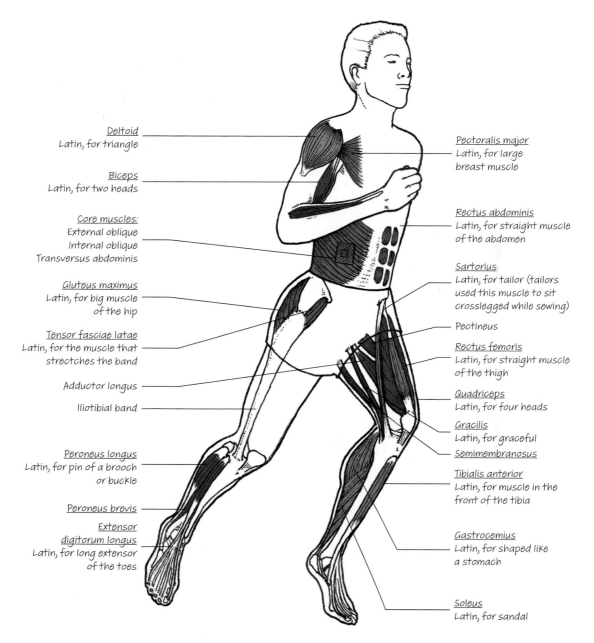

Deltoid
Latin, for triangle

Biceps
Latin, for two heads

Core muscles:
External oblique
Internal oblique
Transversus abdominis

Gluteus maximus
Latin, for big muscle
of the hip

Tensor fasciae latae
Latin, for the muscle that
stretches the band

Adductor longus

Iliotibial band

Peroneus longus
Latin, for pin of a brooch
or buckle

Peroneus brevis

Extensor
digitorum longus
Latin, for long extensor
of the toes

Pectoralis major
Latin, for large
breast muscle

Rectus abdominis
Latin, for straight muscle
of the abdomen

Sartorius
Latin, for tailor (tailors
used this muscle to sit
crosslegged while sewing)

Pectineus

Rectus femoris
Latin, for straight muscle
of the thigh

Quadriceps
Latin, for four heads

Gracilis
Latin, for graceful

Semimembranosus

Tibialis anterior
Latin, for muscle in the
front of the tibia

Gastrocemius
Latin, for shaped like
a stomach

Soleus
Latin, for sandal

Fig. 1.7. *Muscle anatomy (front view).*

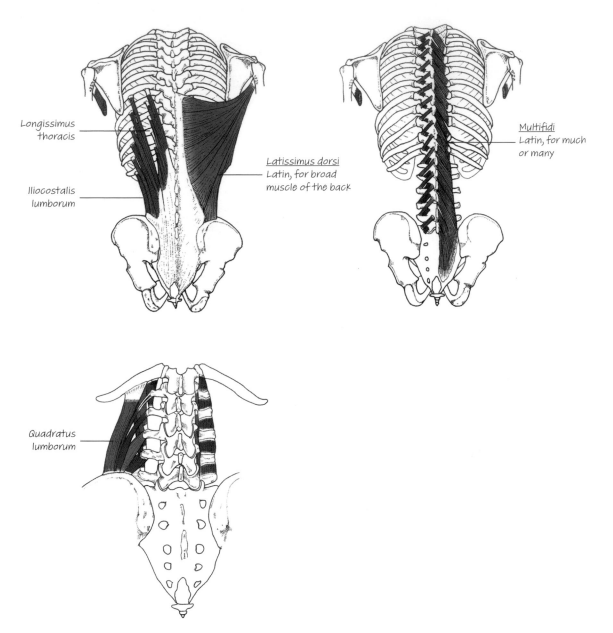

Longissimus thoracis

Iliocostalis lumborum

Latissimus dorsi
Latin, for broad
muscle of the back

Multifidi
Latin, for much
or many

Quadratus lumborum

Fig. 1.8. *Muscles of the back.* *The iliocostalis and longissimus muscles are important while running, since they prevent excessive forward lean of the torso. Collectively, these muscles are referred to as the "erector spinae" (Latin for "erect the spine"). The quadratus lumborum and the multifidi are powerful stabilizers of the spine and are exercised while performing side and conventional planks.*

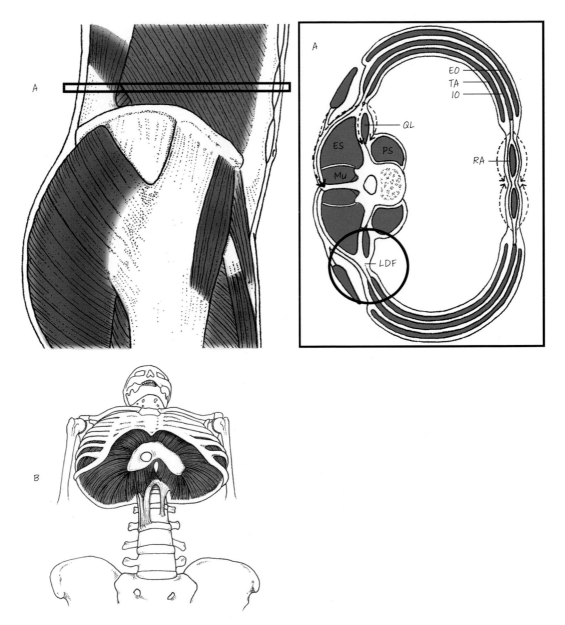

Fig. 1.9. *Core muscles.* *These important muscles wrap around the torso, connecting our rib cage to our pelvis. The force created by the internal oblique (**IO**), external oblique (**EO**), and transversus abdominis muscles (**TA**) gets transferred through the lumbodorsal fascia (**LDF**) to help stabilize the entire lower spine (**A**). Though rarely discussed, the pelvic floor (not shown) and diaphragm (**B**) are also important core muscles. The diaphragm fires with the transversus abdominis to help stabilize the core and plays an important role in running, particularly sprinting. (Muscle abbreviations: **ES** = erector spinae; **Mu** = multifidi; **PS** = psoas; **QL** = quadratus lumborum; **RA** = rectus abdominis [the six-pack muscle].)*

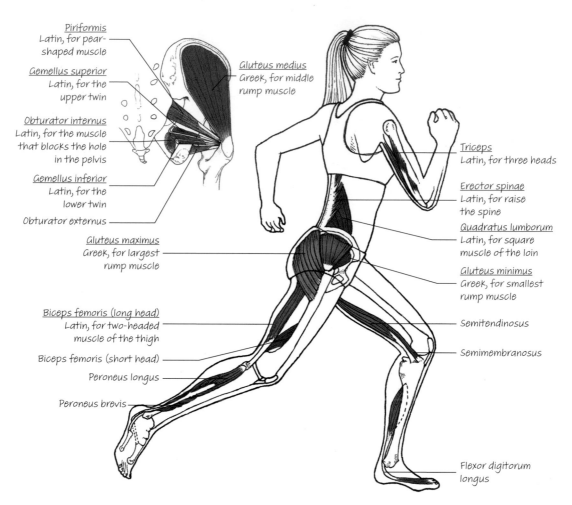

Piriformis
Latin, for pear-
shaped muscle

Gemellus superior
Latin, for the
upper twin

Obturator internus
Latin, for the muscle
that blocks the hole
in the pelvis

Gemellus inferior
Latin, for the
lower twin

Obturator externus

Gluteus maximus
Greek, for largest
rump muscle

Biceps femoris (long head)
Latin, for two-headed
muscle of the thigh

Biceps femoris (short head)

Peroneus longus

Peroneus brevis

Gluteus medius
Greek, for middle
rump muscle

Triceps
Latin, for three heads

Erector spinae
Latin, for raise
the spine

Quadratus lumborum
Latin, for square
muscle of the loin

Gluteus minimus
Greek, for smallest
rump muscle

Semitendinosus

Semimembranosus

Flexor digitorum
longus

Fig. 1.10. *Muscle anatomy (side view).*

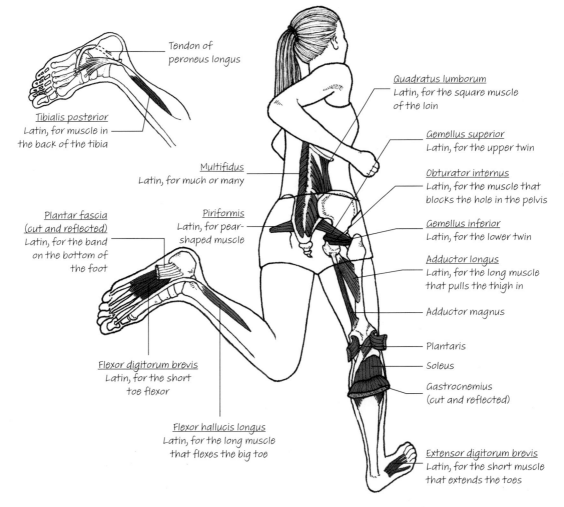

Tendon of
peroneus longus

Quadratus lumborum
Latin, for the square muscle
of the loin

Gemellus superior
Latin, for the upper twin

Obturator internus
Latin, for the muscle that
blocks the hole in the pelvis

Tibialis posterior
Latin, for muscle in
the back of the tibia

Multifidus
Latin, for much or many

Gemellus inferior
Latin, for the lower twin

Plantar fascia
(cut and reflected)
Latin, for the band
on the bottom of
the foot

Piriformis
Latin, for pear-
shaped muscle

Adductor longus
Latin, for the long muscle
that pulls the thigh in

Adductor magnus

Plantaris

Soleus

Gastrocnemius
(cut and reflected)

Flexor digitorum brevis
Latin, for the short
toe flexor

Flexor hallucis longus
Latin, for the long muscle
that flexes the big toe

Extensor digitorum brevis
Latin, for the short muscle
that extends the toes

Fig. 1.11. *Muscle anatomy (back view).*

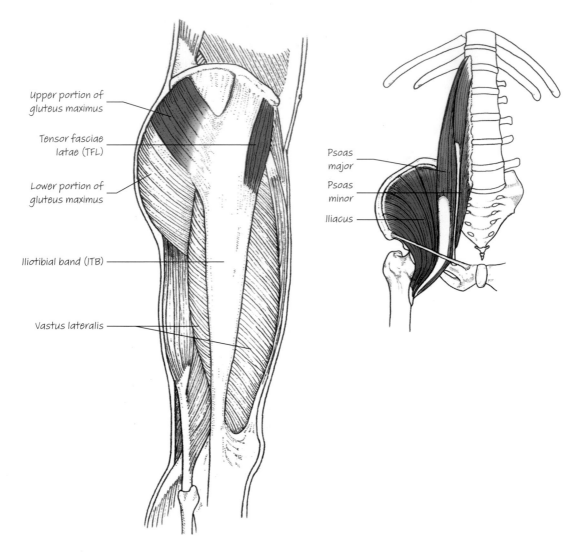

Fig. 1.12. *The iliotibial band (ITB) and the iliopsoas.* *The ITB behaves as a broad tendon that transfers the force generated in the gluteus maximus and tensor fascia latae muscles to the leg and thigh. It has multiple attachments to the femur and plays an important role in preventing the opposite side of your pelvis from dropping too much while you run. The iliopsoas is a powerful hip flexor, and because of its multiple attachments to the lumbar spine, the psoas acts as a spinal stabilizer.*

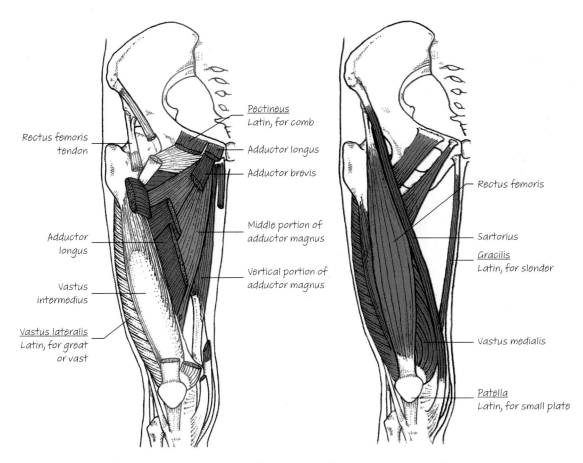

Fig. 1.13. ***Muscles of the front of the thigh.*** *The adductors consist of the adductor longus, adductor brevis, adductor magnus, gracilis, and pectineus. The vertical portion of the adductor magnus is also called the "ischiofemoral portion," since it runs from the ischium of the pelvis to the lower portion of the femur. The quadriceps consist of four different muscles: vastus lateralis, vastus intermedius, vastus medialis, and rectus femoris. The vastus lateralis is by far the largest of these muscles and plays an important role in shock absorption while running. The rectus femoris is the only quadriceps muscle to cross the hip joint, and it is one of the few hip muscles to possess a tendon that rotates appreciably. The rotation of the rectus femoris tendon allows it to store energy while your leg is extended behind you, and return that energy in order to bring your swinging leg forward.*

Located in the quadriceps tendon, the patella is the body's largest sesamoid bone. Sesamoid bones are located inside various tendons all over the body, especially ones requiring high force output. They essentially act to pull the muscle's tendon farther away from the joint's axis of motion, thereby improving the mechanical efficiency of the muscle. Think about a doorknob: If a doorknob is located close to the hinge, it is difficult to open the door. However, as the doorknob moves farther away from the hinge, less force is required to open the door. That's essentially what sesamoids do. Sesamoid is Latin for "sesame seed."

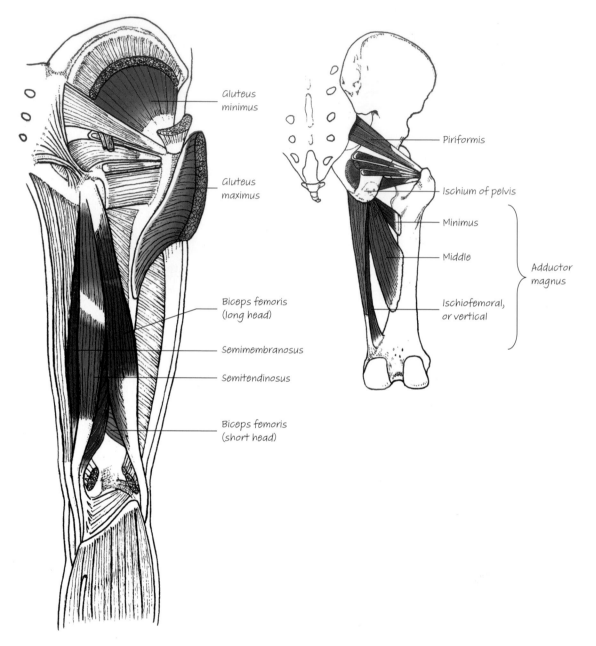

Fig. 1.14. ***Muscles of the back of the thigh.*** *The hamstrings are subdivided into the semimembranosus, semitendinosus, and biceps femoris (which contains a long head and a short head). Because it attaches so low on the femur, the vertical component of the adductor magnus behaves as a hamstring. The hip rotators are also important while running, as they prevent the entire lower limb from twisting inward too much.*

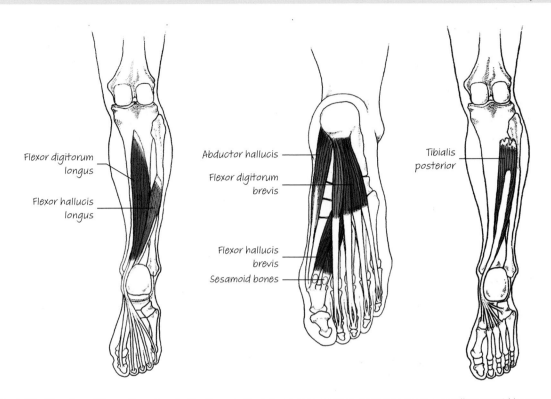

Fig. 1.15. *Muscles of the calf and arch.* *The flexor hallucis brevis is important, as it contains two small sesamoid bones, which often cause problems in runners. Weakness of the muscles of the arch is an extremely common cause of injury: Abductor hallucis weakness correlates with the development of bunions, while a weak flexor digitorum brevis is a common cause of plantar fasciitis. The tibialis posterior plays an important role in supporting the arch, as it possesses numerous attachment points to the center of the arch.*

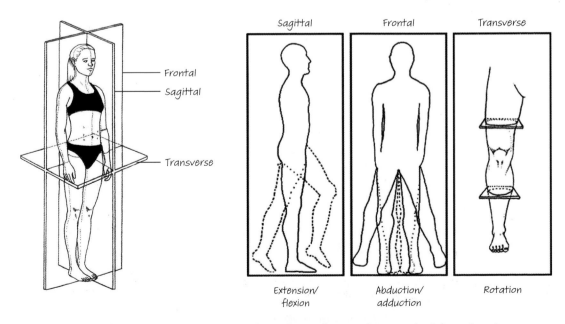

Fig. 1.16. *To describe motion, the body is divided into three reference planes: sagittal, frontal, and transverse.*

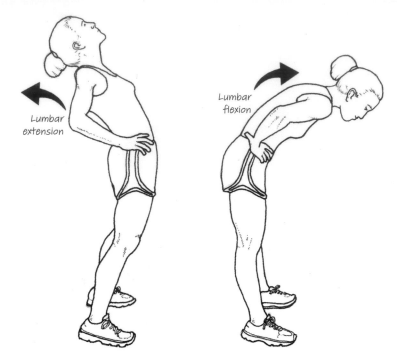

Lumbar extension

Lumbar flexion

Fig. 1.17. *Sagittal plane motion of the spine.*

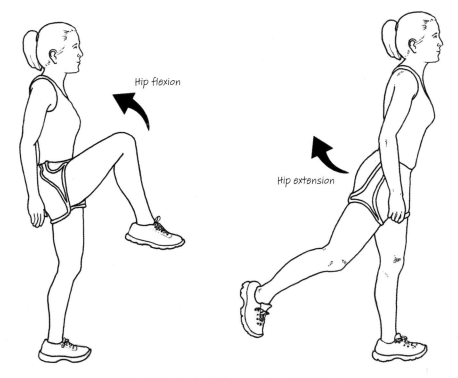

Hip flexion

Hip extension

Fig. 1.18. *Sagittal plane motion of the hip.*

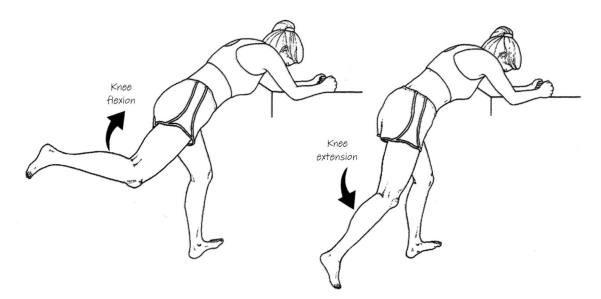

Fig. 1.19. *Sagittal plane motion of the knee.*

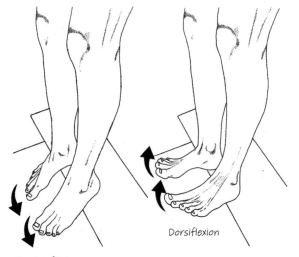

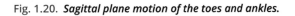

Fig. 1.20. *Sagittal plane motion of the toes and ankles.*

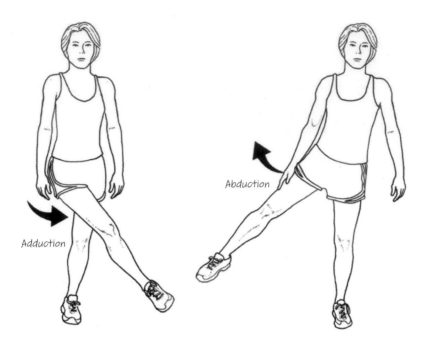

Abduction

Adduction

Fig. 1.21. *Frontal plane motion of the hip.*

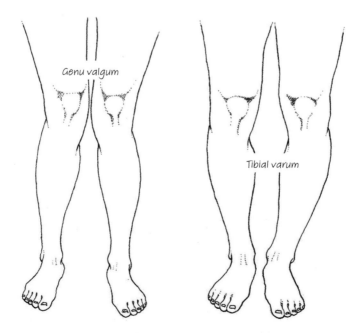

Genu valgum

Tibial varum

Fig. 1.22. *Fixed frontal plane positions of the knees.*

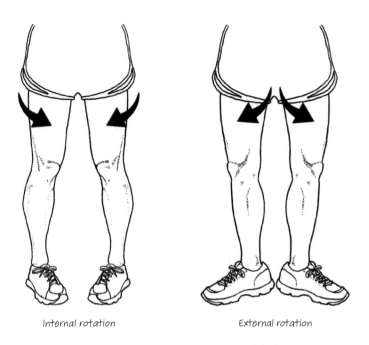

Internal rotation   External rotation

Fig. 1.23. *Transverse plane motion of the hips.*

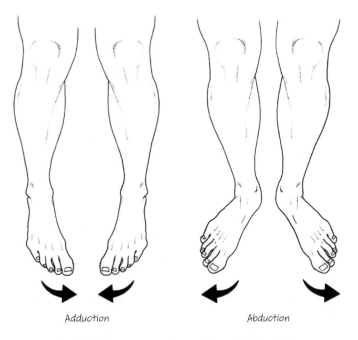

Adduction   Abduction

Fig. 1.24. *Transverse plane motion of the forefeet.*

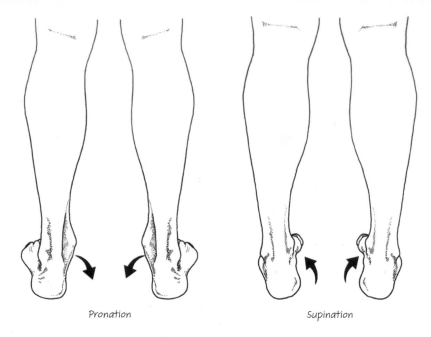

Pronation   Supination

Fig. 1.25. *Pronation and supination occur in all planes and represent lowering and elevation of the arch, respectively.*

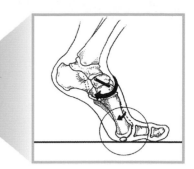

CHAPTER 2

THE BIOMECHANICS OF WALKING AND RUNNING

In order to understand what it takes to be a great runner (and remain injury free), it's important to understand exactly what's going on while we're upright and moving around. To accurately describe the various anatomical interactions occurring while we walk and run, researchers have come up with the term "gait cycle." Traced back to the 13th-century Scandinavian word *gata* for "road or path," one complete gait cycle consists of the anatomical interactions occurring from the moment the foot first contacts the ground until that same foot again makes ground contact with the next step.

The gait cycle consists of two distinct phases: stance phase, in which the foot is contacting the ground; and swing phase, in which the lower limb is swinging through the air preparing for the next impact (Fig. 2.1). Because of the complexity of stance phase motions, this portion of the gait cycle has been subdivided into contact, midstance, and propulsive periods. Although running is also divided into the same three periods, the increased speed and the need for a more forceful propulsive period changes the timing of the events: The contact and midstance periods are slightly shorter, and the propulsive period is longer (Fig. 2.2).

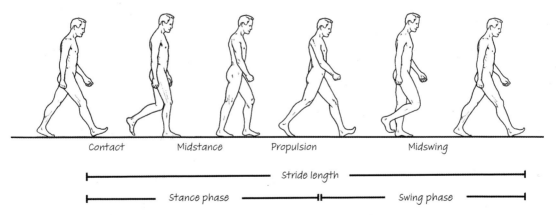

Fig. 2.1. ***Gait cycle of the right leg.*** *Stance phase begins when the heel hits the ground and ends when the big toe leaves the ground. Swing phase continues until the heel again strikes the ground. Stance phase is subdivided into contact, midstance, and propulsive periods. Important components of the gait cycle are step length, stride length, and cadence. "Step length" refers to the distance covered between the right and left foot in a single step, while "stride length" refers to the distance covered by a single foot during the entire gait cycle; i.e., the distance covered during two steps. "Cadence" (or step frequency) is the number of times your feet make ground contact per minute. While walking, the typical person takes 115 steps per minute with an average stride length equal to 0.8 times body height.*

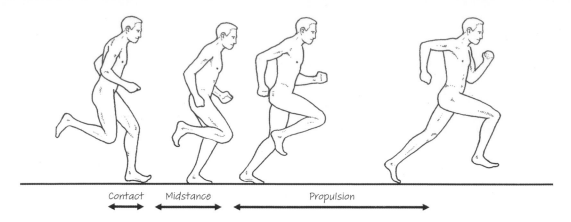

Contact   Midstance   Propulsion

Fig. 2.2. *Stance phase while running.* *Although running is divided into the same phases as walking, there is tremendous variation in stride length and cadence depending upon running speed. While recreational runners have stride lengths of about 6½ feet (2 m) and cadences of 165 steps per minute, the world's fastest marathon runners have stride lengths of more than 10 feet and cadences of around 200 steps per minute. In contrast, Usain Bolt set the world record in the 100-meter sprint by running with a stride length of 16 feet (4.8 m) and a cadence of 265 steps per minute!*

The neurological mechanisms necessary to complete the gait cycle are unusual in that swing phase motions are reflexive and present at birth (e.g., an unbalanced toddler will immediately swing the lower extremity into a protected position), while movements associated with stance phase represent a learned process. This statement is supported with the clinical observation that children born without sight make no spontaneous attempts to stand up and walk on their own and will only do so when physically guided.

As soon as we become toddlers, we begin experimenting with a wide range of walking and running patterns, subconsciously analyzing the metabolic expense associated with each variation in gait. This is a time-consuming process, and perfecting the musculoskeletal interactions necessary to become metabolically efficient can take up to a decade to master. Even when adjusting for size differences, the average three year old consumes 33% more oxygen when traveling at a fixed speed than an adult. By the age of six, children continue to burn more calories while walking and running. Fortunately, by age 10,

mechanical efficiency is equal to that of an adult, and after almost a decade of practice, children are finally efficient at getting around on two legs.

WHAT IS PERFECT RUNNING FORM?

Despite the controversy among coaches as to what constitutes perfect running form (they'll tell you to modify everything from the position of your wrist to the angle of your torso), the actual answer is pretty simple and can be traced back to a 1953 article published in the *Journal of Bone and Joint Surgery* (1). In this article, a team of orthopedic specialists conclude that in order to be efficient, we must learn to "move our center of mass through space along a path requiring the least expenditure of energy." (Located in the middle of the pelvis, the center of mass represents the point about which our bodies would rotate if we were to flip in the air.)

We minimize energy expenditure by modifying the positions of our joints in such a way that the pathway of the center of mass through space is flattened (Fig. 2.3). For example, if we were

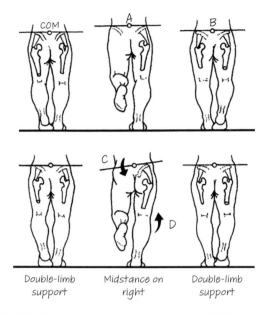

Double-limb support | Midstance on right | Double-limb support

Fig. 2.3. *Movement of the center of mass (COM).* *If we walk with our hips and knees stiff, the COM moves up and down through a large range of motion (compare the height of **A** and **B**). The excessive up-and-down movement of the COM is metabolically expensive because muscles have to work hard to move the COM up and down. By dropping the opposite hip (**C**), flexing the knee (**D**), and moving the ankle, we can keep our COM moving along a straight line.*

to walk with our knees locked and our pelvis stiff (e.g., with a Frankenstein-like gait), the body's center of mass would move up and down through a series of abruptly intersecting arcs, which would significantly increase the metabolic cost of locomotion because specific muscles would tense to accommodate the exaggerated up-and-down motions.

Try taking a few paces mimicking Frankenstein's gait and you will quickly feel yourself accelerate downward before reversing direction and suddenly accelerating upward. The rapid acceleration/deceleration is made more apparent by trying to walk while holding a glass of water: The water in the glass splashes forward the moment the heel strike occurs, and moves backward as you accelerate. The extreme

version of this gait occurs when trying to walk while wearing stilts, when the abrupt transitions between low and high points become more obvious.

Considering the inefficiency associated with excessive up-and-down motions, you would think that the ideal gait would be one in which the pathway of the center of mass was flattened into a straight line: This is often suggested by many running experts who claim the most efficient gait is the one with the least vertical oscillation. The problem is that flattening the progression of the center of mass too much can be just as costly as not flattening it at all. For example, try walking in a manner similar to the comedian Groucho Marx (you can find videos of him walking on *YouTube*). Although excessive flexion of the knees and hips associated with this style of gait will flatten the pathway of the center of mass, it is metabolically expensive because the caloric cost associated with exaggerated knee flexion is high. In fact, research has shown that walking with a "Groucho gait" results in a 50% increase in oxygen consumption (2). Excessive flattening of the pathway of the center of mass accomplished by flexing our limbs explains why small mammals are so inefficient compared to large mammals; e.g., on an ounce per ounce basis, a mouse consumes 20 times more energy than a pony (3).

It turns out that moderately flattening our center of mass allows us to maximize efficiency while walking and running. The catch is that the precise movement patterns we need to incorporate in order to adjust the pathway of our center of mass so that we are maximally efficient change depending upon whether we are walking or running. At slower speeds, we are most efficient when our legs are stiff and inflexible, but at higher speeds, we must increase the degree of knee and hip flexion in order to improve shock absorption. These findings correlate with the clinical observation that walking feels more comfortable when moving slowly, while running is more comfortable as speeds increase.

To determine exactly which gait pattern is most efficient at a specific speed of locomotion (there are hundreds of options regarding the selection of specific joint movements), scientists from the robotics laboratory at Cornell University created a computerized mathematical model to evaluate metabolic efficiency associated with every possible type of gait (including odd patterns such as the Groucho gait), the results of which are published in an article in the prestigious journal *Nature* (4). As expected, at slow speeds of locomotion, walking was most efficient with the knees relatively stiff and nearly locked (remember the quadriceps are expensive muscles to fuel), while at higher speeds, sprinting with an extended airborne phase was most efficient (Fig. 2.4, A and B).

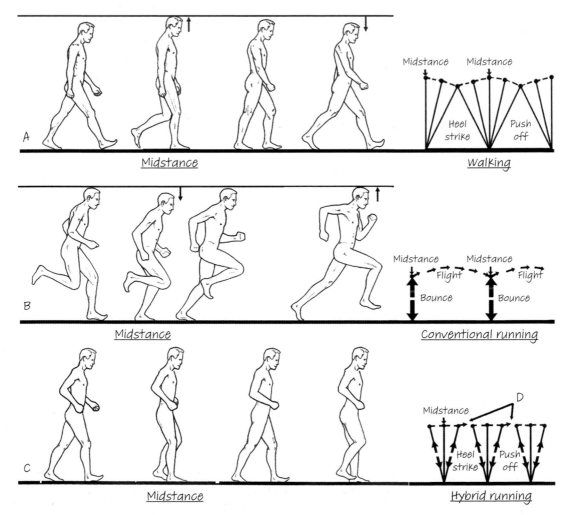

Fig. 2.4. *Walking and sprinting.* *Notice that while walking (**A**), the center of mass is highest during midstance and lowest when both legs are on the ground. When sprint running (**B**), the center of mass is highest during swing phase and lowest during midstance. With hybrid running (**C**), the stride length is shortened, there is a brief airborne phase, and knee stiffness prevents excessive up-and-down movement of the center of mass. As with conventional running, the center of mass reaches its highest point during the airborne phase while hybrid running (**D**).*

HYBRID RUNNING: THE IDEAL RUNNING FORM

The most important result of the computerized model created by the Cornell researchers was that walking and sprint running were only used at the extremes of speed: walking at low speeds and sprinting at high speeds. For all in-between speeds, the computer model suggested that people would choose an intermediate gait referred to as "pendular running." In this gait pattern, which I like to call "hybrid running," the stride length is shortened, the airborne phase is reduced, and the lower limbs are stiff for brief periods during stance phase (Fig. 2.4, C). The stiff legs allow you to efficiently store and return energy associated with subtle up-and-down movements of the center of mass. The lead foot in slow hybrid runners hits the ground only a few inches in front of their center of mass and initial ground contact is made along the outer side of the heel. In contrast, faster hybrid runners cover ground quickly but lose efficiency, as their longer stride lengths require greater knee and hip motions to absorb the significantly increased impact forces (Fig. 2.5).

Unlike sprinting, hybrid running requires metabolic efficiency with minimal displacements of the center of mass. At slow speeds, hybrid runners have short stride lengths (0.9 times their height) and keep their knees stiff at impact. Their knees remain stiff throughout stance phase, flexing only an additional 7° by midstance. With both slow and fast hybrid running, the leg typically strikes within 3° of vertical, and the foot is angled only 5° to the ground.

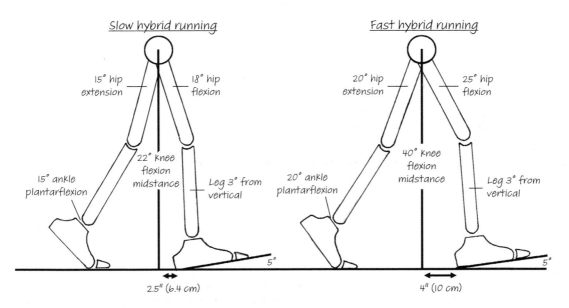

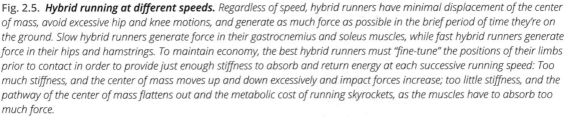

Fig. 2.5. **Hybrid running at different speeds.** Regardless of speed, hybrid runners have minimal displacement of the center of mass, avoid excessive hip and knee motions, and generate as much force as possible in the brief period of time they're on the ground. Slow hybrid runners generate force in their gastrocnemius and soleus muscles, while fast hybrid runners generate force in their hips and hamstrings. To maintain economy, the best hybrid runners must "fine-tune" the positions of their limbs prior to contact in order to provide just enough stiffness to absorb and return energy at each successive running speed: Too much stiffness, and the center of mass moves up and down excessively and impact forces increase; too little stiffness, and the pathway of the center of mass flattens out and the metabolic cost of running skyrockets, as the muscles have to absorb too much force.

In slow hybrid running, the initial point of contact is almost always the outer heel, which makes initial contact only 2½ inches (6.35 cm) in front of the center of mass. This contrasts with fast running, where stride lengths increase to 1.3 times body height, and the initial contact occurs 4 inches (10.15 cm) in front of the center of mass. The world's fastest distance runners make ground contact with the foot more than 12 inches (30.5 cm) in front of the center of mass and have strides lengths greater than twice their height.

Notice in fast hybrid running how the ranges of hip flexion and extension increase (Fig. 2.5), which allows for the longer stride lengths necessary to run fast. To keep the center of mass relatively flat, the knee has to be flexed 40° during midstance while fast hybrid running. Although this illustration makes hybrid running seem complicated, it's actually very simple. *Think of slow hybrid running as a shuffle run in which you generate force by moving your hips in a scissors-like action while moving your knees through a small range of motion. Spend as little time on the ground as possible and focus on rapidly pushing off with your calf muscles to initiate a brief airborne phase. Almost all force associated with slow hybrid running comes from your calves and Achilles tendons.*

Because your stride length is so short, you don't hit the ground very hard, and ground contact is typically made with the outside of the heel, with your foot only a few inches in front of you. To run fast while hybrid running, gradually increase your stride length and try to spend as little time on the ground as possible (you hit the ground like a bouncing ball, rapidly storing and returning energy). Your knees and hips are still moderately stiff but move through larger ranges of motion,

since you have to absorb more impact force as stride lengths increase.

To perform fast hybrid running correctly, your leg must be within a few degrees of vertical when you make initial ground contact, and your hips and knees can't move through excessive ranges of motion. Unlike in slow hybrid running, almost all the force involved in fast hybrid running comes from your hips, quads, and hamstrings (5). The precise form associated with fast hybrid running is described in detail in Chapter 4, where specific drills for learning hybrid running are also reviewed.

Notice that in all of these illustrations, the primary difference between walking and running is that the center of mass is at a low point during midstance when running, and at a high point during midstance when walking. The location of the center of mass during midstance is important because it serves as the only accurate indicator to signal when we transition from walking to running. Unfortunately, the overwhelming majority of running researchers continue to use the presence of an airborne phase as a way to differentiate walking from running. The improper use of the airborne phase to define running was pointed out more than 30 years ago by the Harvard biologist Tom McMahon (6), who noted that slow runners often make contact with their lead foot before their push-off foot has left the ground; i.e., there is no airborne phase. Non-airborne phase running is not uncommon in nature, as ostriches, quails, and gibbons lack an airborne phase while running. In a great paper titled "Running biomechanics: what did we miss?", Shorten and Pisciotta (7) note that 16% of marathon runners lack an airborne phase while running. Non-airborne phase running, also referred to as "ground running," occurs exclusively in slow runners.

GROUND RUNNING: THE IDEAL GAIT FOR INJURY PREVENTION

Given the popularity of running, it's surprising that until recently no one has ever looked into the biomechanics of ground running. In 2019, the first scientific paper on ground running appeared in *Medicine and Science in Sports and Exercise* (8). Bonnaerens et al. took 30 male runners and had them switch from conventional slow airborne, or aerial running to ground running by instructing them to "run without a flight phase." The training protocol was that simple. The researchers then measured a wide range of running parameters, including stride length, cadence, tibial acceleration, metabolic rate, and impact intensity as the runners ran at the same speed (approximately 12.8 minute/mile pace) performing either ground running or conventional airborne running. To get a better idea of how ground running relates to conventional running, the researchers repeated their measurements as runners increased their pace to 8.4 minutes/mile. Table 2.1 summarizes the outcomes of this study. Notice how stride length and cadence are nearly identical in ground running and slow aerial running, but stride length increased from 5⅖ feet (1.6 m) while running slowly to 7⅗ feet (2.3 m) with faster running. The most important finding of this research was that switching from slow aerial running to ground running reduced impact intensity by 35% and musculoskeletal loading by 34%.

Interestingly, runners increased their metabolic rate by 5% by switching to ground running, confirming that ground running is an excellent way to both stay fit and avoid injury. Unlike other gait retraining protocols, switching to ground running is incredibly simple, as runners can transition to ground running with a simple verbal cue: "Run without a flight phase." The researchers emphasize that ground running is an excellent option for older runners, especially if they are overweight or have arthritis. A separate study by Gazendam & Hof showed that nearly one-third of runners prefer ground running over slow aerial running with a flight phase when running slower than a 13 minute/mile pace (9).

Table 2.1. ***Differences between ground running, slow aerial running, and fast running.***

Gait Parameters	Ground Running @ 12.8 min/mile pace	Slow Aerial Running @ 12.8 min/mile pace	Fast Aerial Running @ 8.4 min/mile pace
CADENCE	151	150	163
STRIDE LENGTH	5⅗ feet (1.6 m)	5⅗ feet (1.6 m)	7¾ feet (2.35 m)
STANCE TIME	.39 sec	.32 sec	.25 sec
GRF BW = BODY WEIGHT	1.8 x BW	2.26 x BW	2.57 x BW
MAX TIBIAL ACCELERATION	2.25	3.46	5.72
MAX VILR	32.49	46.73	75.27

*Notice how stride length remains the same for both ground running and slow aerial running, which averages 0.9 times body height (stride length while walking is 0.8 times height). Stride length increased to 1.3 times height while running at an 8.4 minute/mile pace. The significant reductions in ground reaction force, tibial acceleration, and instantaneous load rate explains why ground runners have such low injury rates. (**GRF** = ground reaction force; **Max VILR** = maximum vertical instantaneous load rate.)*

TRANSITIONING BETWEEN DIFFERENT RUNNING STYLES

The various types of gait available during locomotion are made apparent by stepping onto a motorized treadmill and gradually increasing your speed. At first, conventional walking is very comfortable but as you press the button to increase speed, you're quickly unable to match the speed of the treadmill, so you respond by increasing the frequency of your steps (i.e., cadence). Increasing your step frequency is only comfortable for a short time because the metabolic cost of rapidly accelerating and decelerating the lower limbs is too high, so you eventually respond by increasing your stride length. While professional racewalkers are capable of greatly increasing stride lengths by hyperextending their knees and exaggerating pelvic and ankle motions (often achieving walking speeds of 6 minutes/mile), the average person rapidly reaches a length of stride that becomes difficult to maintain. At this point, most people transition into ground running. The precise point at which you will transition into a slow, non-airborne phase run varies, as each person has his or her own unique transition speed (the average transition to running occurs at a little over 4 mph).

The reason each person has a unique transition speed has been the topic of debate until recently. By embedding special sensors into the calf muscles of test subjects while measuring force beneath their forefeet, researchers have determined that people transition into a slow run in order to lessen strain on their gastrocnemius and soleus muscles: As our stride length increases, the muscles in the back of our calves become so overstretched that they are no longer able to generate sufficient force to push us forward (10) (Fig. 2.6).

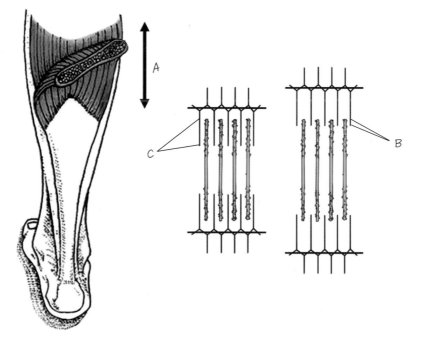

Fig. 2.6. *When the gastrocnemius and soleus muscles are stretched (A), the muscle filaments responsible for creating strength are separated (compare contact areas B and C) and are unable to generate force.*

At this point, and it's slightly different for everyone, we immediately transition into slow hybrid running because the shorter stride lengths associated with non-airborne running allow the calf muscles to work in a more midline position. The fact that an overstretched muscle is unable to generate significant force is apparent while attempting to do a push-up: At first, it feels impossible to lift yourself off the floor, but when you pass the first few inches, the push-up becomes easier because your pectoral muscles are in a more midline position.

Once you've initiated ground running, continuing to increase the speed button on the treadmill will force you to increase your stride length and you will quickly begin slow hybrid running. Impact forces increase and you can feel the strain on your quadriceps as your knees stiffen to flatten the pathway of the center of mass. Although metabolically slightly more expensive, running with an airborne phase allows you to increase your speed simply by increasing your stride length. If you were to accelerate into fast hybrid running and then a full-out sprint, you'd reach an optimal stride length while running at about 80% of full speed, and you'd achieve your fastest possible sprint speed by increasing your cadence after your stride length was maxed out. Remember, legs are heavy and they are metabolically expensive to move back and forth, so you only increase your cadence when you have to; i.e., to reach top sprinting speed. Importantly, by analyzing all methods of increasing the speed of fast running (i.e., increasing stride length, cadence and/or increasing the time you're in the air), Weyand and colleagues (11) determined that the world's fastest runners don't spend more time in the air—they spend less time on the ground and generate more force during that shorter time period. This interesting research confirms that if you want to run faster, you have to generate a lot of force in the very short period of time you're on the ground. The ability to generate explosive force requires strong muscles and flexible tendons.

Since the increased aerial phase associated with fast running results in a fivefold increase in ground reaction force, the body must immediately choose from several different biomechanical options in order to dissipate these amplified forces. For example, the increased impact forces can be dampened by making initial ground contact with the forefoot, lowering the opposite hip, and/or by excessively flexing the knee and hip. The exact combination of biomechanical options chosen is highly variable, as each person has significant differences in strength, bony architecture, and flexibility. Even prior injury may influence which joint movements are incorporated. By experimenting with every biomechanical option, people select a specific running pattern that is metabolically most efficient for them. This explains why runners, unlike walkers, present with such a wide range of running styles. It also explains why any attempt to appreciably modify a runner's self-selected stride length results in a metabolically less efficient gait. According to the exercise physiologist Tim Anderson (12), runners are able to critically evaluate all factors associated with "perceived exertion to arrive at a stride length which minimizes energy cost." It doesn't take long for a runner to learn his or her own ideal stride length, as inexperienced and experienced runners have equally efficient stride lengths.

Because understanding exactly what's going on in the body while running is helpful when trying to figure out the best ways to improve performance and avoid injury, the following sections review the more important biomechanical events occurring during the gait cycle.

STANCE PHASE

While walking is a relatively simple process in which we strike the ground with our heel and smoothly pole vault over our stance phase limb, running presents a greater challenge because of the significantly amplified impact forces. To emphasize the difference between these two activities, if a 150-pound (68 kg) man were to walk one mile (1.6 km), his feet would hit the ground 115 times per minute, impact forces would be 110% of his body weight, and a force of 9.5 tons (8.6 tonnes) would be applied to his feet every 60 seconds. If the same man were to run one mile, his feet would hit the ground 175 times per minute, impact forces would increase to three to five times his body weight, and his feet would have to absorb a force in excess of 52 tons (47 tonnes) of impact force every minute.

Dissipating such large forces is no easy task, and we learn to incorporate nearly every muscle and joint in the body in order to remain injury free. Just before we contact the ground, our body aligns itself so the shock-absorbing muscles are in midline positions (muscles are strongest when neither stretched nor shortened) and each joint is ideally aligned to manage the impending impact. While walking and running slowly, we almost always make initial contact along the outer aspect of the heel, and to keep our stride short, we bend our knees slightly. Fast running is different because in order to run fast, we have to significantly increase our stride lengths. (Remember, sprinters have stride lengths of up to 16 feet (4.9 m).) To produce these long strides while running at full speed, we rotate our pelvis forward, flex our hips and knees through larger ranges of motion, and make initial ground contact with the forefoot. By contacting the ground with the forefoot, we can immediately pull the contact leg back to accelerate us forward.

The biomechanics of sprinting and distance running are very different. Sprinters couldn't care less about efficiency and their only concern is achieving top speeds. Conversely, efficiency is everything to a marathon runner. One of the key distinctions between fast and slow distance runners is that while slow runners almost always make initial contact along the outer side of the heel, fast distance runners will strike the ground pretty much anywhere they want: along the heel, midfoot, or forefoot. Although the reason fast runners choose such varied contact points is unclear, it is more than likely influenced by a variety of factors, including foot architecture, bony alignment, muscle flexibility, and even prior injuries. The perfect example of how bony alignment can influence strike patterns is the great marathon runner Bill Rogers. In order to compensate for a large discrepancy in the lengths of his legs, Bill contacts the ground with the forefoot on the side of the short limb and with the heel on the side of the long limb. The asymmetrical contact points level his pelvis and more than likely reduce his risk of low back injury.

Should You Make Initial Ground Contact with Your Heel, Midfoot, or Forefoot?

Despite the fact that 95% of recreational runners instinctively strike the ground with their heels, many running experts claim that all runners should strike the ground with a more forward initial contact point. Proponents of the more forward contact point suggest that a midfoot strike pattern is "more natural," because experienced lifelong barefoot runners immediately switch from heel to midfoot strike patterns when transitioning from walking to running. The switch to a more forward contact point is theorized to improve shock absorption (lessening our potential for injury) and to enhance the storage in, and the return of energy to, our tendons (making us faster and more efficient). Advocates of Chi and Pose Running have gone so far as to say that runners who continue to strike the ground with their heels are reducing running efficiency and increasing their potential for injury. Something as fundamental as which part of your foot should hit the ground first while running should not be controversial.

To evaluate the effect different foot strike positions has on impact force, researchers from the University of Wisconsin measured foot contact angle and vertical impact forces in 170 healthy NCAA Division I cross-country runners (13). After studying these runners during a variety of running speeds, the authors concluded that impact forces were actually highest in runners who struck the ground with their midfoot, and lowest in runners who struck the ground with their ankles dorsiflexed more than 20° or plantar flexed more than 15° (Fig. 2.7). The authors state: "Encouraging rearfoot strikers to transition to a midfoot strike is very likely to result in an increase, and not a reduction, in loading rate."

In a 2017 literature review examining the merits of the various foot contact points, Joe Hamill and Allison Gruber (14) looked at every published paper addressing the controversy and came to the conclusion that "changing to a mid-or forefoot strike does not improve running economy, does not eliminate an impact at the foot-ground contact, and does not reduce the risk of running-related injuries." Prior research confirms that changing foot contact positions doesn't alter overall force—it just changes which part of the body absorbs the force; e.g., heel strikers absorb more force with their knees, while forefoot strikers absorb more force with their calves. It's the biomechanical version of "nobody rides for free" and explains why heel strikers are more prone to knee pain and why forefoot strikers so often develop chronic plantar fasciitis.

Foot Strike and Metabolic Efficiency at Different Running Speeds

In an important paper published in the *Journal of Experimental Biology*, scientists calculated joint torque, mechanical work performed, and muscle activity associated with altering initial contact points at various speeds of walking and

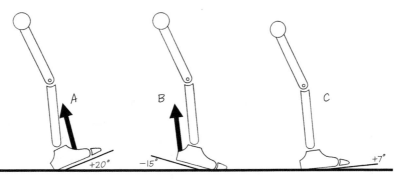

Fig. 2.7. *Runners who strike the ground with their ankles dorsiflexed 20° (A) or plantar flexed 15° (B) have significantly lower impact rates than runners who strike the ground with their ankles near neutral (C).* Note that the reduced impact forces don't necessarily correlate with efficiency, as the tibialis anterior and the gastrocnemius/ soleus muscles work harder to dampen impact forces in **A** and **B**, respectively (**arrows**). Because the hips and knees are far and away the most important shock absorbers, the ability of the foot and ankle to absorb shock is relatively limited.

running (15). The results of this study confirmed that running with a mid/forefoot contact provided no clear metabolic advantage over a heel-first strike pattern. In contrast, walking with a heel-first strike pattern reduced the metabolic cost of walking by a surprising 53%. That's a huge difference in efficiency and explains why almost all recreational runners make initial ground contact with their heels. While some elite runners are efficient while landing on their forefeet, the overwhelming majority of regular runners are more efficient with a heel-first strike pattern.

The big question is, since the world's fastest runners often strike the ground with their forefeet while slow runners strike with their heels, at exactly what speed do you lose the metabolic efficiency associated with heel strike? In a computer-simulated study evaluating efficiency, researchers from the University of Massachusetts showed that while running at a 7:36 minute/mile pace, heel striking was approximately 6% more efficient than midfoot or forefoot striking (16). Some experts believe that the 6 minute/mile pace is the transition point at which there is no difference in economy between heel and midfoot strike patterns.

Given the clear metabolic advantage associated with heel striking at all but the fastest running speeds, it's not surprising that when asked to rate comfort between heel and midfoot strike patterns, recreational runners state that a rearfoot strike pattern is significantly more comfortable (17). Improved efficiency also explains why approximately 35% of recreational runners transitioning into minimalist footwear continue to strike the ground with their heels, despite the amplified impact forces: Heel striking is too efficient to give up (18).

Evolution of the Calcaneus

Our preference for rearfoot strike patterns dates back millions of years, as a laser analysis of the 1.5-million-year-old *Homo erectus* footprints found in Ileret, Kenya, revealed that our most efficient hominid ancestor made initial ground contact with the heel (19). The reason for this is simple: Seven million years of evolution have molded the heel bone (aka the "calcaneus") into a shape that is perfectly suited to absorbing the forces associated with heel strike. One of the most important factors making the heel effective at stress dissipation is its size: The average 100-pound human female has a larger calcaneus than a 350-pound gorilla.

Another factor improving the calcaneus's ability to absorb shock is the somewhat incongruous finding that, despite being exposed to large impact forces during contact, it possesses an extremely thin outer layer of bone (i.e., the cortical bone is paper thin). The inner supporting bone (spongy bone) is also thin, but it is reinforced with an extensive supply of blood vessels that function to assist in the repair of damaged bone. The combination of the thin outer layer of bone and the extensive internal supply of blood vessels results in the formation of a nearly hollow structure that functions like an overblown cushion at heel strike; i.e., the heel expands and contracts like a rubber ball bouncing off the ground. Clinically, the fact that the calcaneus has such a thin layer of cortical bone is helpful when trying to diagnose possible stress fractures in the heel: A light squeeze to the sides of the heel produces significant pain when a stress fracture is present. If the heel's cortical bone were thick (as it is in the vast majority of bones), even a vise-like squeeze would barely be noticed. This simple test can save you or your insurance company about $1,400 on an MRI because the squeeze test is extremely accurate for diagnosing calcaneal stress fractures.

The World's Best Shock Absorber

The final factor making the calcaneus effective at stress dissipation is that it is protected by an incredibly well-designed fat pad. With an average thickness of ¾ inch (19 mm) in the typical adult male, the fat pad of the heel is comprised of spiral chambers of sealed fat surrounded by whorls of fibroelastic material (Fig. 2.8).

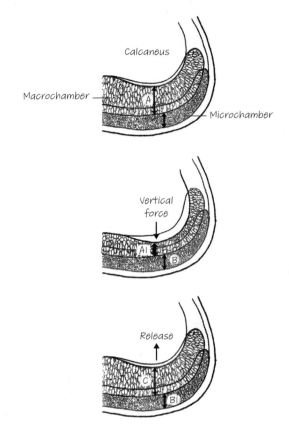

Fig. 2.9. *The normal fat pad is composed of a deep macrochamber and a surface microchamber.* When exposed to impact forces, the macrochamber compresses significantly (compare *A* and *A1*), while the microchamber remains unchanged (compare *B* and *B1*). When impact forces are removed, the macrochamber springs back to its original shape, returning a significant amount of energy.

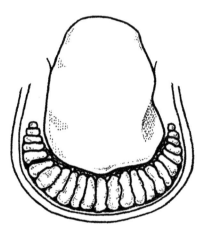

Fig. 2.8. *The calcaneal fat pad.*

Ultrasound evaluation reveals that the fat pad is divided into a deep, thick, highly deformable inner chamber (macrochamber), and a thin, superficial, nondeformable outer chamber (microchamber). Because it maintains its shape upon compression, the outer chamber functions as a protective cup that serves to contain the inner chamber beneath the heel. In contrast, the inner chamber functions as the major shock absorber, quickly deforming and rebounding with the application of force (Fig. 2.9). The heel pad is remarkably effective at absorbing impact forces and was recently shown

to be more than two times better at absorbing shock than Sorbothane, which is considered the most effective commercial shock absorber available.

When you stand upright, the fat pad functions to reduce peak pressure points beneath the heel by distributing pressure evenly over the entire surface of the calcaneus. The heel pad also plays a role in reducing heat loss to the environment. Although I wouldn't recommend it, if you were to run barefoot in the snow for a period of time, you'd realize the heel pad provides significant insulation and reduces heat loss from the body into the ground. The pad is also unusual in that it retains almost all of its shock-absorbing properties even in subzero temperatures. The ability of the heel pad to function in cold environments is due to the higher percentage of polyunsaturated fats present in the pad. Unlike conventional fatty tissue with a polyunsaturated-to-saturated fat ratio of 2.5:1, the typical human heel pad contains 4.5 times more polyunsaturated fats. The increased prevalence of polyunsaturated fat improves function because it reduces heel pad viscosity, allowing the heel pad to be more stable at low temperatures.

Using fluoroscopy and a special optical display, researchers have evaluated exactly how the fat pad functions while we walk (20). During initial contact, the fat pad compresses very rapidly to a deformation of about 40%, dissipating approximately 20% of the forces associated with heel strike. Although effective at dampening forces while walking, the three- to fivefold increase in vertical forces associated with heel strike while running produces a jarring impact capable of damaging the walls of the heel pad chambers. In a study of heel pad compression in barefoot and shod running, researchers from the Netherlands (21) demonstrated that barefoot running produces a 60% deformation of the heel pad, compared to the 35% reduction when wearing running shoes. The reduction with running shoes is comparable to the 40% deformation associated with walking barefoot (20).

The Dutch studies confirm that running while wearing running shoes produces about the same fat pad compression as walking barefoot (an activity the heel pad was designed to tolerate). Conversely, barefoot running, or heel-strike running while wearing minimalist shoes (which often occurs in slow runners), may produce a level of compression capable of permanently damaging the heel pad. Maintaining a healthy heel pad is important because thinning of the heel pad is a proven predictor of chronic heel pain. As our hominid ancestors rarely lived past the age of 35, and more than likely didn't run that much, maintaining the integrity of the heel pad was not much of a concern to them (they had more pressing things to worry about). Since we're currently expected to live into our late 70s (and runners are expected to live up to six years longer), maintaining a healthy heel pad is extremely important for the long-term health of our feet.

Because the forces of running are so great, the degree of shock absorption provided by the heel pad is helpful, but the amplified impact forces associated with running are better managed by our powerful muscles, which actively lengthen to absorb shock. To understand how important muscle lengthening is for absorbing shock, picture yourself catching a fastball with your bare hands: To prevent injury, you reflexively extend your arms while you're about to catch the ball, so your elbows can quickly flex while you're in the process of catching it. Flexing your elbows allows your triceps to absorb shock and reduce the risk of hand injury. The faster the ball is thrown, the more you flex your elbows. Another great example is an egg-catching contest: The farther an egg is thrown, the more the person exaggerates body motions while trying to catch it in order to allow the muscles more time to reduce impact forces on the egg's shell.

Options for Ground Contact

If you choose the heel as your initial contact point, the muscles in the front of the leg assist in shock absorption by slowly lowering the forefoot to the ground (Fig. 2.10).

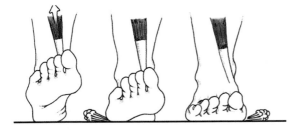

Fig. 2.10. *During the contact period, the muscles in the front of the leg smoothly lower the forefoot to the ground.*

The tibialis anterior is particularly well suited to lowering the forefoot because its muscle architecture is arranged in such a way that it is almost impossible to damage, even with repeated forceful contractions (22).

If a midfoot strike pattern is your preferred contact point, you should strike on the outer side of your midfoot, so the tibialis posterior can slowly lower the inner foot to the ground. This muscle is also specially designed to handle impact forces because its tendon rotates almost 45° before it attaches, allowing it to absorb shock like a spring (23).

Lastly, if a forefoot strike pattern is chosen, the gastrocnemius and soleus muscles slowly lower the heel to the ground, and impact forces are absorbed by the large muscles of the calf. While forefoot contact points are very effective in absorbing shock, the gastrocnemius is not very well designed for lowering the heel to the ground, because it crosses both the ankle and the knee (Fig. 2.11).

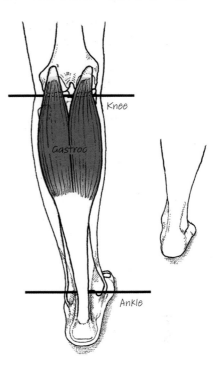

Fig. 2.11. *The gastrocnemius crosses both the knee and the ankle, and has no direct attachment to the tibia.*

Several studies have shown that muscles that cross more than one joint are more likely to be damaged while lengthening under tension (22, 24). The relative weakness of two-joint muscles explains why heel strikers who switch to forefoot contact points frequently complain of delayed onset muscle soreness in their gastrocnemius muscles. Unlike the tibialis anterior, which can tolerate even the most forceful contractions without being damaged, the gastrocnemius is a strong but sensitive muscle and should not be used by slow long-distance runners.

Vibrating Bones

Once impact forces pass the ankle, they travel through the leg toward the knee. By embedding special sensors in the tibia, researchers proved that these forces travel at speeds exceeding 200 mph, creating horizontal oscillations that cause the tibia to vibrate at approximately 40 to 50 cycles per second (23). In order for you to remain injury free, these potentially dangerous vibrations must be dampened.

In an intriguing study of contact forces in horses, researchers determined that when a galloping horse's leg strikes the ground, the impact causes the horse's leg to vibrate rapidly (25). By evaluating all possible ways that horses can dampen these dangerous vibrations, the investigators concluded that the digital flexor muscle plays the most important role in dampening the harmful bony vibrations. The ability of the digital flexor to do anything important came as a surprise because it was previously believed that this muscle was a useless evolutionary remnant of when horses had toes. Also, because the digital flexor has extremely short muscle fibers and a long, thin tendon, it was believed that it was incapable of producing motion. From an evolutionary point of view, it appeared that the digital flexor was slowly disappearing.

It turns out that although useless for creating joint movement, the horse's digital flexor is ideal for dampening bony vibrations, since its short muscle fibers angle sideward to absorb and distribute the bony vibrations that occur upon impact. To understand how this muscle dampens vibration, imagine taking an aluminum baseball bat and striking a metal signpost: The vibrations would be felt through your entire body. Now picture yourself tightly wrapping the bat with a wet towel before hitting the same signpost. The towel would muffle the impact, and the vibrations would be significantly reduced. The wet towel in this analogy does the same thing

the flexor muscle does in horses: It dampens the dangerous vibrations by absorbing them with its short, angled muscle fibers.

In an attempt to understand which muscles dampen vibrations in humans, scientists examined bony oscillations while subjects ran on hard and soft surfaces and compared the results to EMG studies evaluating muscle activation patterns when running on different surfaces (26). Using this elaborate technique, the researchers determined that the lateral head of the gastrocnemius and the outer hamstring muscle (biceps femoris) were the major contributors to dampening the lower extremity vibrations associated with heel strike.

Because impact vibrations occur so quickly following ground contact, reflex muscular activation is unable to provide protection, and the vibration-dampening muscles, to be effective, must be preactivated prior to the foot contacting the ground. This explains the research confirming that running on concrete produces the same bony vibrations as running on dirt: Your body anticipates the increased impact forces associated with concrete, and preactivates muscles to manage the resultant bony oscillations more effectively. Amazingly, animal studies confirm that variation in surface hardness is accommodated by altered muscle function within a single stride length.

The Knee

After impact forces have passed through the tibia, they come upon the knee, which is by far the body's most effective shock-absorbing system. While we walk, the knee is relatively straight and most of the impact force is absorbed by the ankle and hip. In contrast, the impact forces associated with running are so high that the knee often flexes more than 40°. Knee flexion allows the quadriceps to absorb force, as these muscles rapidly lengthen under tension. The role of the quadriceps while running is similar to the role the triceps play when catching a fastball: As soon as the ball hits their glove, the catcher flexes their elbows, allowing force that would otherwise go into the hand to go into the triceps.

Interestingly, not all of the quadriceps muscles absorb force equally. Using specialized shear wave ultrasonography, researchers from Hong Kong demonstrated that the outer portion of the vastus lateralis lengthens to absorb force more than any of the other quadriceps muscles. If the vastus lateralis is tight, it is unable to effectively absorb force by lengthening, causing a significant amount of pressure to be transferred into the kneecap and patellar tendon. This important paper explains why foam rolling your outer quadriceps muscles before running is so important, and why a tight vastus lateralis correlates with the development of patellar tendinopathy (27).

To improve the ability of the entire quadriceps muscles to absorb shock, the body incorporates a large bone, the patella (aka the "kneecap"), directly inside the quadriceps tendon. As mentioned in Chapter 1, the patella belongs to a group of bones called "sesamoids," which are strategically positioned inside tendons to improve mechanical efficiency by pulling the tendon farther away from the joint's axis of motion (Fig. 2.12). Unlike conventional sesamoid bones, which tend to be small and oval (*sesamoid* is Latin for "sesame seed"), the patella is broad and flat (*patella* is Latin for "small

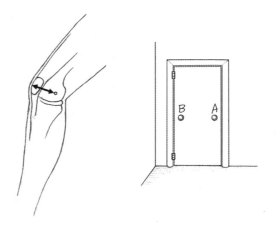

Fig. 2.12. ***The patella belongs to a group of bones called "sesamoids," which move tendons farther away from their joint's axis of motion (double arrow).*** *Moving the tendon farther away from the axis of motion improves efficiency because the muscle now works through a longer lever arm. The classic example of this is the standard doorknob. Because the typical knob is located farther away from the hinges (**A**), it doesn't take a lot of force to open the door. In contrast, it takes significantly more force to open the door when the doorknob is located close to the hinges (**B**).*

plate"). By some estimates, the patella improves efficiency of the quadriceps by more than 50%.

As the knee flexes, contact points on the back of the patella constantly shift (Fig. 2.13). When peak flexion occurs while running, pressure is distributed along the middle portion of the patella, an area possessing the thickest cartilage in the body.

To help the quadriceps absorb shock at peak knee flexion, the body actually shifts the knee's axis of motion ⅜ inch (9.5 mm) backward at the precise moment the knee reaches maximum flexion while running (Fig. 2.14).

This sudden shifting of the axis was proven in an interesting study in which researchers evaluated the knee's axis of motion as subjects ran through specially designed MRIs (28).

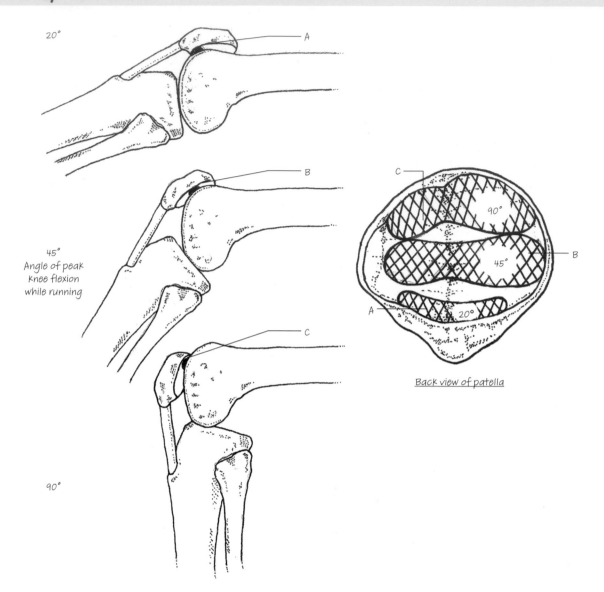

Fig. 2.13. ***When the knee is straight (A), the patella has minimal contact with the femur.*** *When the knee is bent 45° (**B**), the center of the patella contacts the femur. With the knee bent 90° (**C**), the upper portion of the patella contacts the femur. At angles greater than 90°, the outer portions of the kneecap contact the femur. Note that the cartilage in area **B**, which is the area of peak knee flexion while running, possesses the thickest cartilage in the body.*

The rapid and completely unexpected shift of the knee's axis of motion temporarily increases the quadriceps' lever arm at the exact moment that peak knee flexion occurs while running. Although only reported in one study, this amazing shifting of the axis prevents countless injuries by lessening the strain on the quadriceps at just the right time.

The Hip

While not as important as the knee for absorbing shock, the hip, with its powerful muscular support and significant surface area, also contributes appreciably to dampening impact forces associated with running. At slower speeds of running, the gluteus medius plays

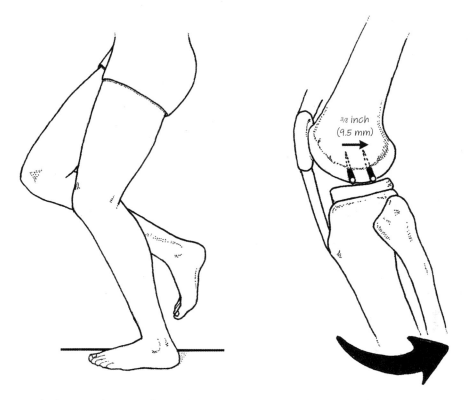

Fig. 2.14. *Just as the knee reaches peak flexion during stance phase, the knee's axis of motion rapidly displaces ⅜ inch (9.5 mm) backward.*

an important role by smoothly lowering the opposite pelvis to the ground (Fig. 2.15). This method of shock absorption is not that effective, and as speeds of running increase, the gluteus maximus plays a more important role in both absorbing shock and providing stability. Interestingly, the gluteus maximus is almost completely inactive while walking but fires vigorously while running.

Because the gluteus maximus controls movement in all three planes of motion, it functions to prevent lowering of the opposite hip (i.e., assisting the gluteus medius) while simultaneously decelerating hip flexion and inward rotation of the thigh (Fig. 2.16). These latter actions are essential for absorbing shock and preventing inward collapse of the knee while running.

Although not essential for shock absorption, the piriformis and lower gluteus medius muscles play a key role in protecting the femoral neck from fracturing. While most orthopedic surgeons claim the piriformis is vestigial and unimportant while running, the paleoanthropologist Owen Lovejoy proved otherwise. After meticulously reconstructing Lucy's pelvis from more than 40 pieces, Lovejoy confirmed the piriformis and gluteus medius muscles function to create a compressive force along the entire femoral neck that prevents it from bending (Fig. 2.17).

In fact, the piriformis and gluteus medius are so effective at reinforcing the femoral neck that modern humans possess significantly less cortical bone than either Lucy or a

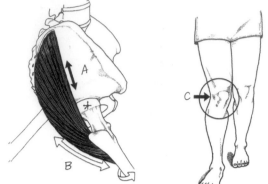

Fig. 2.16. *Because the gluteus maximus is such a large muscle, its upper fibers assist the gluteus medius in keeping the pelvis level (A), while its lower fibers prevent the knee from turning inward (B).* By limiting inward rotation, the gluteus maximus plays an important role in protecting the knee from excessive inward collapse (**C**).

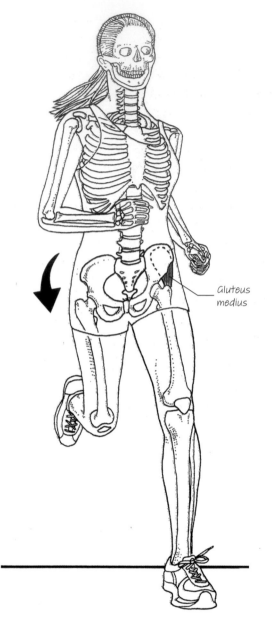

Gluteus medius

Fig. 2.15. *At slow speeds of running, the gluteus medius improves shock absorption by lowering the opposite pelvis toward the ground (arrow).*

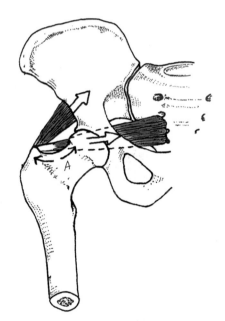

Fig. 2.17. *The piriformis and gluteus medius muscles create a powerful compressive force that prevents the femoral neck (A) from fracturing.*

modern chimpanzee (Fig. 2.18). (Lovejoy used this fact to prove that Lucy was only occasionally upright.)

Since stress fractures of the upper femoral neck are notorious for progressing into full-blown

fractures, maintaining strength in the hip abductors and external rotators is essential for the well-being of the hip. After reading Lovejoy's article, I began treating femoral neck stress fractures with the piriformis and

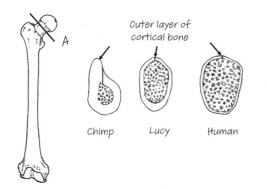

Fig. 2.18. ***Cross-sections through the femoral neck (A) in chimpanzees, Lucy, and modern humans.*** *Because the piriformis and gluteus medius muscles in Lucy and in modern humans prevent the femoral neck from bending, the cortical bone in their femoral necks is extremely thin compared to chimpanzees*

gluteus medius exercises illustrated in Fig. 2.19 and have had great results. Unfortunately, many orthopedic surgeons continue to cut the piriformis from its attachment in an attempt to reduce compression of the sciatic nerve. (Because the piriformis sits on top of the sciatic nerve, excessive tension in this muscle can cause sciatica in runners.) Surgical sectioning of the piriformis can have disastrous consequences for the long-term health of the femoral neck.

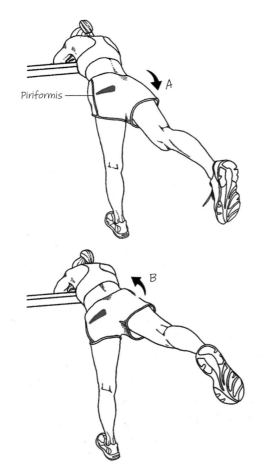

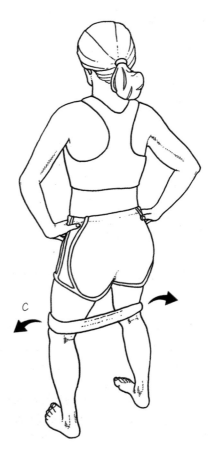

Fig. 2.19. ***While standing on the involved leg, use your piriformis to raise and lower the opposite hip (arrows A and B).*** *Another exercise is to wrap a TheraBand around your lower thighs and move your knees in and out (**arrows** in **C**).*

The Sacrum and Lumbar Spine

Once past the hip, impact forces travel through the sacroiliac joints into the sacrum and lumbar spine. Compared to the sacrum of a chimpanzee, the past seven million years of evolution have formed our sacrum into a keystone-shaped structure that becomes more stable with the application of impact forces (Fig. 2.20).

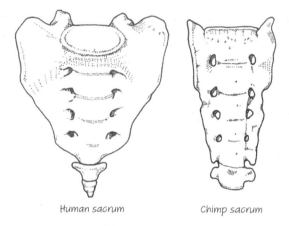

Human sacrum   Chimp sacrum

Fig. 2.20. *Compare the keystone-shaped human sacrum with the rectangular chimpanzee sacrum.*

The sacrum has also changed in that there has been a marked increase in the surface area of the sacroiliac joint, which allows this joint to assist in shock absorption more effectively (Fig. 2.21).

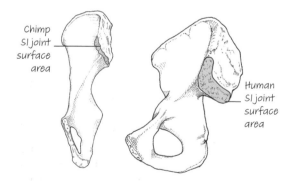

Chimp SI joint surface area

Human SI joint surface area

Fig. 2.21. *The surface area of the sacroiliac joint in chimpanzees is greatly reduced compared to the human sacroiliac joint (shaded areas).*

Notice in Fig. 2.22 that when the foot hits the ground, the pelvis extends backward while body weight causes the sacrum to rock forward. This subtle shifting allows the ligaments of the sacroiliac joint to absorb energy during early stance and to uncoil to return this energy when we go into the propulsive period.

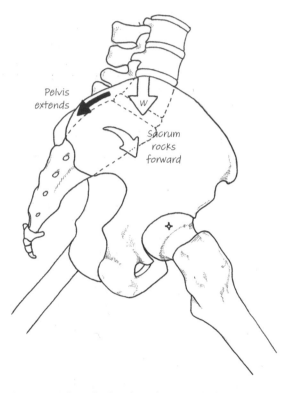

Pelvis extends

W

Sacrum rocks forward

Fig. 2.22. *When the foot hits the ground while running, the weight of the spine (W) causes the sacrum to rock forward (white arrow) while the pelvis extends back (black arrow).* This subtle action is important for shock absorption and protects the lower discs from excessive impact forces.

To stabilize the sacroiliac joint and assist in the storage of energy, our outer hamstring muscle tenses just before we strike the ground. In addition to reducing bony vibrations, tensing the outer hamstring muscle increases tension on the sacrotuberous ligament, which plays an important role in limiting the degree to which the sacrum rocks forward (Fig. 2.23).

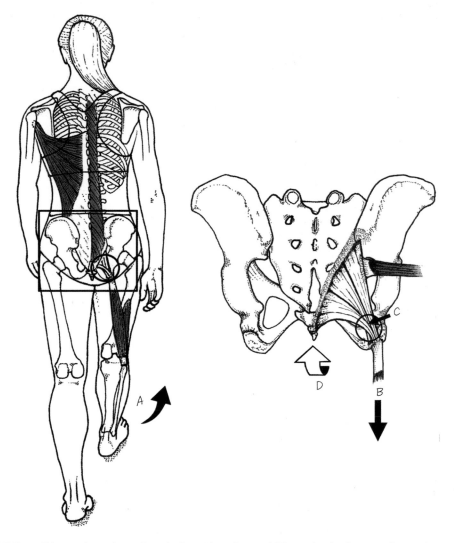

Fig. 2.23. *While walking and running, when the leg swings forward (A), tension in the outer hamstring muscle (B) pulls on the sacrotuberous ligament (C), which stops the sacrum from rocking forward excessively (D).*

Recent dissections of this important ligament show that it spirals in a spring-like manner to effectively control movement of the sacrum.

After being slightly dampened by the sacroiliac joint, impact forces enter the lumbar spine. Just as the sacrum has widened to tolerate the forces associated with walking and running, the lumbar spine has also evolved to manage the forces associated with running by becoming gradually wider when moving from top to bottom

(Fig. 2.24). The greater surface areas present in the lower vertebrae allow for improved pressure distribution.

To enhance shock absorption following ground contact, the lumbar spine quickly bends forward, allowing the back muscles to absorb shock by lengthening. In a comparable way to the quadriceps absorbing shock while the knee flexes, decelerating spinal flexion allows the back muscles to dampen impact forces by

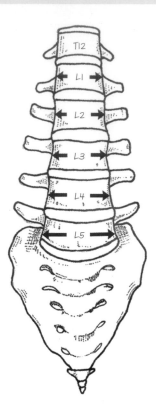

Fig. 2.24. *The lumbar vertebrae become gradually wider when moving toward the bottom of the lumbar spine (L1 to L5).*

absorbing energy as they lengthen. In a study in which spinal motions (flexion, rotation, and side bending) were evaluated at different speeds of locomotion, the degree of spinal flexion present following initial ground contact increased in a linear manner with speed, while rotation and side bending remained unchanged (emphasizing the importance of a slight forward bend to the spine following impact) (29).

In a different study, evaluating efficiency in runners, researchers determined that the most economical runners made ground contact with the spine flexed forward 5.9°, while the least efficient runners made ground contact with the spine almost vertical (30). Although most coaches suggest you make ground contact

with a straight spine, maintaining a slightly flexed spine at impact appears to be advantageous, both for improving shock absorption and for increasing efficiency.

Contrary to popular belief, the discs of the lumbar spine play almost no role in shock absorption. As discussed in his textbook *Low Back Disorders: Evidence-Based Prevention and Rehabilitation*, Stuart McGill points out that because intervertebral discs are composed of a contained liquid, they are unable to absorb shock, since a contained fluid does not compress (31). According to McGill, it is the end plates of the vertebral bodies, not the discs, that absorb shock while running, by rapidly bulging inward with the application of impact forces. Dissections of vertebral bodies confirm that the end plates are made from extremely thin bone (i.e., less than 1/50 in. [0.50 mm] thick) that rapidly deforms with the application of impact forces (Fig. 2.25). The inward bulging allows the upper and lower portions of the vertebral bodies to absorb shock like a trampoline, while the heights of the intervertebral discs remain unchanged.

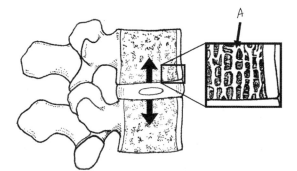

Fig. 2.25. *Side view of the lumbar vertebrae, demonstrating how the thin vertebral end plates bulge in and out (arrows), allowing impact forces to be absorbed by the specially designed bone present inside the vertebral bodies (inset).* The bone inside the vertebral bodies contains long vertical supports (**A**) that bend with the application of impact forces.

When properly functioning, the lumbar spine is remarkably resistant to the forces associated with running. In fact, McGill claims that it is almost impossible to herniate a disc while running, since almost all disc injuries occur when the lumbar spine is flexed forward. I've noticed that if a runner does present with a herniated disc, it is more likely to have occurred while doing a kettlebell workout in a CrossFit class than while running long distances.

The Midstance Period

With forces associated with the contact period absorbed, the runner begins a brief midstance period. Throughout this period, the body attempts to hold onto the energy absorbed during initial contact in order to return it during the propulsive period. By some estimates, the storage and return of energy during midstance reduces the metabolic cost of running by as much as 40%.

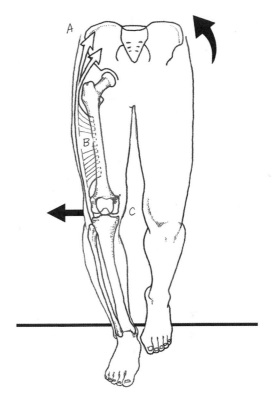

Fig. 2.26. *Different actions of the iliotibial band (see text).*

The ITB and a Level Pelvis

In the hip, the iliotibial band (ITB) plays a role in storing energy by preventing the opposite pelvis from dropping (Fig. 2.26, A). The ITB uses this stored energy to protect the thigh and knee from the bending strains present during midstance: A recently discovered band of connective tissue extends from the ITB to reinforce the femur. This extensive soft tissue support creates a compressive force that stops the femur from bending (Fig. 2.26, B).

Though rarely included in rehab programs, femoral shaft stress fractures in runners should be treated with aggressive strengthening exercises for the gluteus maximus and tensor fasciae latae muscles. By protecting the femoral

shaft from bending, the iliotibial band functions in a manner similar to the way the piriformis protects the femoral neck from bending.

Because the ITB crosses the knee, it also creates a protective compressive force that stops the knee from bowing inward (Fig. 2.26, C). The band is so effective at reducing the inward bow of the knee that individuals with inner knee arthritis rarely complain of pain as long as the muscles controlling the ITB are strong.

The Hips as Motors and the Legs as Springs

While the ITB plays a role in storing energy and providing stability, the muscles of the hip are really designed to be the body's force generators: They possess long powerful muscle fibers with short inelastic positional tendons that allow for maximum force generation. In contrast, the muscles of the foot and leg are perfectly designed to store and return energy because they possess short, angled muscle fibers and long, flexible energy-storing tendons that stretch with the application of force (see Fig. 1.2).

When you run, the muscles of the hip generate force, while the energy-storing tendons of the foot and leg act like large rubber bands that store and return energy. Prosthetic researchers took advantage of this knowledge when creating the artificial legs used by Paralympic athletes (Fig. 2.27). Because the prosthetic limbs possess the perfect degree of flex, they absorb force generated by the hips by bending during early stance and return the force by springing back during late stance. Creating the perfect limb requires tuning the degree of flex so forces are absorbed and returned at just the right time.

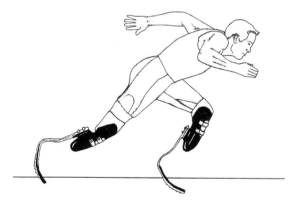

Fig. 2.27. *Prosthetic limbs on a Paralympic athlete.*

The muscles and ligaments of the human foot and leg are also designed to absorb and return energy generated by the hip. Although counterintuitive, muscle lengths present in the foot and leg during midstance remain relatively unchanged, while the corresponding tendons stretch and rebound back through significant

ranges, comparable to the prosthetics used by Paralympic athletes. The nearly isometric contraction of muscles allows tendon elasticity to perform most of the work, while muscle activity is significantly reduced (saving precious calories).

By placing special sensors in the muscles and tendons of turkeys and evaluating them as they ran on treadmills, researchers from Brown University confirmed that even though the turkeys' joints moved through large ranges while they ran, there was little change in the lengths of the muscles (32). In contrast, the tendons of the turkeys were shown to move through large ranges, stretching and recoiling back to return stored energy. In fact, certain tendons were so efficient that they were able to return 93% of the work performed while stretching them. Interestingly, animal studies also confirm that the capacity of tendons to store and return energy decreases with age (i.e., running economy is significantly reduced in older adults because muscles are unable to compensate for the stiffer tendons) and in immature tendons (explaining the metabolic inefficiency present in children). The reduced elasticity present in older tendons explains why the perceived effort associated with running increases as we age (and why we slow down so much). The good news is that researchers are coming up with ways to improve tendon flexibility, and these new techniques are reviewed in chapter 3.

Tendon Resiliency and Energy Return

In humans, for tendons to store and return energy effectively, they must be stretched through very specific ranges. Because excessive stretching can damage a tendon and too little stretching can limit the storage of energy, it is important for a tendon to be moved through a very specific range. Think of the tendon as a rubber band. If you stretch a rubber band too far it will break. Alternately, if you stretch the same rubber band too little, it won't shoot very far. (Remember, even energy-storing tendons can only lengthen 11%.)

To determine the ideal degree of tendon stretch necessary to maximize efficiency in runners, a group of exercise physiologists decided to evaluate the precise degree the medial arch lowers while running. Because lowering of the arch stretches tendons, measuring the deflection of the arch is an easy way to quantify tendon stretch. After carefully measuring arch motions, researchers determined the typical medial arch lowers ¼ to ⅜ inch (7 to 10 mm) while running (33).

A separate study of the effect of surface stiffness on running efficiency proved that this exact distance results in the fastest running times. By having subjects run over experimental tracks made from different materials, researchers determined that an overly flexible track absorbs too much energy, while a rigid track absorbs too little, causing running speeds to be diminished in both situations. In their quest to identify the perfect amount of track flexibility, scientists determined a track that flexes ¼ inch (7 mm) vertically will return more than 90% of the energy stored following foot strike, allowing for the fastest possible running speeds. Because this distance is identical to the degree of motion present as our arch flattens, it is suggested that a ¼ inch (7 mm) lowering of the medial arch stores the perfect amount of energy in the tendons and muscles of the foot and ankle. The authors speculate that when moving through this precise range, the tendons in the arch can return up to 17% of the energy absorbed during early stance.

To evaluate the exact degree of joint motion associated with deflection of the arch, scientists surgically embedded metal pins into nine bones of the foot and ankle while subjects walked and then ran over level terrain (34, 35). Not surprisingly, the joints of the midfoot moved through the largest ranges of motion, with the medial cuneiform moving as much as the ankle (Fig. 2.28).

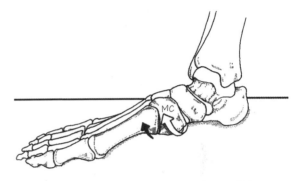

Fig. 2.28. *While walking and running, the medial cuneiform (MC, white arrow), moves upward as much as the ankle.* The first metatarsal moves about half that distance (**black arrow**).

What really made these papers interesting was that joint motions were significantly greater in all subjects while walking than during slow running. The clinical implication of this research is that contrary to popular belief, slow running is often easier on the joints of the feet and ankles than walking.

Muscular Control of the Foot and Ankle During Midstance and Propulsion

Although difficulties in quantifying energy storage make it impossible to determine exactly which tissues of the arch are responsible for specific amounts of energy storage, it is likely that the tibialis posterior, flexor digitorum brevis, and plantar fascia play key roles in storing and returning energy (Fig. 2.29).

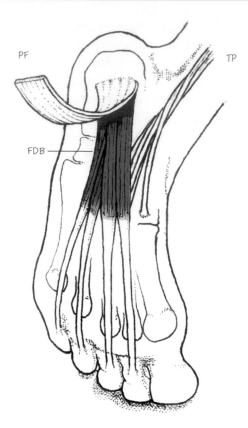

Fig. 2.29. *The tibialis posterior (TP), flexor digitorum brevis (FDB), and plantar fascia (PF) all store and return energy during propulsion.* *The TP is particularly effective at storing and returning energy because its fibers rotate nearly 45°, allowing it to function like a spring.*

The tibialis posterior is especially important because when utilized properly, this muscle can actually produce a structural change in the height of the medial arch (i.e., convert a low arch into a neutral arch). Increased tone in the tibialis posterior possibly explains why individuals running in minimalist shoes frequently report a gradual elevation in height of the medial longitudinal arch. The increased muscle activity in response to barefoot activity is theorized to enhance the ability of this muscle to store and return energy.

While the tibialis posterior is important during midstance, the flexor digitorum brevis

is especially important during the propulsive period, as it fires to offload the plantar fascia. In a clever study of the role of the intrinsic arch muscles while running, researchers used nerve blocks to paralyze the arch muscles of 24 people before they got on a treadmill and began running (36). Surprisingly, in spite of being paralyzed in their flexor digitorum brevis, there was little change in height of the longitudinal arch during midstance. In contrast, there was a huge increase in stress beneath the forefoot, causing the runners with paralyzed arches to shorten their stride length and increase their cadence markedly. They essentially performed a rapid ground run, spending most of their time in midstance and almost completely avoiding the propulsive period. This research explains why there is such a strong connection between weakness of the flexor digitorum brevis and plantar fasciitis: Tension in the flexor digitorum brevis creates a compressive force that stops the plantar fascia from being stretched during the propulsive period.

By increasing tone in response to stress, the flexor digitorum brevis may behave as a variable-length spring that functions to reduce stress on the plantar fascia if forces become too high. The downside is that this muscle can fire with so much force that it actually results in the formation of a heel spur at the muscle's attachment to the base of the heel.

As the heel leaves the ground during propulsion, the leg continues to pivot over the talus, and the energy stored in the muscles and tendons is used to propel us forward. The talus is perfectly designed to function as a pivot point because more than 70% of its surface is covered with cartilage, allowing it to function as a nearly frictionless ball bearing (Fig. 2.30).

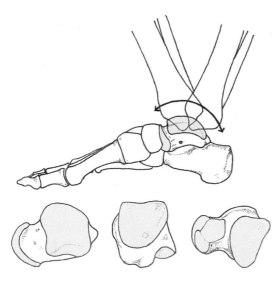

Fig. 2.30. *Because so much of its surface is covered with cartilage (shaded areas), the talus functions like a frictionless ball bearing, allowing the lower leg to glide over its upper surface (arrow).*

To stabilize the talus during the push-off phase, the muscle that goes to the big toe (the flexor hallucis longus) pulls the fibula downward (Fig. 2.31). Downward motion of the fibula serves to deepen the ankle mortise and protects against lateral ankle sprains. As a result, in addition to conventional ankle exercises, runners with recurrent ankle sprains should consider mobilizing the fibula and/or strengthening the flexor hallucis longus (all exercises are reviewed in Chapter 3).

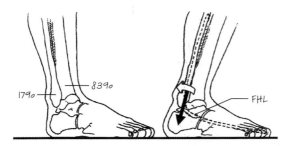

Fig. 2.31. *During early stance, the fibula supports less than 17% of body weight while the tibia supports 83%.* *The fibula plays a more important role during propulsion, when the flexor hallucis longus muscle (**FHL**) pulls the fibula downward. Pulling the fibula downward deepens the ankle socket and makes the ankle less likely to be sprained.*

The Achilles Tendon

By far, the most important tendon for storing and returning energy is the Achilles. Putting aside its significant length and thickness, the Achilles tendon is uniquely designed to store and return energy because the lower portions of the tendon rotate approximately 90° before attaching to the heel (Fig. 2.32). This extreme rotation allows the Achilles tendon to return more than 35% of the energy used to stretch it.

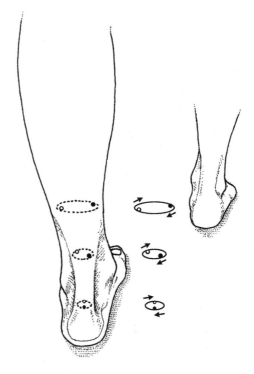

Fig. 2.32. *Rotation of the Achilles tendon.* *When moving top to bottom, the inner fibers move backward (**black dots**) while the outer fibers move forward (**white dots**). This results in a 90° twisting of the Achilles tendon.*

Surprisingly, research has demonstrated that the gastrocnemius and soleus muscles perform relatively little work during the propulsive period because they isometrically tense just before the initiation of propulsion. Rather than rapidly shortening to propel the body forward (which is how most muscles function to produce movement), it appears the primary role of these muscles while running is to produce an "isometric impulse" that anchors the Achilles tendon so that the tendon itself can store and return energy.

In the previously mentioned study of turkeys forced to run on treadmills, Roberts and colleagues (32) show that when turkeys run at progressively faster speeds, their gastrocnemius muscles remain relatively stationary, while their Achilles tendons stretch through large ranges before snapping back to return the stored energy. The nearly isometric contraction of the gastrocnemius and soleus muscles significantly lessens the metabolic expense of running by reducing the work performed by the muscles (which consume calories, generate heat, and require removal of waste products, such as lactic acid). In order to perfectly time the isometric impulse, the gastrocnemius and soleus muscles receive information regarding changes in muscle length and acceleration from an unusual muscle called the "plantaris."

Located between the gastrocnemius and soleus muscles (see Fig. 1.11), the plantaris is too thin to function in force production, but it was recently proven to contain a large number of special sensory nerve receptors that provide the central nervous system with detailed information regarding length changes in the gastrocnemius and soleus muscles. The additional sensory information improves our ability to precisely time the exact point the isometric impulse should be applied in order to allow the Achilles tendon to return energy more efficiently.

In addition to propelling the body forward, the rapid return of energy associated with the snapping action of the Achilles tendon

significantly lessens strain on the hip flexors. As demonstrated by researchers from the Rehabilitation R&D Center in Palo Alto, California, plantar flexion of the ankle during propulsion allows the gastrocnemius to function as a powerful hip flexor by driving the knee up and forward during the initiation of swing phase (37) (Fig. 2.33). By driving the knee up and forward, a strong gastrocnemius will greatly reduce the risk of injuring the hip flexor muscles while running.

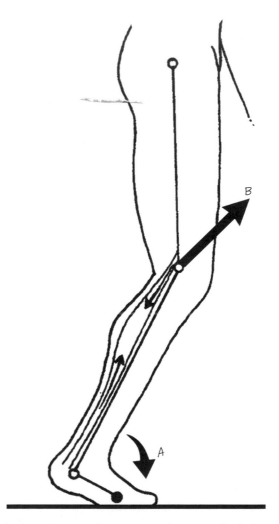

Fig. 2.33. *Because the gastrocnemius crosses both the ankle and the knee, plantar flexion of the ankle during propulsion (A) drives the knee up and forward (B), significantly reducing strain on the hip flexors.*

Once the heel has left the ground, a considerable amount of stress is transferred directly into the forefoot. To protect the forefoot from the extreme forces present during propulsion, pressure receptors present in the skin beneath the forefoot cause the flexor muscles to tense, creating a stabilizing force in the toes that reduces pressure beneath the metatarsal heads. To determine the exact degree of protection provided by the toe muscles, researchers measured pressure changes beneath the forefoot while using pneumatic clamps to duplicate the effect of toe muscle activity (38) (Fig. 2.34).

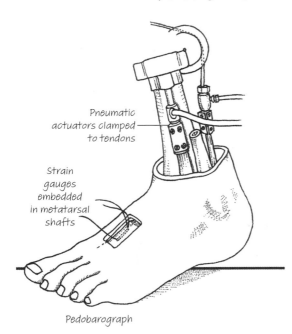

Fig. 2.34. *Cadaveric experiment evaluating the pressures beneath the forefoot and the metatarsal bending strains present during propulsion.*

Strain gauges were also embedded into the metatarsal shafts to evaluate the bending forces present in the bone with and without simulated muscle contraction. This elaborate laboratory experiment confirmed that reflex activation of the toe muscles markedly reduces pressure beneath the central forefoot and prevents buckling of the metatarsal shafts. The authors of the study state that the toe muscles could play a key role in the redistribution of pressure throughout the forefoot and in the prevention of metatarsal stress fractures.

The Sesamoid Bones

In a separate study of forces acting on the foot during propulsion, an orthopedic researcher from Switzerland determined that when you push down with your big toe, you transfer a significant amount of pressure away from the center of the forefoot onto the toe (39). As a result, to avoid developing a range of forefoot injuries (such as metatarsal stress fractures and/or interdigital neuritis), it is very important that runners be capable of generating significant force in the flexor muscles attaching to the big toe. To that end, the body places two sesamoid bones in the tendon of the flexor hallucis brevis muscle (Fig. 2.35).

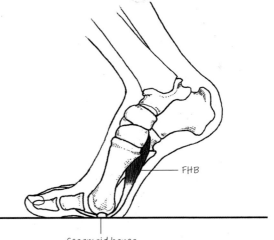

Fig. 2.35. *Two sesamoid bones are located in the tendon of the flexor hallucis brevis (FHB).*

Similarly to how the relationship between the kneecap and the quadriceps tendon works, the sesamoid bones increase muscular efficiency, thereby stabilizing the big toe during propulsion. Unfortunately, they also become weight-bearing points and can be a chronic source of pain in runners. (Treatment of this condition will be discussed in Chapter 6.)

Peroneus Brevis and Running Speed

While the Achilles tendon is important for storing and returning energy, the peroneus brevis plays an important role in allowing us to run faster. In a paper published in the *American Journal of Sports Medicine*, researchers evaluated leg muscle activity as subjects ran at different speeds, and concluded that the transition to the faster running speeds was associated with significant increases in peroneus brevis activity, with little change in activity of the gastrocnemius and soleus muscles (40). The peroneus brevis can be exercised by running back and forth on slightly inclined surfaces. The peroneus brevis is important in fast running because it everts the heel, thereby allowing push-off to occur through the transverse axis of the metatarsal heads (Fig. 2.36). According to the anatomist Bojsen-Moller (41), use of the transverse axis by means of peroneus brevis contraction represents the final evolutionary change in the process of producing a fast, efficient propulsion.

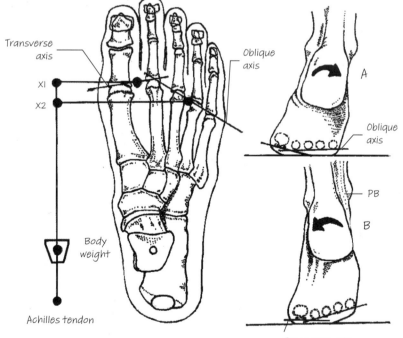

Fig. 2.36. *Because the second metatarsal is longer than the remaining metatarsals, it serves as a pivot point allowing the foot to choose between two different push-off options.* When the rearfoot supinates (*A*), push-off occurs through the oblique axis, which has a shorter lever arm to the ankle joint (compare *X1* and *X2*). This lessens strain on the Achilles and is often used when running uphill. Because of the shorter lever arm, use of the oblique axis is called a "low gear push-off." When greater force is needed (e.g., in sprinting), the peroneus brevis (*PB* in *B*) everts the rearfoot (*B*), thereby forcing the foot onto the transverse axis. Because of the longer lever arm, use of the transverse axis is referred to as a "high gear push-off," and this axis is used when faster speeds are required.

SWING PHASE

Once the foot has left the ground, the leg and hip swing forward in anticipation of the next ground contact. To increase stride length, runners rotate their pelvis forward on the side of the swing leg. To counter the forward motion of the pelvis, the upper body and arms rotate in the opposite direction. Because these rotations are equal in magnitude and occur in opposite directions, some coaches suggest that rotational arm motions are necessary to maximize efficiency because they counteract horizontal motions in the pelvis. A few world-class coaches have gone so far as to have their endurance athletes modify the positions of their thumbs while running.

Unfortunately, the belief that arm motions actively counterbalance pelvic motion, and are therefore necessary to improve efficiency, is incorrect. Research in 2009 confirmed that the arms act as passive dampeners that reduce the amount of torso and head rotation, not active force generators necessary to counteract pelvic motions (42). The negligible effect that arm motions have on efficiency is supported by the fact that ostriches are among the most efficient bipeds on the planet even though they do not move their wings to counter pelvic rotations. Fortunately for ostriches, they possess long necks that reduce head oscillation without upper extremity involvement.

Arm Motions

Essentially, arm motions in distance runners act in a manner similar to the vibration dampeners placed on the bows of Olympic archers (Fig. 2.37): They dampen bow vibration while having no effect on the speed of the arrow.

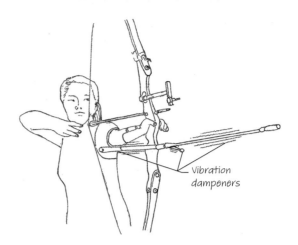

Fig. 2.37. *Vibration dampeners used in archery reduce vibration of the bow while having no effect on arrow speed.*

The incorrect assumption that arm motions play an important role in improving efficiency while distance running may come from the fact that sprinters incorporate exaggerated forward/backward arm motions to maximize acceleration. Although important for sprinting, endurance runners need to avoid excessive forward/backward motion of the arms, and their upper extremities should remain relaxed. Several studies confirm that the most economical distance runners present with low amplitude arm movements (30, 43). Exaggerated arm motions should always be discouraged because it takes muscular effort to accelerate and decelerate these motions, which can lessen efficiency.

To improve performance, distance runners should try to incorporate arm motions that minimize wrist excursions and reduce excessive forward/backward motions at the shoulders. They should keep their arms relaxed with their elbows bent in a comfortable position. Because subtle asymmetries in arm motions are not correlated with inefficiency, long-distance runners can move their arms through any movement pattern that is comfortable for them, as long as the motions are not excessive.

The questionable significance of making slight changes in arm motions while endurance running is obvious when you look at the world's best runners. In the Olympic women's 10K in Athens, Xing Huina from China won a gold medal while running with her arms held straight at her sides. In contrast, Khalid Khannouchi set a world record in the Chicago marathon with his hands positioned near his chin. Additionally, the former world record holder in the women's marathon, Paula Radcliffe, often runs with her arms abducted and her wrists moving through asymmetric motions. If these asymmetric arm motions were metabolically inefficient, Paula would never have been able to shatter the world record with a 2:15:25 marathon. Although asymmetric arm motions may occasionally be a sign of a biomechanical problem elsewhere in the body (e.g., a tight left hip can cause the right arm to cross over more), as demonstrated by Paula Radcliffe, subtle side-to-side variation in arm motions in an endurance runner is not always correlated with reduced efficiency and/or biomechanical problems.

The Hamstrings

While arm motions play a relatively unimportant role during swing phase, the hamstrings play a key role in improving efficiency because they isometrically tense just before your foot hits the ground, allowing you to store some of the energy used to swing the leg forward. In a study of hamstring activity present while sprinting, researchers noted that during the late swing phase of sprinting, contraction of the hamstrings slowed considerably while their tendons lengthened

(storing the elastic energy associated with decelerating the forward motion of the foot and leg) (44). Again, the body attempts to reduce the metabolic cost of running by isometrically tensing muscles in a fixed position, while the tendons store and later return the free energy. According to some experts, this is a learned response, and the ability to store and return energy can improve with practice. As will be discussed later, the incorporation of specific plyometric and agility drills may be the key to optimizing the storage and return of energy.

Until recently, no one could figure out why the outer hamstring muscle, the biceps femoris, was the hamstring muscle that was strained almost exclusively in runners. Different theories were proposed suggesting that because two different nerves innervate the biceps femoris, it is less coordinated than the other hamstring muscles and therefore prone to injury. The real reason for the high injury rate in the biceps femoris is that it attaches lower on the leg than the other hamstring muscles. The lower attachment point increases the lever arm the biceps femoris works against, which increases the strain absorbed by this muscle.

By calculating the strain associated with the lower attachment point, it was determined that the biceps femoris lengthens 9.5% during late swing phase, while the other hamstrings lengthen less than 8% (45). The amplified strain associated with the lower attachment point increases the potential for injury, but it also improves the ability of the biceps femoris to store and return appreciable amounts of energy. As previously mentioned, this important muscle also plays a key role in dampening bony vibrations following heel strike, and helps the sacroiliac joint absorb shock by limiting excessive tilting of the sacrum (see Fig. 2.23).

The Braking Phase: The Most Overlooked Cause of Running-Related Injuries

Just before the end of swing phase, the runner begins to rotate the pelvis backward in an attempt to minimize the braking phase associated with making ground contact (Fig. 2.38). The braking phase is that brief period of deceleration that occurs immediately following ground contact.

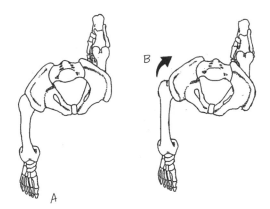

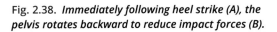

Fig. 2.38. *Immediately following heel strike (A), the pelvis rotates backward to reduce impact forces (B).*

To understand the braking phase, imagine yourself walking across a room while carrying a full bowl of soup: Every time your foot strikes the ground, the soup shifts forward. The soup moves because the forward motion of your body is temporarily decelerated when your front foot strikes the ground. Remember Newton's first law: *Bodies in motion tend to stay in motion.* When your foot hits the ground, forward motion of your body is decelerated by the sudden ground contact, but the soup continues to stay in motion. While running, the braking phase is a common and overlooked cause of a wide range of impact-related injuries because it can create dangerous shockwaves that travel up the foot and leg.

To determine the effect of excessive braking force, researchers from Vancouver, Canada,

measured vertical loading rates, instantaneous vertical loading rate, active peak, vertical impulse, and peak braking force as 65 healthy female runners ran on treadmills (46). These athletes were then asked to participate in a 15-week half-marathon training program. By the time they finished the training program, nearly 35% of the runners were injured, and peak braking force was the only variable that correlated with the development of running injuries. In fact, runners with high peak braking forces were five to eight times more likely to be injured than runners with low braking force. Prior research demonstrated that peak braking force increases as your stride length increases and you place your foot progressively farther forward at initial contact (47).

Should You Shorten Your Stride Length?

Even though runners self-select stride lengths based on their individual efficiency, it is occasionally necessary to reduce a runner's preferred stride length in order to decrease the risk of injury. As will be discussed in Chapter 4, my favorite way to determine if you should change your stride length is to evaluate the position your leg is in when you initially make ground contact. Ideally, your leg should be near vertical with your ankle and foot in a near midline position. If your contact knee is nearly straight and your leg is angled more than 10° to the vertical, definitely shorten your stride. At first, running with a shorter stride may slightly impair performance, but over time, you adapt to the new running style and will more than likely become faster and more efficient as the braking forces are reduced. While not an option for fast runners, the forces present during the braking phase can easily be reduced in slower recreational runners by transitioning to ground running. Albeit slow, avoiding the aerial phase by switching to ground running is the single best way to avoid injury.

The Best Way to Reduce the Braking Phase Forces

Although ground running and/or making initial ground contact with the vertical leg decreases the forces associated with the braking phase, nothing compares to using posterior rotation of the pelvis. After evaluating all possible ways to reduce the braking phase forces, researchers determined that backward rotation of the pelvis during initial ground contact plays the greatest role in limiting the magnitude of these forces (48). Apparently, the best runners learn to markedly reduce impact forces associated with the braking phase by pulling their pelvis back at just the right time. While it may occasionally be necessary to shorten your stride (especially if your contact leg is not vertical), the preferred approach would be to run with your naturally selected stride length and learn to efficiently reduce the braking phase forces by incorporating specific movements of the pelvis, knees, and ankles. In order to effectively absorb force through posterior rotation of the hip, you have to have flexible hip rotators. My favorite way to improve hip flexibility is with the muscle energy stretch illustrated in Fig. 2.39. Additional hip rotator stretches are described in the piriformis section of Chapter 6. In my experience, runners with strong flexible hips rarely get injured.

GRAPHIC SUMMARY OF MUSCLE ACTIVITY DURING THE GAIT CYCLE

Understanding when muscles fire while running is important for both performance and injury

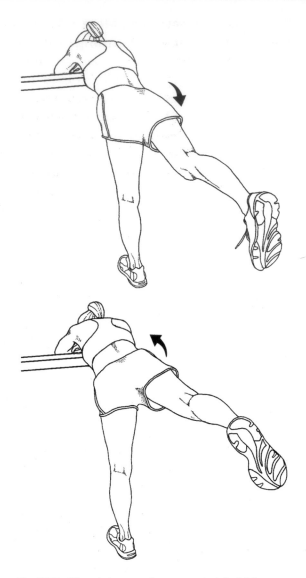

Fig. 2.39. *Hip rotator muscle energy stretch. While standing on one leg, lean forward to rest on a stable surface. From that position, raise and lower the opposite hip, moving through progressively greater ranges of motion (**arrows**). Try doing 2 or 3 sets of 25 repetitions as part of your pre-run warm-up.*

prevention. The graphs in Fig. 2.40 summarize muscle function on the basis of EMG studies. The following section summarizes this research.

The gluteus maximus is an especially important muscle during early stance phase, as it prevents

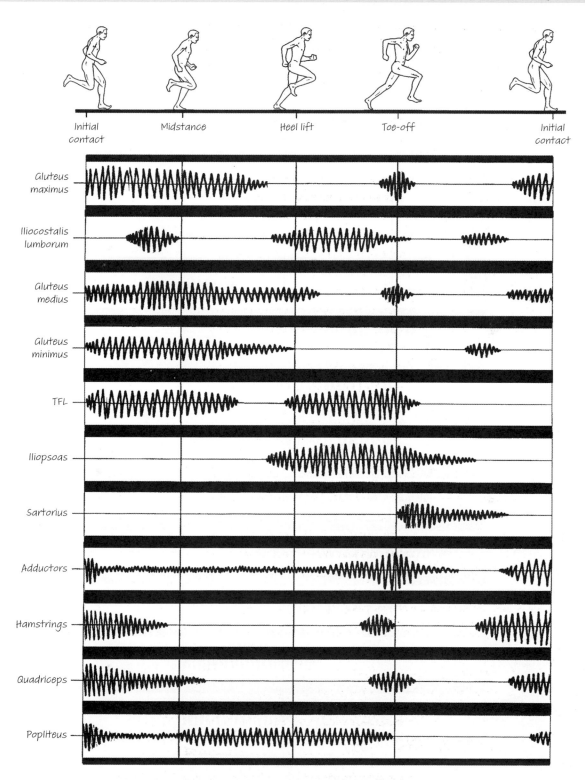

Fig. 2.40. *Graphic summary of muscle function during the gait cycle.*

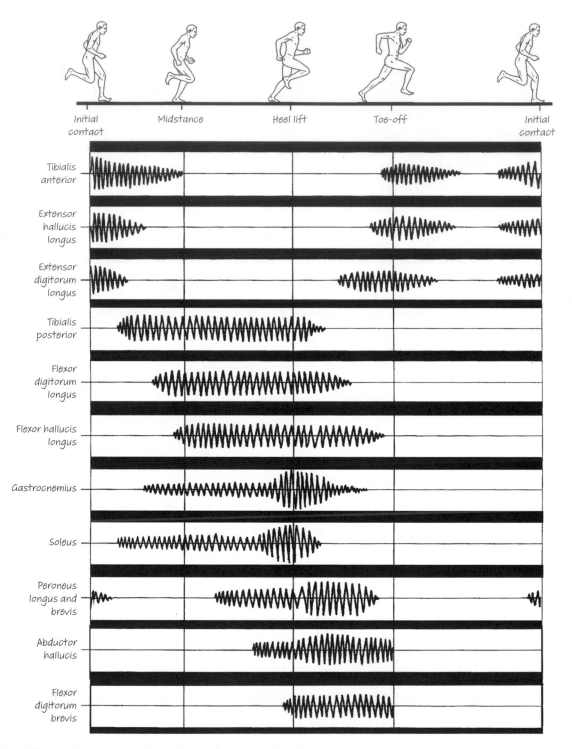

Fig. 2.40. *Graphic summary of muscle function during the gait cycle. (continued)*

the limb from rotating in too far, and works with the hip rotators to absorb forces associated with the braking phase. The upper fibers of this muscle work to prevent the opposite hip from lowering, while the lower fibers control rotation. Because the largest portion of the gluteus maximus inserts directly into the iliotibial band, this muscle provides significant stability to the hip and knee during midstance while running.

The gluteus medius plays a huge role while running, as it prevents the opposite pelvis from dropping down during midstance. The anterior fibers of this muscle are slightly active during toe-off and early swing phase, when they work to keep the femur from twisting outward during propulsion. The gluteus minimus is also important while running, as it opposes the action of the gluteus medius, which is necessary in order to maintain a constant pressure throughout the hip socket.

The tensor fascia latae contracts with significant force during propulsion, and it assists the iliopsoas in flexing the hip. The iliopsoas demonstrates peak activity during late stance in early swing phase, when it assists the adductors, tensor fascia latae, rectus femoris, and sartorius in flexing the hip. The momentum gained by rapid thigh flexion during early swing phase plays an important role in accelerating the center of mass up and forward during late swing phase.

The adductors, as a group, demonstrate peak activity during toe-off, when they flex the hip and help control rotation of the femur. With the exception of a brief quiet period during midswing, the adductor magnus fires constantly throughout the running cycle. In contrast, the hamstrings demonstrate peak activity at the end of swing phase, when they eccentrically contract to decelerate forward motion of the rapidly extending leg. Strong hamstrings are extremely important while running, as they prevent overstriding and help store and return energy. During propulsion, there is a brief burst of activity in the hamstrings, as these muscles assist the gastrocnemius in flexing the knee.

The quadriceps muscles pre-tense during late swing phase, as they're getting ready to absorb forces at the knee during initial ground contact. These muscles are important shock absorbers, particularly when running fast, as they work hard to absorb the increased impact forces associated with fast running (which is evidenced by the increased range of knee flexion present at high running speeds). Slower recreational runners move through small ranges of knee flexion, and shock absorption is not as important, which reduces stress on the quadriceps muscles. In fact, slower runners are more efficient when they use quadriceps muscles to keep their knees stiff.

The popliteus is important while running, as it prevents forward motion of the femur on the tibia during initial ground contact. The muscle concentrically contracts during initial contact, to allow the tibia to internally rotate, which is necessary for smooth flexion.

The anterior compartment muscles demonstrate peak activity immediately following heel strike. Activity in these muscles is greatly reduced during midfoot strike patterns, and is almost completely absent during forefoot contacts. As a result, switching to a more forward ground contact can offload the anterior compartment muscles and is an effective method for managing anterior compartment syndromes.

The tibialis posterior functions during early stance phase and works to prevent excessive pronation of the midfoot. It is also important during propulsion, when it assists the gastrocnemius and soleus muscles in creating a rapid force to push us forward. The long toe muscles are also important during push-off, as they assist in lifting the heel during propulsion and in stabilizing the metatarsal shafts to protect them from excessive bending forces.

Both the gastrocnemius and the soleus demonstrate peak activity during propulsion, when they function to produce heel lift. The soleus prevents forward motion of the leg, while the gastrocnemius flexes the knee and raises the heel. The gastrocnemius also drives the knee up and forward, offloading the hip flexors. During initial contact, the soleus decelerates internal rotation of the tibia, while the gastrocnemius controls inward rotation of the femur. These dual actions reduce the buildup of torsional strain at the knee during early stance and are essential for remaining injury free.

Just prior to initial contact, the peroneal muscles (aka the fibularis muscles) play an important role in preventing ankle injury by keeping the heel vertical. The peroneus longus is also important during propulsion, when it works with the tibialis posterior to stabilize the midfoot, while the peroneus longus and brevis muscles play a crucial role in fast running by shifting the body weight toward the great toe.

Lastly, the abductor and adductor hallucis muscles function almost exclusively during propulsion to stabilize the big toe against the ground. The exception to this rule is in flat-footed individuals, where the abductor hallucis fires constantly during stance phase to prevent lowering of the arch. Because these muscles control alignment of the big toe, they are important in preventing the formation of bunions. The other intrinsic muscles of the arch are important for storing and returning energy, and for diverting pressure away from the metatarsal heads toward the tips of the toes.

REFERENCES

1. Saunders JB, Inman VT, Eberhart HT. The major determinants in normal and pathological gait. *J Bone Joint Surg.* 1953;5813:153.
2. McMahon T, Valiant G, Fredrick E. Groucho running. *J Appl Physiol.* 1987;62:2326–2337.
3. Taylor C. Relating mechanics and energetics during exercise. *Adv Vet Sci Comp Med.* 1994;38A:181–215.
4. Srinivasan M, Ruina A. Computer optimization of a minimal biped model discovers walking and running. *Nature.* 2006;439:72–75.
5. Schace A, Doran T, Williams G, et al. Lower-limb muscular strategies for increasing running speed. *J Orthop Sports Phys Ther.* 2014;44:813.
6. McMahon T. The spring in the human foot. *Nature.* 1987;325:108–109.
7. Shorten MR, Pisciotta E. Running biomechanics: what did we miss? *ISBS Proc Arch.* 2017;35(1):34–37.
8. Bonnaerens S, Fiers P. Galle S, et al. Grounded running reduces musculoskeletal load. *Med Sci Sports Exerc.* 2019;51: 708–715.
9. Gazendam MG, Hof AL. Averaged EMG profiles in jogging and running at different speeds. *Gait Posture.* 2007;25:604–614.
10. Neptune R, Sasaki K. Ankle plantar flexor force production is an important determinant of the preferred walk-to-run transition speed. *J Exp Biol.* 2005;208:799–808.
11. Weyand P, Sternlight D, Belizzi J, Wright S. Faster top running speeds are achieved

with greater ground forces not more rapid leg movements. *J Appl Physiol.* 2000;89:1991–1999.

12. Anderson T. Biomechanics and running economy. *Sports Med.* 1996;22:76–89.

13. Stiffler-Joachim M, Wille C, Kliethermes S, et al. Foot angle and loading rate during running demonstrate a nonlinear relationship. *Med Sci Sports Exerc.* 2019;51:2067–2072.

14. Hamill J, Gruber A. Is changing foot strike pattern beneficial to runners? *J Sport Health Sci.* 2017;6(2):146–153.

15. Cunningham C, Schilling N, Anders C, et al. The influence of foot posture on the cost of transport in humans. *J Exp Biol.* 2010;213:790–797.

16. Miller R, Russell E, Gruber A, et al. Foot-strike pattern selection to minimize muscle energy expenditure during running: a computer simulation study. *Proc Am Soc Biomech. Ann. Meet.* 2009, State College, PA.

17. Delgado T, Kubera-Shelton E, Robb R, et al. Effects of foot strike on low back posture, shock attenuation, and comfort in running. *Med Sci Sports Exerc.* 2013;45(3):490–496.

18. Goss D, Lewek M, Yu B, et al. Accuracy of self-reported foot strike patterns and loading rates associated with traditional and minimalist running shoes. Human Movement Sci Res Symp. 2012, U North Carolina, Chapel Hill.

19. Bennett M, Harris J, Richmond B, et al. Early hominin foot morphology based on 1.5-million-year-old footprints from Ileret, Kenya. *Science.* 2009;323:1197–1201.

20. Gefen A, Megido-Ravid M, Itzchak Y. *In-vivo* biomechanical behavior of the human heel pad during the stance phase of gait. *J Biomech.* 2001;34:1661–1665.

21. DeClercq D, Aerts P, Kunnen M. The mechanical behavior characteristics of the human heel pad during foot strike in running: an in vivo cineradiographic study. *J Biomech.* 1994;27:1213–1222.

22. Hasselman C, Best T, Seaber A, et al. A threshold and continuum of injury during active stretch of rabbit skeletal muscle. *Am J Sports Med.* 1995;23:65–73.

23. Roukis T, Hurless J, Page J. Torsion of the tibialis posterior. *J Am Podiatr Med Assoc.* 1995;85:464–469.

24. Garrett W. Muscle strain injuries. *Am J Sports Med.* 1996;24(6):S2–8.

25. Wilson A, McGuigan M, Su A, et al. Horses damp the spring in their step. *Nature.* 2001;414:895–899.

26. Lake M, Coyles V, Lees A. High frequency characteristics of the lower limb during running. *Proc 18th Congr Int Soc Biomech.* 2001:200–201.

27. Zhang Z, Ng G, Lee W, et al. Increase in passive muscle tension of the quadriceps muscle heads in jumping athletes with patellar tendinopathy. *Scand J Med Sci Sports.* 2016;10:1099–1104.

28. van den Bogert A, Reinschmidt C, Lundberg A. Helical axes of skeletal knee joint motion during running. *J Biomech.* 2000;41:1632–1638.

29. Callaghan J, Patla A, McGill S. Low back three-dimensional joint forces, kinematics and kinetics during walking. *Clin Biomech.* 1999;14:203–216.

30. Williams K, Cavanagh P. Relationship between distance running mechanics, running economy, and performance *J Appl Physiol.* 1987;63:1236–1246.

31. McGill S. *Low Back Disorders: Evidence-Based Prevention and Rehabilitation.* Champaign, IL: Human Kinetics Publishing 2002.

32. Roberts T, Marsh R, Weyand P, et al. Muscular force in running turkeys: the economy of minimizing work. *Science.* 1997;275:1113–1115.

33. Ker R, Bennett M, Bibby S, et al. The spring in the arch of the human foot. *Nature.* 1987;325:147–149.

34. Arndt A, Wolf P, Liu A, et al. Intrinsic foot kinematics measured in vivo during the stance phase of slow running. *J Biomech.* 2007;40:2672–2678.

35. Lundgren P, Nester C, Liu A, et al. Invasive in vivo measurements of rearfoot, mid and forefoot motion during walking. *Gait Posture.* 2008;28:93–100.

36. Farris D, Kelly L, Cresswall A, et al. The functional importance of human foot muscles for bipedal locomotion. *PNAS.* 2019;116:1645–1650.

37. Neptune R, Kautz S, Zajac F. Contributions of individual ankle plantar flexors to support, forward progression and swing initiation during walking. *J Biomech.* 2001;34:1387–1398.

38. Ferris L, Sharkey N, Smith T, et al. Influence of extrinsic plantar flexors on forefoot loading during heel rise. *Foot Ankle Int.* 1995;16:464–473.

39. Jacob H. Forces acting in the forefoot during normal gait: an estimate. *Clin Biomech.* 2001;16:783–792.

40. Reber L, Perry J, Pink M. Muscular control of the ankle in running. *Am J Sports Med.* 1993;21:805–810.

41. Bojsen-Moller F. Calcaneocuboid joint and stability of the longitudinal arch of the foot at high and low gear push off. *J Anat.* 1979;129:165–176.

42. Pontzer H, Holloway J, Raichlen D, Lieberman D. Control and function of arm swing in human walking and running. *J Exp Biol.* 2009;212:523–534.

43. Anderson T, Tseh W. Running economy, anthropometric dimensions and kinematic variables (abstract). *Med Sci Sports Exerc.*1994;26(5 Suppl.):S170.

44. Thelen D, Chumanov E, Best T, et al. Simulation of biceps femoris musculotendon mechanics during the swing phase of sprinting. *Med Sci Sports Exerc.* 2005;37:1931–1938.

45. Thelen D, Chumanov E, Hoerth D, et al. Hamstring muscle kinematics during treadmill sprinting. *Med Sci Sports Exerc.* 2005;37:108–114.

46. Napier C, MacLean C, Maurer J, et al. Kinetic risk factors of running-related injuries in female recreational runners. *Scand J Med Sci Sport.* 2018;28:2164–2172.

47. Heiderscheit BC, Chumanov ES, Michalski MP, et al. Effects of step rate manipulation on joint mechanics during running. *Med Sci Sports Exerc.* 2011;43:296–302.

48. Pandy M, Berme N. Quantitative assessment of gait determinants during single stance via a three-dimensional model: Part 1. Normal gait. *J Biomech.* 1989;22:717–724.

CHAPTER 3

RISK FACTORS PREDISPOSING TO RUNNING INJURIES

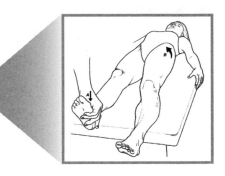

Even with perfect running form, odds are that sooner or later you're still going to get injured. In many situations, the cause of an injury can be traced back to a specific training error (e.g., running more than 40 miles per week is a proven predictor of injury). Other times, running injuries can be related to problems with bony alignment, flexibility, strength, and/or prior injury. In many cases, the potential for developing an injury (or reinjury) can be greatly reduced with specific rehabilitative techniques. The classic example of this is hamstring injuries. With an annual reinjury rate of more than 70%, hamstring injuries are considered one of the worst soft tissue injuries a runner can get. However, a paper published in the *Journal of Orthopedic and Sports Physical Therapy* shows that when certain rehabilitative exercises are performed, the annual reinjury rate for hamstring strains drops from 70% to 7.7% (1). If these exercises were performed routinely by all runners, the potential for developing hamstring strains could be significantly reduced.

Another modifiable risk factor for developing running injuries is tightness in the gastrocnemius. In a clever paper in which ankle range of motion was related to a variety of midfoot and forefoot injuries, researchers demonstrated that individuals with tight gastrocnemius muscles were three times more likely to develop metatarsalgia, plantar fasciitis, and metatarsal stress fractures (2). The authors suggest that tightness in the gastrocnemius causes the heel to leave the ground prematurely, transferring a greater percentage of force into the forefoot (Fig. 3.1).

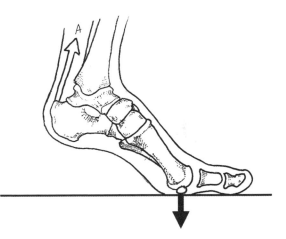

Fig. 3.1. *Tightness in the gastrocnemius (A) causes a premature lifting of the heel, driving the forefoot into the ground with more force (arrow).*

The potential for injury with a tight gastrocnemius really skyrockets if the toe muscles are weak. Strong toes have been proven to protect against the development of plantar fasciitis and metatarsal stress fractures, particularly in the presence of a tight calf. If runners would routinely lengthen the gastrocnemius by performing straight leg calf stretches, they could reduce their potential for developing a range of serious injuries. The remainder of this chapter reviews the causes and treatments for the more common biomechanical factors associated with injury.

HEIGHT OF THE MEDIAL LONGITUDINAL ARCH

A long-held belief in the running community is that arch height is a predictor of injury. The basic premise is that low-arched runners tend to pronate, or roll in excessively, and this excessive inward rolling has been blamed for the development of a variety of injuries, ranging from bunions to low back pain (Fig. 3.2). Conversely, high-arched runners don't pronate enough, and the lack of inward rolling predisposes them to ankle sprains and stress fractures. To protect themselves from the perils of pronation and supination, runners have spent millions on running shoes and custom orthotics designed to lessen their potential for developing injury.

While the correlation between arch height and foot function is clear to the average sports medicine practitioner with more than a few years of experience, the respected researcher Benno Nigg published a paper suggesting that arch height and pronation/supination are in no way correlated (3). By using calipers to measure height of the medial arch, Nigg and his colleagues performed three-dimensional imaging on 30 subjects and found no connection between arch height and foot function: Individuals with

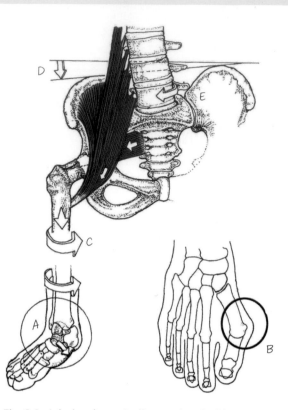

Fig. 3.2. *Injuries theoretically associated with excessive pronation. Excessive inward rolling of the foot (**A**), is often blamed for the development of bunions (**B**). Because pronation causes the leg to twist inward (**C**) and drop downward (**D**), excessive pronation has been blamed for the development of hip flexor tendinitis and external rotator strain. The downward drop associated with excessive pronation has also been implicated in the development of low back pain (**E**).*

high arches frequently pronated excessively, while low-arched individuals often supinated excessively. Even though this paper was published more than 20 years ago, Dr. Nigg's research continues to be referenced in the mainstream literature. *The New York Times* (4) published an article in which Dr. Nigg was quoted as saying: "Arches are an evolutionary remnant, needed by primates that gripped trees with their feet. Since we don't do that anymore, we don't really need an arch." The main point of the article was that since arch height does not correlate with altered movement, there is no need to correct the "perceived biomechanical defect" of being flat-footed by means of an arch support or a running shoe.

A major shortcoming of the belief that arch height does not affect function is that it's based on the findings from one study. While Dr. Nigg used very sophisticated machinery to measure motion, he and his team of researchers made a very basic error in that they identified people as having high or low arches using store-bought calipers, and the resultant arch measurements were never checked against true arch height as determined using weight-bearing x-rays. If they had, they would have found that because each person's arch has a unique curve, it's impossible to pick the precise point along the curve of the arch that actually correlates with true arch height. Because their caliper measurements did not accurately identify true arch height, Dr. Nigg's research provided little insight into the connection between arch height and motion.

In 2001, the controversy regarding arch height and three-dimensional motion was resolved. By using the highly reliable method of quantifying arch height by creating a ratio between the length of the foot and the top of the arch (which is extremely reproducible and has been proven to correlate with x-ray measurements of arch structure), Williams and McClay (5) performed three-dimensional motion analysis on high- and low-arched runners and conclusively demonstrated that arch height and foot function are indeed correlated: People with low arches pronate more rapidly through larger ranges of motion, while people with high arches hit the ground harder and pronate through very small ranges.

In a follow-up study using the same measuring techniques (6), the authors determined that arch height was also predictive of injury: Low-arched runners exhibited more soft tissue injuries and a greater prevalence of injuries along the inside of their leg (especially at the knee and ankle), while high-arched runners had a greater prevalence of bony injuries (e.g., they had twice as many stress fractures). High-arched runners also had more injuries along their outer leg (e.g., iliotibial band friction syndrome and ankle sprains were particularly common). Overall, the low-arched runners had a much greater tendency for inner foot injuries (such as injuries to the sesamoids beneath the big toe), while the high-arched runners had a greater tendency for outer forefoot injuries (such as stress fractures of the fifth metatarsal).

More recently, researchers from Virginia evaluated three-dimensional motion and impact forces in 10 high-arched and 10 low-arched runners. The participants ran at their self-selected running pace, and were then later asked to drop down from a 12 inches (30 cm) platform to evaluate differences and impact forces. The authors concluded that high-arched runners place a greater reliance on their skeletal structures for shock absorption, potentially increasing the risk of stress fractures.

Combined, these three papers confirm what everyone in the sports community has always known: Arch height not only predicts whether your foot pronates or supinates excessively, but also predicts the location of future injuries. One of the nicest things about this research is that the measuring technique used to identify arch height is simple to perform and can be done at home (Fig. 3.3).

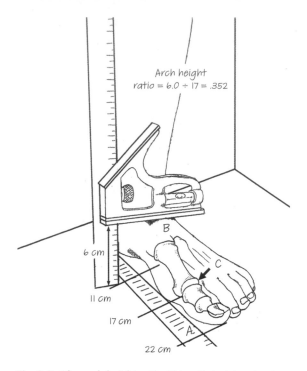

Arch height
ratio = 6.0 ÷ 17 = .352

6 cm

11 cm

17 cm

22 cm

Fig. 3.3. *The arch height ratio. This ratio is determined by measuring the length of the foot to the tip of the big toe (**A**). This number is divided by two, and the height on the top of the foot is measured at this point (**B**). The arch height ratio is determined by dividing the height at the top of the foot by the length of the foot measured at the base of the big toe (**C**). It is usually easy to find the base of the big toe by feeling for a small bump at the end of the metatarsal head (**arrow**). If the resultant number is less than 0.275, the arch is characterized as low. Runners with high arches present with an arch height ratio greater than 0.356.*

Arch Height and the Potential for Injury

While the arch height ratio illustrated in Fig. 3.3 provides information regarding the location of potential injuries, it does not predict the probability of sustaining an injury. To evaluate the relative risk of injury with different arch heights, researchers from Denmark measured arch heights in 927 novice runners before beginning a one-year running program (7). At the end of the year, 33% of the runners with very low arches and 25% of the runners with very high arches were injured. Runners with slightly high arches and neutral feet suffered the same injury rate, around 18%, while only 13% of runners with slightly low arches were injured. In addition to a lower injury rate, the runners with slightly low arches suffered fewer overall injuries, suggesting that a little bit of pronation may actually be protective, probably because slightly low arches are excellent shock absorbers.

This research is important because it shows that only runners with excessively high and low arches have an increased potential for being injured. The runners with the lowest arches in this study were especially prone to injury, as they were unable to run more than four miles per week throughout the year before dropping out because of injury.

If you happen to have very low or very high arches, there are a few simple things you can do to decrease your potential for injury. Because low arches distribute more pressure to the inner side of the foot, it is important that the muscles of the arches remain strong. The easiest way to strengthen the arch muscles is with the exercises described at the end of this chapter. An alternate method to strengthen the arch muscles is to wear minimalist shoes while performing daily activities.

While not recommended for long-distance running because lightweight running shoes are notorious for producing plantar fasciitis in low-arched runners, minimalist shoes allow the toes to move through larger ranges of motion and can very effectively strengthen the muscles of the arch when worn routinely throughout the day. To prove minimalist shoes can strengthen your arches, researchers from Brigham Young University and the Spaulding National Running Center had 57 runners wear minimalist shoes throughout the day (8). During the first two weeks, these runners were told to walk 2,500 steps per day, and by the eighth week, they gradually increased usage of their lightweight shoes to the point they were walking 7,000 steps per day. At the end of the study, the authors showed that in addition to significant gains in arch strength, there were also increases in the cross-sectional area of the most important arch muscles, including the flexor hallucis brevis, abductor hallucis, and flexor digitorum brevis. This paper is significant, as new research shows that people with excessively pronated feet are much less likely to be injured when their feet are strong (9). In an interesting study evaluating the effect of foot strengthening exercises on running performance, researchers from Poland (10) demonstrated that when runners were given the same exercises, low-arched runners had significantly greater improvements in running performance than runners with neutral arches. Again, this confirms that low-arched runners require more muscle strength to remain injury free and perform well.

Custom and Over-the-Counter Orthotics

The most popular method for treating flat feet is to wear either over-the-counter or custom orthotics. Although the precise reason for their success remains obscure (i.e., you will continue to pronate the same amount whether or not you wear orthotics), several studies have shown that orthotics can reduce your potential for being injured. In a paper published in 2011 in the *American Journal of Sports Medicine*, researchers performed a randomized controlled trial of 400 military recruits during basic training, and determined that the trainees wearing orthotics specifically designed to reduce pressure points along the bottom

of their feet were 49% less likely to develop overuse injuries than the control group that did not wear orthotics (11).

Despite the fact that orthotics do not appreciably alter range of motion, they may lessen your potential for injury by distributing pressure away from the heel and forefoot into the arch. Increased skin contact with the edges of the orthotic may also reduce your potential for injury by enhancing sensory feedback, which is thought to improve balance.

An alternate theory to explain why orthotics may lessen your potential for injury is that even though they don't alter the overall range of pronation, they reduce the velocity of the pronating joints (12). According to some experts, the speed of pronation is more likely to produce injury than the overall range of pronation.

The Best Way to Treat High-Arched Runners

Unlike flat-footed runners, high-arched runners rarely require orthotics (why support an already elevated arch?). Because high-arched runners are forced to manage large impact forces, they should avoid minimalist shoes and wear running shoes with cushioned heels. An alternate way for high-arched runners to reduce impact forces is to do gait retraining to learn how to run quietly, a technique that will be discussed in Chapter 4. In every situation, runners with high arches should be discouraged from making initial ground contact with the forefoot because this contact point increases the potential for ankle sprain. Regardless of how ground contact is made, ankle sprains are so prevalent in high-arched runners that they should consider using ankle rock boards to preventively strengthen their ankles (Fig. 3.4).

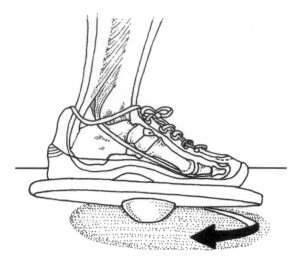

Fig. 3.4. **The Two-to-One Ankle Rockboard.** *Unlike conventional rock boards that tilt equally in each direction, this rock board has an off-center pivot point that allows your foot to tilt the way it does in real life: Your foot will invert twice as much as it everts, which comes in handy when managing people with high arches.*

One study from the Netherlands showed the regular use of a balance board reduced the frequency of ankle sprains by 47% (13).

Arch Height and Balance

Besides increasing range of motion and strengthening the muscles of the leg, ankle rock boards can also improve balance. In an interesting evaluation of balance in people with high and low arches, researchers from the University of North Carolina at Chapel Hill determined that compared to people with neutral arches, people with high and low arches have impaired balance, but for different reasons (14). People with high arches have poor balance because the bottom of their feet make less contact with the ground, and the pressure receptors located in the skin supply less information regarding the distribution of pressure. The reduced sensory feedback associated with lessened contact with the ground

makes it difficult for high-arched runners to maintain balance. Low-arched runners were also shown to have impaired balance, possibly because their overall joint laxity makes it harder for their muscles to control the rapid and often extreme joint movements. As a result, ankle rock board exercises can be helpful for both high- and low-arched runners.

Pronation and Knee/Hip/Back Injuries: A Questionable Connection

An important point regarding the effect of high and low arches is that pronation and supination are more likely to injure the foot and/or ankle than injure the knee, hip, and/or back. As a rule, the farther you get away from the foot, the less likely pronation and supination are responsible for producing an injury. For example, while low arches have frequently been blamed for the development of low back pain, a study in 2007 proved that excessive pronation and low back pain are in no way connected (15). In my opinion, as with running injuries in general, slightly low arches may actually protect the hip and low back because a little extra pronation improves shock absorption.

Until recently, it was believed that excessive pronation caused the leg to twist inward an excessive amount, transferring the rotation up the entire lower extremity. The belief that exaggerated pronation causes the knee and hip to rotate excessively is related to a mitered hinge analogy developed over 60 years ago. In this model, which is still taught in medical schools, pronation of the foot is converted into inward rotation of the leg with a 1:1 movement ratio; e.g., 8° of pronation causes the leg to twist inward 8° (Fig. 3.5).

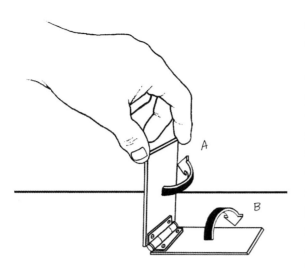

Fig. 3.5. *Mitered hinge analogy.* If you twist the top of a mitered hinge (**A**), the bottom of the hinge will twist the same amount (**B**).

Since low-arched people pronate more, it makes perfect sense that they would have greater ranges of leg rotation. However, evaluation of three-dimensional motion shows that this is not the case: The legs of low-arched pronators rotate inward the same degree as the legs of high-arched supinators (16). The equal ranges of leg rotation present in low- and high-arched runners explains why orthotics produce more consistent outcomes when treating foot and ankle injuries than when treating knee and hip injuries.

Recent research confirms that the mitered hinge analogy is all wrong. Even though low-arched people pronate through larger ranges of motion, the joints of their feet absorb most of this motion and they transmit less rotation into their legs. Conversely, high-arched individuals pronate less but their feet transfer a greater degree of rotation into their legs. The end result is that both high- and low-arched runners transmit the same rotation into their legs even though they pronate different amounts. This is nature's way of accommodating variation in arch height so the

structures above the ankle are not affected by the different degrees of pronation.

The bottom line is that while arch height may predispose runners to certain injuries (especially in the feet), slightly high or low arches rarely require treatment unless an injury is present. On the other hand, to deal with the stresses associated with high-mileage running, experienced runners frequently wear orthotics to lessen their potential for injury regardless of their arch height. As mentioned, orthotics do not work by altering the overall range of pronation; their effectiveness is more than likely related to their ability to distribute pressure, decelerate joint movements, and improve balance. These are good things whether you have high, neutral, or low arches.

Rather than investing in expensive custom orthotics right off the bat, you should first try running with a pair of over-the-counter orthotics. Even though custom orthotics have been shown to distribute pressure more effectively than over-the-counter orthotics, there is no evidence that custom orthotics are superior to prefabricated orthotics for injury prevention (17). Nonetheless, lifelong orthotic users often prefer custom orthotics because of their durability (graphite orthotics can last up to 15 years) and versatility (any of a dozen different modifications can be added to an orthotic). Over time, despite their initial cost, custom orthotics eventually become less expensive than over-the-counter orthotics because they are replaced so infrequently.

Varus and Valgus Posts: An Inexpensive Alternative to Orthotics

While custom and over-the-counter orthotics are great for treating and preventing a wide range of injuries, an equally effective and significantly less expensive treatment option for high- and low-arched runners is to use valgus or varus posts (Fig. 3.6). These posts are placed directly beneath the insole of your running shoe and are very easy to get used to.

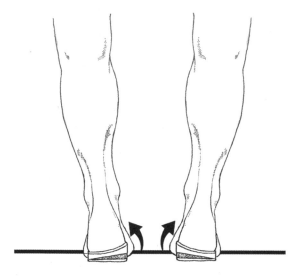

Fig. 3.6. *Varus posts elevate the inner side of your foot and effectively control excessive pronation.* Valgus posts are placed beneath the outer side of the foot and are helpful when treating high-arched runners.

While early cadaveric studies showed that varus posts could significantly reduce strain on the plantar fascia, studies on valgus posts showed that they could reduce knee pain in patients with arthritis, especially if they had high arches. In 2019, researchers from Brazil (18) took a group of runners who pronated excessively and gave them standard insoles, or an insole with a varus post. The researchers then measured three-dimensional motion and determined that compared to the runners with the standard insole, runners who wore the posted insole pronated less and had significantly less inward twisting of their legs and knees. This research is important because excessive inward rotation of the leg has been linked to a wide range of running injuries and is one of the more difficult movement patterns to change with gait retraining. My favorite over-the-counter varus posts are the slimline posts, as they are lightweight and the self-stick back allows you to easily attach it to the bottom of your insole.

What About the Transverse Arch of the Foot?

While the medial longitudinal arch is the most important arch of the foot, recent research shows that the midfoot arches from side to side, creating a transverse arch that is important in storing and returning energy (Fig. 3.7).

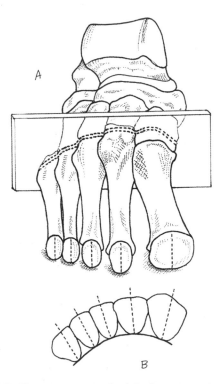

Fig. 3.7. *The transverse arch of the foot.* Notice that when sectioned at the midfoot (**A**), the bones of the midfoot create a functional arch (**B**) that stabilizes the foot during push-off. While the medial arch receives most of its support from the plantar fascia and the intrinsic muscle of the arch, the transverse arch is primarily controlled by the tibialis posterior.

Although not as important as the medial longitudinal arch for absorbing shock, the transverse arch improves running efficiency by stiffening the midfoot during the propulsive period. Because great apes lack this midfoot locking mechanism, they are less efficient during propulsion, as their midfoot buckles. The tibialis posterior is instrumental in maintaining the transverse arch, as it attaches to nearly all the bones of the midfoot, effectively stabilizing the transverse arch. Because the tibialis posterior rotates 45° before it attaches and is made from energy-storing collagen, it acts as a spring to store energy during contact while running, and return it in order to lock and stabilize the midfoot during propulsion.

LIMB LENGTH DISCREPANCY (LLD)

Surprisingly, almost everyone has legs that are within a fraction of an inch of being the same length. In a study of limb symmetry in rural Jamaica, researchers determined that while arm length differs markedly from side to side, only one in 1,000 people have leg length discrepancies greater than ⅜ inch (10 mm) (19). The authors attribute the reduced frequency of lower extremity limb length discrepancies to natural selection favoring lower limbs of equal lengths; i.e., because the muscles on the side of the long limb work harder while walking and running, individuals with large limb length discrepancies have to spend more calories getting around. As a result, they would have less energy left for reproduction and would therefore be quickly removed from the gene pool.

While moderate limb length discrepancies rarely cause problems in the general population, even small limb length discrepancies can injure a runner. To dramatize this point, the podiatrist

Steve Subotnick came up with the threefold rule: Because the forces associated with running are three times greater than the forces associated with walking, a ⅙ inch (4 mm) discrepancy in the legs of a runner (which is present in about 30% of the population) produces the same symptoms as a ½ inch (12 mm) discrepancy in a non-runner (which is present in about one in 2,000 people).

Structural Versus Functional Discrepancies

An important factor to consider is that many runners possess functional limb length discrepancies in which tightness in certain muscles and/or asymmetric pronation can make limbs that are actually of equal length appear to be different (Fig. 3.8). This is a significant distinction because functional discrepancies, unlike structural discrepancies, are not treated with heel lifts, since the bones of the lower extremity are the same length. When a functional discrepancy is the result of muscle tightness, stretching the affected muscles is the appropriate treatment. Conversely, asymmetric pronation is treated with arch supports.

The Long Limb and Stress Fractures

When a true limb length discrepancy is present and there is a short tibia and/or femur (referred to as a "structural LLD"), the longer limb is much more likely to develop stress fractures because it is exposed to greater impact forces (20). This is consistent with a study of Norwegian military recruits showing that 73% of the recruits fractured a bone on the side of the long limb and 16% on the side of the short limb, while only 11% of stress fractures occurred in recruits with equal limb lengths (21). The long limb hip is also prone

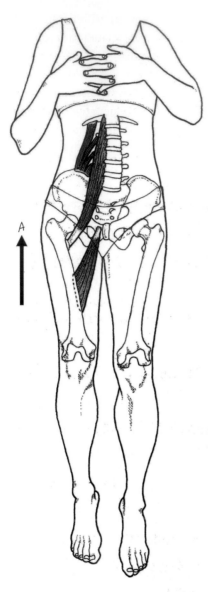

Fig. 3.8. ***Functional limb length discrepancies.*** *Tightness in certain muscles can pull the limb up on one side (**A**), causing one leg to appear shorter than the other.*

limb has a longer distance to fall while walking and slow running, people often attempt to modify their gait by slowly lowering the shorter limb to the ground by using their long limb hip abductors. This frequently results in chronic strain of the gluteus medius and may cause injury to the lumbar spine, since the lumbar vertebrae tilt sideward toward the long limb (Fig. 3.9). Long before symptoms develop, the runner presents with increased tightness in the gluteus medius on the long limb side.

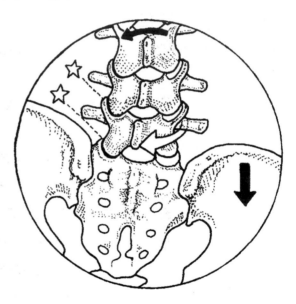

Fig. 3.9. ***The lumbar spine tilts away from the side of the short limb, rotating and compressing the joints in the low back (stars).***

to injury. In a study of 100 patients presenting for total hip replacement, 84% of the patients had arthritis on the side of the long limb (22).

The hip abductors on the side of the long limb are especially prone to injury. Because the short

In addition to stress fractures and hip injuries, the patella on the structurally long limb side is also more likely to be injured. Because the most effective way a runner can level the pelvis is by flexing the long limb knee, the knee on that side is subjected to greater force and therefore prone to breaking down. Individuals with limb length discrepancy often walk with the long knee flexed, which strains both the patella and the quadriceps tendon.

The Short Limb

While the majority of injuries occur on the side of the long limb, it is also possible for a runner to get injured on the side of the short limb. In an attempt to stabilize against the tendency to drop sideward toward the short limb, some runners turn their leg out prior to making ground contact. Although this protects you from falling toward the side of the short limb, it increases the potential of a fibular stress fracture because running with your foot pointing out increases the transfer of forces through the fibula (23). This is consistent with Friberg's study of military recruits: Although the long limb tibia was more prone to developing stress fractures, the fibula on the side of the short limb was more likely to fracture (21).

An alternate pattern of compensation for a short limb occurs when the runner hyperextends the knee on that side. While this movement may be helpful in bringing the heel closer to the ground during late swing phase, hyperextension of the knee impairs the ability of the quadriceps to absorb shock, possibly explaining why runners more frequently develop knee arthritis on the side of the short limb.

The sacroiliac joint is also prone to injury on the side of the short limb, as, in an attempt to level the sacrum, the pelvis tilts forward on that side (Fig. 3.10). Because of the limited range of motion available to this joint, the compensatory tilting greatly stresses the sacroiliac joint, possibly impairing its ability to absorb shock. This may explain why the sacroiliac joint on the side of the short limb shows earlier and more extensive arthritis than the sacroiliac joint on the side of the long limb (24).

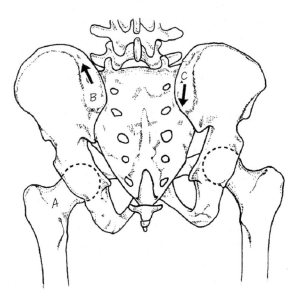

Fig. 3.10. *Pelvic compensation for a limb length discrepancy.* To keep the spine vertical, the pelvis on the side of the short limb (*A*) tilts forward (*B*), while the pelvis on the side of the long limb tilts backward (*C*).

Evaluating Limb Length Discrepancies

Given the clear association between structural limb length discrepancy and injury, it is important for runners to know whether or not their limbs are the same length. Because functional and structural limb length discrepancies are treated differently, it is important to differentiate a true structural limb length discrepancy (in which the bones are of different lengths) from a functional limb length discrepancy (which most often results from asymmetric muscle tightness). An experienced rehab specialist can easily differentiate structural and functional discrepancies by measuring the distance between the outer pelvis and the inner ankle with a tape measure (Fig. 3.11).

While some experts claim CAT scans are necessary to identify true asymmetry in bony

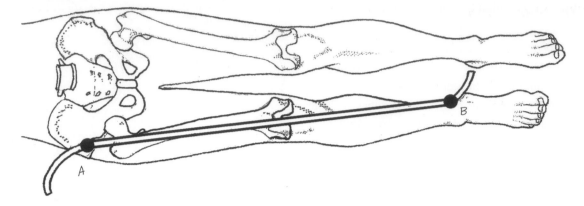

Fig. 3.11. *Measuring limb length discrepancies.* *By running a tape measure from the anterior superior iliac spine (ASIS) of the pelvis (**A**) to the medial malleolus of the ankle (**B**), it is possible to evaluate limb lengths very accurately.*

limb length, a study in 2013 comparing tape measurements to CAT scans confirmed that the tape measurement has an accuracy of 98% relative to the expensive and dangerous CAT scans (25) (CAT scans emit ionizing radiation, a proven carcinogen).

Consulting a Specialist

Before casually incorporating a heel lift based upon information obtained from a single measurement, your sports specialist should have fully evaluated respective tibial and femoral lengths in a variety of positions, checked for soft tissue contracture that might be twisting the pelvis, and carefully evaluated foot function to determine whether asymmetric arch height is contributing to a functional limb length discrepancy (Fig. 3.12).

Prior to wearing a heel lift, you can perform a simple test on yourself to confirm the presence of a structural limb length discrepancy. Shift your weight back and forth between your right and left leg for about 30 seconds and then stand on the leg that feels more comfortable.

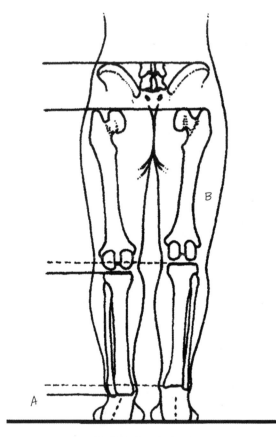

Fig. 3.12. *Evaluating limb length discrepancies.*
*A functional limb length discrepancy on the left, which is secondary to asymmetric pronation (**A**), coupled with a structural limb length discrepancy of the right femur (**B**), gives the appearance of symmetric limb lengths.*

When a structural limb length discrepancy is present, the pelvis levels when you stand on your short limb, so 99% of runners with true limb length discrepancy will stand on their short limb. If you find it's more comfortable to stand on what has been diagnosed as your long limb, you should think twice about wearing a heel lift. This test is surprisingly accurate, and runners with true limb length discrepancies stand on the short limb with almost no hesitation.

If you do have a structural limb length discrepancy, the height of the lift is determined by placing lifts of various sizes beneath the short limb and evaluating alignment. The ideal lift will level the iliac crest and, more importantly, bring the lumbar spine closer to vertical. Because of conflicting research regarding the degree of discrepancy necessary to justify treatment, the use of a lift should be based upon physical examination and the runner's symptoms; e.g., strain of the right gluteus medius responds

well to a left heel lift, while right sacroiliac pain responds well to a right heel lift.

When a limb length discrepancy is clear upon gait evaluation, and the location of the symptoms match with the side of the discrepancy, it is suggested that runners with limb length differences greater than $\frac{1}{6}$ inch (4 mm) be treated with the appropriate lift. On occasion, high-mileage runners often do well with lifts as small as $\frac{1}{12}$ inch (2 mm). Since the pelvis compensates for structural limb length discrepancies by tilting back on the side of the long limb and forward on the side of the short limb (26), individuals with structural limb length discrepancy should perform the stretches illustrated in Fig. 3.13. Because of the effect they have on the entire body, runners with structural limb length discrepancies often respond best to a comprehensive program that includes specific stretches, exercises, and/or chiropractic adjustments to restore symmetric flexibility.

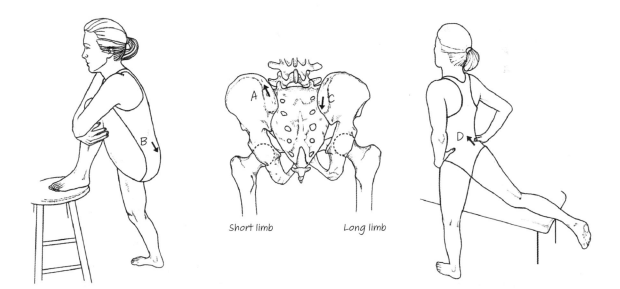

Short limb   Long limb

Fig. 3.13. *Home stretches to correct soft tissue imbalances associated with a limb length discrepancy.* Because the pelvis on the side of the short limb tilts forward (**A**), you should pull your knee toward your chest on that side (**B**). Because the pelvis on the side of the long limb tilts back (**C**), you should stretch the hip flexors on that side by extending the hip back (**D**). The stretches should be held for 20 seconds and performed five times per day.

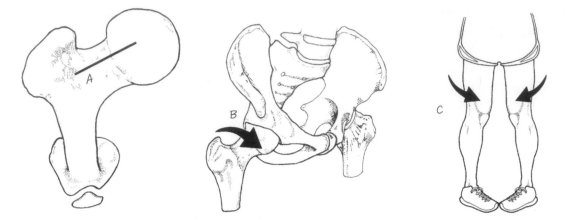

Fig. 3.14. *Typically, the neck of the femur angles only a few degrees forward so people can turn their knees in and out by equal amounts (A).* When the hips are anteverted, the neck of the femur turns in too far *(B)*, allowing the knees to twist in much farther than they can twist out *(C)*.

Anteverted Hips and/or External Tibial Torsion

While pronated feet and limb length discrepancies can occasionally cause problems in runners, in my opinion the most important and overlooked cause of running injuries is the presence of anteverted hips (Fig. 3.14, A). This is especially true when runners also possess external tibial torsion (Fig. 3.16).

From the Latin word for "forward twisting," *anteversion* of the hip represents a bony alignment in which the femur twists forward more than 10°. You can tell if you have anteverted hips by standing up and turning your feet in and out as much as you can. While the typical person can turn their feet in and out about 45° in each direction, people with anteverted hips can turn their feet in almost 80°, while barely being able to turn them out at all (they make terrible ballet dancers). Anteverted hips are often troublesome for runners because they allow the knees to twist inward too far, which greatly stresses the outer kneecaps (Fig. 3.15).

Individuals with anteverted hips often need to strengthen their hips and practice running

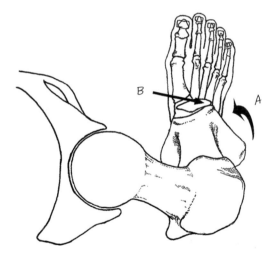

Fig. 3.15. *Anteverted hips allow the knees to twist in excessively (A), causing the outer side of the patella to collide into the femur (B).*

with their knees straight. A simple test you can do to evaluate your hip strength is to slowly step off a stair while looking down to see if your knee twists in (see Fig. 3.35, page 119). If your hip drops or your knee twists in while performing this test, you should do the hip and knee strengthening exercises shown in Fig. 3.36. Runners with anteverted hips need to have strong hip rotators in order to stop their hips from twisting in while they run.

While anteverted hips can increase the risk of hip and knee pain, they are especially problematic when they occur with external tibial torsion. The combination of hip anteversion and external tibial torsion occurs in about 15% of the running population and is responsible for a wide range of running injuries. Unfortunately, most runners who have this combination are unaware of it, as so few healthcare providers even know what external tibial torsion is. To determine if you have external tibial torsion, lie face down and flex your knees 90°. Move your ankles until your feet are horizontal and check to see how your feet align with your thighs: They should be parallel. In people with external tibial torsion, their feet point out relative to their thighs (Fig. 3.16).

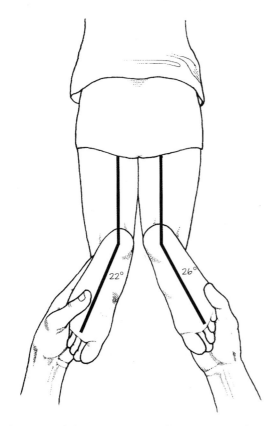

Fig. 3.16. *While lying face down, have someone place your feet in a horizontal position.* Ideally, your feet will parallel to your thighs. The person shown has external tibial torsion.

External tibial torsion causes a great deal of trouble because runners who possess it are frequently told to run with their feet straight, which causes their knees to twist in. This irritates the knee and alters the efficiency of the hip rotators. The hip rotators become so overstretched that control of the lower limb in the transverse plane is lost, resulting in chronic piriformis syndrome, sciatica, and outer knee pain. Unfortunately, while anteverted hips are treated with aggressive strengthening of the hip rotators, there is no way to correct external tibial torsion, as this is a bony alignment pattern that cannot be changed. The only treatment is to do gait retraining that encourages running with the appropriate toe-out gait pattern. This gait retraining program will be discussed in the next chapter.

FLEXIBILITY

In 1986, Rob DeCastella set a course record by running the Boston Marathon in 2:07:51, just 39 seconds off the world record. A few days before the race, I saw Rob in my office and when I checked his hamstring flexibility, I was shocked to see he could barely raise each leg 30° off the table (even tight runners can raise their legs 60°). Having never seen hamstrings that tight, I asked Rob if he ever stretched and he responded: "When I run, that's as far as my legs go forward so that's as far as I want them to go forward."

At the time, it was just assumed that runners had to stretch in order to run fast and remain injury free, but here was one of the world's fastest runners who not only didn't stretch regularly but avoided stretching altogether. According to conventional wisdom, I should have encouraged Rob to stretch, but I didn't. Besides being one of the world's fastest runners, Rob DeCastella knew a lot about exercise physiology and I trusted his judgment.

Years later, research appeared suggesting that tight runners were metabolically more efficient than flexible runners. This is what DeCastella intuitively knew: Tight muscles can store and return energy in the form of elastic recoil, just like a rubber band can stretch and snap back with no effort. Because tight muscles provide free energy (i.e., the muscle fibers are not shortening to produce force so there is no metabolic expense), stiff muscles can significantly improve efficiency when running long distances.

To understand why muscles are able to store and return energy, just take a look at what they are made of. To protect individual muscle fibers from developing too much tension, and to assist in the storage and return of energy, a bundle of muscle fibers is surrounded by a special soft tissue envelope called the "perimysium." These envelopes contain thousands of strong cross-links that traverse the entire muscle (Fig. 3.17). The cross-links are essential for injury prevention because they distribute tension generated on one side of the tendon evenly throughout the entire muscle.

If these cross-links were not present, or if they were excessively flexible, the asymmetric tendon force would be transferred through the muscle fibers only on the side of the tendon being pulled. Because fewer muscle fibers would be tractioned, the involved fibers would be more prone to

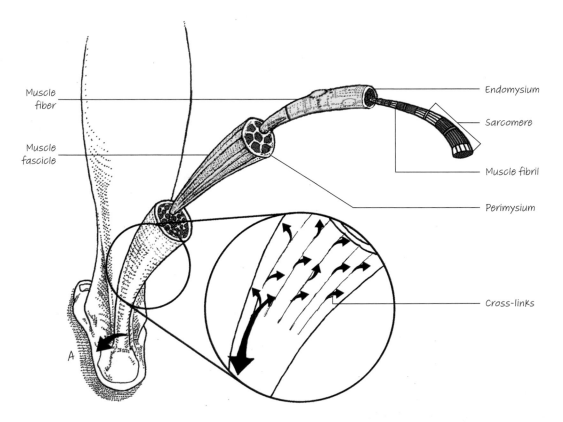

Fig. 3.17. ***The components of a muscle.*** *When the foot pronates (**A**), excessive tension is placed on the inner side of the Achilles tendon (arrow). Small cross-links present in the perimysium distribute pressure generated on one side of the tendon evenly throughout the entire muscle.*

being injured because the pulling force would be distributed over a smaller area. The muscle itself would also be less able to store and return energy simply because fewer fibers would be stretched (the more fibers being pulled, the greater the return of energy). The tight cross-links present in the soft tissue envelopes act as powerful reinforcements that distribute force over a broader area.

Given the improved efficiency associated with tightness, you would think that the world's fastest runners would all be extremely stiff. This isn't the case. Compared to the mid-to-late 1980s, today's elite runners are significantly more flexible. The reason for this is that even though tight muscles can make you more efficient, they are easily strained and are more likely to produce delayed onset muscle soreness after a hard workout (27). Because the best runners currently run more than 130 miles per week with grueling track workouts, increased delayed onset muscle soreness would interfere with their ability to tolerate their rigorous training schedules and would more than likely increase their potential for injury.

To prove that tight muscles are more prone to injury, researchers from Lenox Hill Hospital in New York classified subjects as either stiff or flexible before having them perform repeat hamstring curls to fatigue (27). Following the workout, the stiffer subjects complained of greater muscle pain and weakness. The enzyme marker for muscle damage (CK) was also significantly higher in the stiff group after working out. The authors of the study state that because flexible people are less susceptible to exercise-induced muscle damage, they are able to exercise at a higher intensity for a greater duration on the days following heavy workouts. The catch-22 of muscle tightness is that while a certain degree of tightness increases the storage

and return of energy, excessive tightness can increase your potential for injury.

Muscle Tightness and Injuries: A U-shaped Curve

While excessively tight runners are injury prone, excessively loose runners are also prone to injury because their muscles have to work harder to stabilize joints that are moving through larger ranges of motion. Flexible muscles are also less able to store energy in their epimysium and perimysium so their muscles have to work harder to generate the same force. The end result is that overly flexible runners are just as likely to be injured as stiff runners. It turns out that if you draw a graph of injuries associated with different degrees of flexibility, a U-shaped curve results, with the tightest and loosest runners sustaining a larger percentage of injuries (28) (Fig. 3.18).

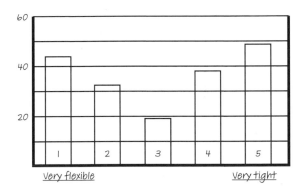

Fig. 3.18. *U-shaped curve of injuries versus flexibility.* *The vertical axis of the graph represents cumulative injury incidence as a percentage. There were the same number of people in each of the five groups.*

The Best Way to Evaluate Your Flexibility

Because runners in the middle of the graph in Fig. 3.18 are typically not prone to flexibility-related injuries, the goal of a rehab program should be to get yourself away from the extreme ends of the curve. A simple test you can do to quickly evaluate flexibility is to bend your thumb back toward your wrist and measure the distance (Fig. 3.19).

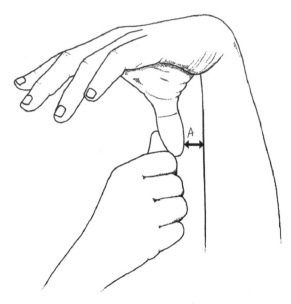

Fig. 3.19. *The thumb to radius index.* Excessive flexibility is present when the thumb can be positioned within 1 inch (2.5 cm) of the forearm (**A**).

Checking the range of motion in your thumb is one of the easiest ways to evaluate overall flexibility because thumb flexibility is a marker for whole body flexibility (just as grip strength is a marker for whole body strength). If you are overly flexible, consider lifting weights to strengthen your muscles and incorporating agility drills to improve coordination.

In contrast, if you happen to fall on the tight side of the spectrum and would like to lessen your potential for injury, consider incorporating specific stretches into your daily routine (Fig. 3.20). This is especially important for tightness of the gastrocnemius, which is an extremely common cause of a variety of forefoot injuries in runners.

Keep in mind that improving flexibility is not that simple. Some great research has shown that when done for just a few weeks, stretching does not alter the ability of a muscle to absorb force because the muscle fibers respond by lengthening slightly to give you the illusion that they're more flexible (29). It's as if the muscle is getting bored with you trying to stretch it so it just separates a few muscle fibers so that you'll leave it alone: You haven't changed the muscle architecture at all, you've just relaxed the muscle a little. Unfortunately, it's still the same muscle and its ability to absorb force has not been altered.

The inability of short-term stretches to improve flexibility explains why there are so many studies showing that stretching does not change injury rates. Because of compliance issues and time constraints, almost every study on stretching and injuries has evaluated stretches over a short duration (probably because so few people would stick with a long-term stretching regimen). That being the case, it's not surprising that while some great research shows that tight muscles are more likely to be injured (27), relatively few studies have ever shown that stretching alters your potential for injury.

In order to produce real length gains, some experts suggest it is necessary to stretch regularly for four to six months. In theory, when a muscle is repeatedly stretched for several months, cellular changes take place within the muscle, allowing for a permanent increase in flexibility. Animal studies have shown that the increased flexibility associated with repeat stretching results from a lengthening of the connective tissue envelope surrounding the muscle fibers (especially the perimysium) and/or an increased number of sarcomeres being added to the ends of the muscle fibers (30) (see Fig. 1.1).

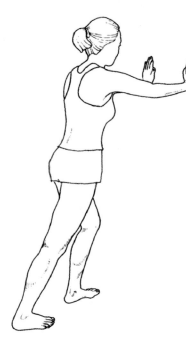

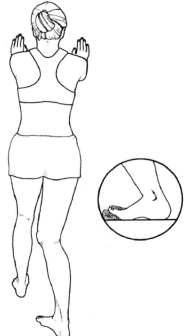

B) Tibialis posterior and inner soleus stretch.

Tibialis posterior and inner soleus stretch. Rotate the
back leg inward while slightly flexing the knee.
To stretch the deep flexors, place a rolled-up
towel beneath the toes (inset).

A) Gastrocnemius stretch.

Keep the knee straight with the hip extended behind you.
To stretch the inner fibers of this muscle, roate the involved
leg inward. To stretch the soleus, bend the knee slightly.

D) An alternate way to stretch the anterior compartment
muscles is to squat down on all fours with a
pillow placed beneath the forefeet (inset).

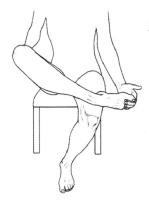

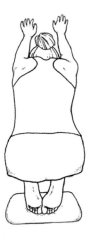

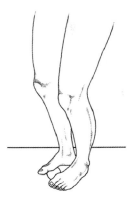

C) Anterior compartment stretches.

While sitting with your leg in a figure 4
position, pull the toes downward.

E) Peroneus longus stretch.

Place a tennis ball beneath your inner forefeet
and slightly flex your knees.

Fig. 3.20. *Common stretches for runners.*

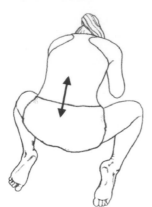

F) Short adductor stretch.
Known as the frog pose in yoga,
get down on all fours with your hips abducted. Move
your pelvis forward and backward so you can
stretch all of the adductor muscles (arrow).

G) Long adductor stretch.
Gracilis and portions of adductor magnus are
stretched by placing your heel on an elevated
surface positioned at your side. By rotating your leg in
and out you can stretch all of the adductor muscles.

H) Hamstring stretch.
Place your heel on elevated surface while keeping a slight
arch in your low back. By pivoting forward at the hips (arrow) the outer
hamstrings are stretched by rotating the leg in, while the inner hamstrings
are stretched by turning the leg out (arrow B). By repeating the stretch with
the knee flexed 30°, 45°, 90°, you can isolate specific areas of tightness
in the upper and lower hamstrings.

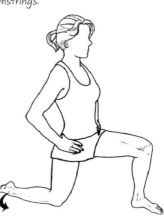

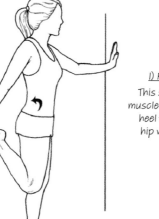

I) Rectus femoris stretch.
This section of the quadriceps
muscle is stretched by pulling your
heel towards the back of your
hip while maintaining a pelvic
tuck (arrow).

J) Hip flexor stretch.
While kneeling on one leg,
shift your weight forward until you feel
slight tension in the front of the groin.
The hip flexors can be isolated by moving the
ankle out slightly (arrow).

Fig. 3.20. *Common stretches for runners.* *(continued)*

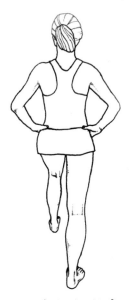

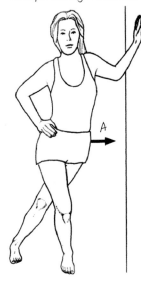

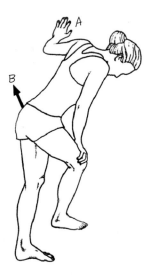

L) Tensor fasciae latae stretch.

The involved leg is positioned behind you while you shift your pelvis towards the wall (A). Your spine should be kept in a midline position while performing this stretch.

K) Standing hip flexor stretch.

An alternate way to stretch the hip flexors is to extend the straight leg behind you while maintaining a neurtral pelvis.

M) Gluteus medius stretch.

The leg you are stretching is positioned behind you, while the hand on that side is resting against a wall (A). To stretch the gluteus medius muscle, move your hip towards the wall (B).

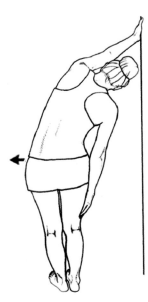

O) Alternate quadratus lumborum stretch.

Kneel back so your hips are over your heels and pull your upper body to the right to stretch the left quadratus lumborum (arrow).

N) Quadratus lumborum stretch.

With your feet touching, grab the side of a door jam and shift your pelvis away from the door (arrow). By grabbing the door at different points while bending forward slightly, specific fibers of the quadratus lumborum can be lengthened.

Fig. 3.20. *Common stretches for runners.* (continued)

Q) Piriformis muscle energy stretch.

To stretch the left piriformis muscle, the hip is flexed 45° while the opposite leg hooks over the knee (A). You then lightly tense the piriformis muscle by pushing the left knee into resistance provided by the right leg. After five seconds, the left piriformis is relaxed and the right leg pulls the left knee inward, stretching the piriformis.

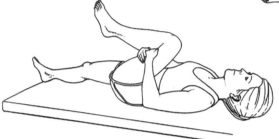

P) Gluteus maximus stretch.

Clasp your hands behind your knee and pull the involved thing towards your shoulder. To stretch the piriformis muscle, pull knee towards the opposite shoulder.

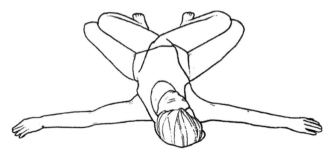

R) Lumbar rotational stretch.

Lie on the ground with your knees and hips flexed with your arms positioned for stability. Gently rock your knees from side to side, moving through gradually larger ranges of motion. Spend about three seconds rocking in each direction for a total of 60 seconds.

S) Standing hyperextension.

Place your hands over the base of the spine and arch back. Your pelvis should remain still while your lumbar spine extends comfortably.

Fig. 3.20. Common stretches for runners. (continued)

To Stretch or Not to Stretch?

Before considering a long-term commitment to stretching, you should be sure it's worth your time and effort. While slower recreational runners running less than 15 miles per week may not want to invest the time, high-mileage runners almost always benefit from regular stretching because it improves their ability to tolerate heavy workouts. Also, runners who are asymmetrically tight should consider committing to a long-term stretching program. To determine if you're asymmetrically tight, perform the stretches illustrated in Fig. 3.20 and compare muscle flexibility on your right and left sides. If one muscle doesn't move as far as the same muscle on the other side, you should definitely stretch the tighter side. Asymmetrical muscle tightness was shown in 2013 to correlate with the development of future injuries (31).

Assuming you decide to begin a long-term stretching routine, determining the ideal frequency and duration that a stretch should be maintained is the subject of debate. Different studies have recommended anywhere from 1 to 20 stretch repetitions with each stretch held for anywhere from 10 seconds to 10 minutes. The amount of force used during a stretch is also a subject of debate, as some studies recommend stretching the muscle to the point of discomfort, while others recommend stretching only to the point where tension is felt.

To identify the ideal stretch frequency and duration, researchers from Duke University placed rabbits on special machines designed to evaluate improvements in muscle flexibility following 10 consecutive 30-second stretches (32). Using this elaborate technique, the authors determined that the majority of length gains associated with stretching occur in the first 15 seconds of a stretch, and that after the fourth 30-second stretch, no appreciable length gains were achieved. This research confirms it is better to perform a few 30-second stretches throughout the day than to spend an extended period of time stretching a specific muscle. (Although if you are pressed for time, stretching just once a day for 30 seconds has been shown to effectively increase range of motion [33].)

Don't Forget Foam Rolling

Self-massage and foam rolling have become increasingly popular over the last 10 years. In part, this is because runners intuitively know that vigorous compression of a muscle stretches individual fibers inside the muscle, enhancing resiliency of the treated area. This is especially true after an injury.

The world-renowned fascial researcher Carla Stecco showed that following injury, the epimysium becomes damaged and fibroblasts lay down collagen cross-links to repair the damaged muscle (34). If excessive damage occurs and the body lays down too much collagen, the epimysial space between muscle fibers becomes greatly reduced, which can interfere with the flow of hyaluronic acid. Hyaluronic acid is your body's natural muscle lubricant, allowing for individual fibers to glide smoothly back and forth over one another. Dr. Stecco used an electron microscope to prove that the epimysial space between muscle fibers is reduced following injury, and that this reduced space correlates with the development of pain.

The reason reduced epimysial space is so troublesome is that it leads to an increase in muscle waste products, such as lactic acid. The increased presence of lactic acid creates an acidic environment that actually thickens your body's hyaluronic acid, which makes it impossible for individual fibers to slide over one another. Small sections of muscle begin to move as a unit, increasing the transfer of force through the tight sections of damaged muscles. Because these regions are stiff and not moving properly, the muscle spindles located on the muscle fibers fail to provide sensory information about position, and the entire muscle becomes less coordinated and more prone to injury.

This is where foam rolling comes into its own. Unlike static stretching, which applies a force to the entire muscle and doesn't target a specific area, foam rolling can be performed specifically over the dense damaged section of muscle. It's easy to find these specific spots by foam rolling immediately after your run. Because lactic acid has accumulated in the dense tight areas, they are sensitive to the touch and can produce significant discomfort as you roll over them.

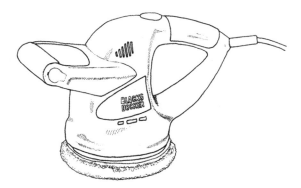

Fig. 3.21. *The Black & Decker car polisher.*

While foam rolling can effectively sort some of these areas out, my favorite way to restore flexibility to damaged sections of muscles is with a Black & Decker car polisher (Fig. 3.21). You can buy one of these for about $30 online and, while leaving the lambswool attachment on, place it directly over the stiffest area of your muscle.

Because the tool vibrates at such a high intensity, it stimulates cutaneous receptors to block pain and allow the muscle to relax. It's called the "gate theory of pain" and it works as follows.

Your central nervous system can only process a limited amount of sensory information at any given time, so it selects the faster moving fibers first (hence the name gate theory). Because nerves that transmit vibration travel at over 100 m/s (225 mph), while pain signals from muscles travel between 5 and 15 m/s (11 and 33 mph), your central nervous system ignores information from the painful muscles and focuses on the vibration stimulus. As a result, the muscles relax as your central nervous system temporarily ignores the pain signals to focus on the incoming vibration stimulus. It's the same mechanism that happens when you scratch a mosquito bite: The itch goes away as your central nervous system blocks it to pay more attention to your cutaneous receptors transmitting rapidly moving sensory stimulation from the skin around the mosquito bite.

The car polisher also creates a frictional force that increases warmth. You can feel this heating sensation after 30 seconds or so, and that increased circulation penetrates deep into the muscle and can enhance the removal of lactic acid while simultaneously breaking down any adhesions present in the perimysium.

The Best Ways to Improve Tendon Flexibility

While improving muscle flexibility is important, without doubt the best way to avoid injury and improve performance is to work on increasing your tendon flexibility. Because tendons don't burn calories like muscles do, they can store and return free energy, making you efficient and resilient.

Some interesting research suggests that it is possible to improve tendon flexibility by performing specific muscle energy stretches. To prove this, Anthony Kay and his colleagues from the UK used ultrasonography to evaluate real-time changes in tendon stiffness as 17 volunteers performed a variety of different stretches, including conventional static stretches and the more complicated contract/relax stretches (35). Not surprisingly, conventional static stretches slightly improved muscle flexibility but had no effect on tendon flexibility. In contrast, stretches using muscle contractions prior to initiating a stretch improved muscle flexibility about the same amount as static stretching, but also increased tendon flexibility by nearly 20%. The authors claim the most effective way to improve tendon flexibility is to place a muscle in a midline position and isometrically tense it for five seconds (isometric contractions involve tensing a muscle with no movement of the joint). This is immediately followed with a ten-second stretch. You then return to the original starting position, tense the muscle again for five seconds, and repeat the stretch for another 10 seconds (Fig. 3.22).

When performed three times, the entire stretching routine takes less than a minute and results in substantial improvements in both muscle and tendon resiliency. Although the illustration depicts the stretch being performed on the Achilles tendon, it can be modified to be done on any tendon. Because the muscle is always tensed while in a midline position, I refer to this stretching technique as "neutral position stretching." The best predictor of a future running injury is a prior running injury; therefore, before beginning your run, this stretching technique should be performed on any muscle you have previously injured.

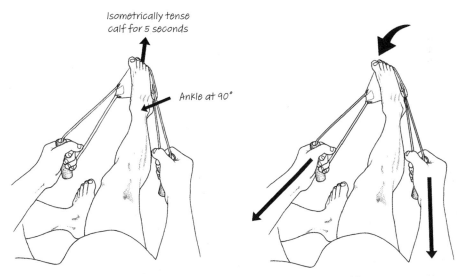

Isometrically tense calf for 5 seconds

Ankle at 90°

Stretch calf for 10 seconds

Fig. 3.22. *Using a belt or strap, place your ankle at a 90° angle to your leg and isometrically tense your calf for five seconds.* Follow the five-second contraction with a ten-second stretch by pulling with your hands (**arrows**).

While neutral position stretching is good for improving tendon flexibility, research in 2011 and 2018 proved that you can significantly increase tendon strength by performing isometric contractions with the muscle maintained in its lengthened position (36, 37). Using the Achilles tendon as an example, stand on the stairway while holding a weight in one hand (or wearing a weighted backpack) and lower your heel so it is positioned slightly below horizontal. You should use enough weight so you are fatigued after 20 seconds. Repeat this maneuver four times on each leg. This exercise routine has been proven to markedly increase tendon resiliency and strength (37) in just a few months.

Apparently, isometrically contracting muscles while they are in a lengthened position stimulates the tenocytes to remodel the tendons, greatly reducing the risk of future tendon injury. In a 2018 review of the literature on the benefits associated with performing isometric contractions with muscles in their lengthened positions, Oranchuk et al. (36) state "long muscle length training results in greater transference to dynamic performance." This research could have a profound effect on improving performance and preventing injury.

A Better Alternative to Static Stretching: Active Dynamic Running Drills

Rather than slowly stretching each muscle statically, many runners prefer active dynamic warm-ups. Popular with elite and sub-elite runners, these drills allow you to warm up specific muscles while simultaneously stretching them. The dynamic drills in Chapter 4 (illustrated in Fig. 4.5) were proven in 2012 to improve performance in sprinters (38). Compared to a control group, runners who performed either 1 or 2 sets of 14 repetitions of each of the exercises were able to run significantly faster sprint times.

Because dynamic stretches can be difficult to master and are time-consuming, slower recreational runners can either incorporate gentler versions of these dynamic stretches or just consider warming up by running slowly with a high cadence and a short stride length. Since older runners tend to be stiffer, the length of time you spend warming up is age-dependent: 30- to 40-year-old runners should consider warming up for 5–10 minutes, while the 50 and older group should run slowly for up to 15 minutes. Each person is different so the length of time you spend warming up is up to you.

In the largest randomized controlled study of stretching to date, Daniel Pereles and colleagues proved in 2012 that runners intuitively know whether or not they should stretch (39). These authors randomly assigned 2,729 recreational runners to either a stretching or a non-stretching pre-run routine. Not surprisingly, there was no significant difference in injury rates between the runners who stretched versus the runners who didn't stretch. However, if a runner who routinely stretched was assigned to the non-stretch protocol, he/she was nearly twice as likely to sustain a running injury. As with almost everything regarding running-related injuries, you are the best judge of choosing which pre-exercise warm-up is right for you.

STRENGTH TRAINING

In the 100th running of the Boston Marathon, Tegla Loroupe was in first place for most of the race with a comfortable lead over Uta Pippig.

At about mile 23, Tegla's back began to hurt and she later said that her left leg felt like it was "dead." Despite the pain, Tegla somehow managed to finish in second place, just 85 seconds behind Uta. She didn't know it at the time but Tegla developed small stress fractures in the base of her spine during the downhill portion of the race. Later that same year, Tegla attempted to run the New York Marathon but the stress fractures hadn't completely healed and this time her back pain became severe. An MRI after the race revealed that she had a fracture in the base of her spine called a "spondylolysis." Frequently present in gymnasts, this type of fracture occurs when the lower lumbar vertebrae repeatedly extend through large ranges of motion, fracturing a section of bone near the spinal joints. To immobilize the spinal fracture, Tegla was fitted with a special brace designed to stop her low back from moving. Unfortunately, the brace compressed a nerve located near the top of her pelvis, causing a decrease in sensation along the outer portion of her thigh.

Core Weakness and Chronic Injury

Because of the progressive loss of feeling in her outer thigh and her continued low back pain, Tegla came to see me for an evaluation. The sensory nerve injury was relatively minor and gradually resolved once the brace was removed. Tegla's real problem became apparent with a test called "Vleeming's test." Developed by a leading spine specialist from the Netherlands, this simple test accurately identifies weakness in the abdominal core muscles. You can do Vleeming's test on yourself by lying on a comfortable surface. With your arms at your sides, raise one leg in the air and have a friend push down on the raised ankle (Fig. 3.23). When the abdominal core muscles are strong, the pelvis remains

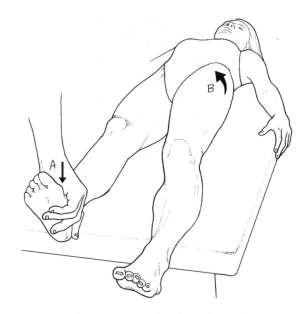

Fig. 3.23. **Vleeming's test.** When the core muscles are weak, pushing down on the elevated leg (**A**) will cause the opposite pelvis to lift (**B**).

horizontal. In Tegla's case, the opposite side of her pelvis lifted right off the table.

Core weakness played a huge role in the chronic nature of Tegla's injury because the core muscles function to lock the vertebrae of the low back together, creating a compressive force that stabilizes the entire lower spine while running. Adequate core strength is especially important while running downhill because the braking phase associated with initial ground contact allows the lower lumbar vertebrae to shift forward upon heel strike (Fig. 3.24).

If the core muscles are weak, this forward shifting is unopposed and the excessive forward motion of the lower lumbar vertebrae creates a shear force in the low back capable of producing a stress fracture. Fortunately, it doesn't take a lot of core strength to prevent injury because the core muscles fire with very low intensities while running.

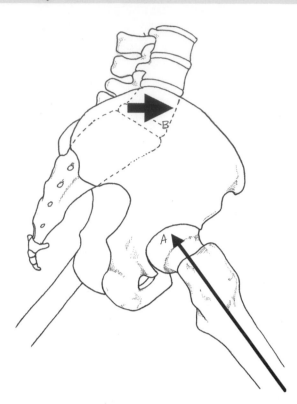

Fig. 3.24. *The braking phase associated with striking the ground (A) causes the lower lumbar spine to shift forward (B).*

Based on her exam results, Tegla was treated with soft tissue manipulation to reduce entrapment of the sensory nerve, stretches to improve the flexibility of her hip flexors and abductors (tight hips can cause the back to arch excessively while running), and gentle mobilization of the stiff spinal joints located above the fracture site. The most important component of Tegla's treatment was an intensive program of core exercises. While many rehabilitation experts recommend complex core strengthening exercises in which special machines are used to provide feedback regarding the successful recruitment of the deep core muscles, research in 2007 confirmed that simple home exercises are just as effective as the expensive and complicated core training

protocols that require special training and access to high-tech machinery (40).

Tegla was consistent with her stretches and home strengthening exercises, and five months later, she set the course record in Rotterdam with a 2:22:07 marathon. She continued with her exercises, and the following year Tegla broke the world record by running a 2:20:47 at Rotterdam. One year later, her chronic low back pain finally resolved, and she set another world record at the Berlin Marathon.

The Diaphragm: The Overlooked Core Muscle

While many runners routinely incorporate sidelying planks, bridges, bird dogs, rollouts, and single-leg raises to strengthen their core muscles, very few of them work on strengthening their diaphragm (Fig. 3.25). This is unfortunate

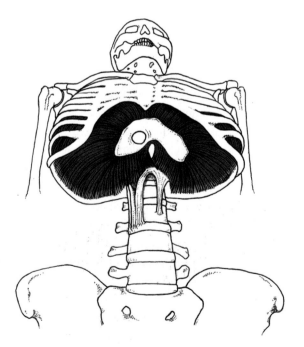

Fig. 3.25. *The diaphragm.*

because the diaphragm is the largest core muscle and plays an important role in injury prevention. Several papers have shown that individuals with weak diaphragms are more likely to develop low back pain and have impaired athletic performance (41, 42).

When you run, the diaphragm's connections to the deep core muscles allow you to maintain a constant intra-abdominal pressure while changing directions, which is particularly important when trail running. More importantly, a weak diaphragm can cause a wide range of problems in runners because the central nervous system prioritizes the delivery of blood to the diaphragm over other neighboring muscles. When the diaphragm fatigues while you run, the central nervous system deliberately decreases blood flow to your low back and legs in order to shunt as much blood as possible to the diaphragm (getting enough oxygen is a big deal to your brain).

Several studies have shown significant reductions in blood flow to the low back and leg muscles when the diaphragm is deliberately exhausted (42, 43). Where this gets interesting is the effect that decreased low back and limb muscle circulation has on your muscle spindles: Because muscle spindles are highly vascular structures, even a slight reduction in blood flow to a spindle (as would occur with premature fatigue of the diaphragm, causing a reflex reduction in blood flow to the low back) would markedly impair muscle coordination in the spine and extremity muscles. Runners with fatigued diaphragms would be much more likely to be injured when blood flow to their lower extremity is impaired, as they would lose the ability to sense where their legs were in space while running. They often complain that their legs feel "dead" at the end of a race.

It's easy to see if your diaphragm is weak with a device called a "K-4 spirometer," which measures diaphragm power, speed, and lung volume. Unfortunately, the machine costs about $400 and not many doctors perform this test. As a result, the easiest solution is to simply assume that your diaphragm is weak and, like all muscles, would benefit from strengthening exercises. The simplest way to strengthen the diaphragm is with a Powerbreathe lung exerciser, which can be purchased for about $35 online. Runners should perform 3 sets of 20 inhale repetitions at 60% full effort (you should be fatigued after finishing the final repetition of each set).

While most yoga instructors encourage deep diaphragmatic breathing to strengthen the diaphragm, this approach has been proven to be ineffective, as high-resistance exercise is necessary in order to strengthen the diaphragm (44). Maintaining a strong diaphragm is essential, as numerous studies have shown that diaphragm strength correlates with improved performance in running, cycling, and even swimming (45–47).

Hip Rotator Strength

In an interesting study published in *Medicine and Science in Sports and Exercise*, researchers from Kentucky and Delaware tested core and hip muscle strength in 140 male and female basketball and track athletes at the start of their season (48). They specifically evaluated endurance in the abdominal and back-extensor muscles, as well as strength in the hip rotators and abductors. By the end of the season, 48 athletes had sustained an injury, and the only predictor of injury was the strength of the hip external rotators. In this study, it was found that the knee was particularly prone to injury, which is not surprising because the hip rotators control rotation.

Using the same protocol to measure hip strength, researchers from Iran repeated this study by measuring hip rotator strength in 501 competitive athletes participating in various sports (49). After only one season, the athletes who were unable to generate 20% of their body weight with the seated hip rotator test were seven times more likely to tear their anterior cruciate ligament. It's easy to quantify strength deficits in the hip external rotators using the testing device illustrated in Fig. 3.26.

If you're handy, you can perform this test on yourself using a luggage scale. Position the scale against your inner ankle and if you can't generate 20% of your body weight in the test position, you need to do the exercises listed in Table 6.3 and set a three-month goal to reach your target strength. Again, I strongly feel that hip rotator weakness is one of the most overlooked causes of running-related injuries, especially in women with anteverted hips and/or external tibial torsion.

Toe Strength

Strengthening specific small muscles of the foot and ankle can play a huge role in performance enhancement and injury prevention. Numerous studies have shown that foot/ankle strengthening exercises can improve balance (50), increase arch height (51), enhance jump performance (52), and make you run faster (53), particularly if you have flat feet (10). Because the toe and arch muscles provide stability during the push-off phase while jumping and running, weakness in these muscles may lead to a variety of injuries, including plantar fasciitis, stress fractures, bunions, and Achilles tendinitis. Maintaining strong toes is especially important in trail runners, as the ability to change direction rapidly is determined to a large extent by toe strength (54).

Despite their strong connection with performance enhancement and injury prevention, toe strengthening exercises are rarely included in conventional rehab programs. To add to the problem, the most commonly prescribed foot strengthening protocols have significant

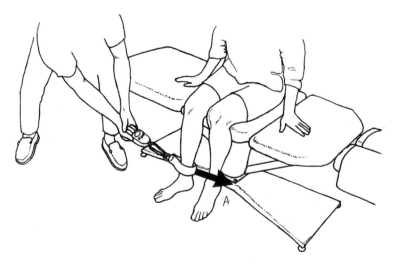

Fig. 3.26. *Testing strength of the hip rotators with a dynamometer.* A strap is placed around the ankle and the person holding the testing device measures hip strength while the seated person pulls inward. You should be able to generate 20% of your body weight during this test.

drawbacks in that they work the toe and arch muscles in their midline or downward positions, which decreases their effectiveness because this is not how these muscles are used in real life. Because strength gains while exercising are angle specific (55) (i.e., strength gains are greatest when muscles are exercised in the joint angles used while exercising), in order to be effective, foot exercises must duplicate the positions in which muscles are used while walking and running.

The importance of exercising the toes in their functional positions was demonstrated in an evaluation of strength gains associated with short foot exercises. Houck et al. (56) had 18 adults perform short foot exercises for four weeks and determined that this popular foot exercise in no way improved the ability of the toes to push down while walking. This is consistent with the findings of Spink et al. (57), who had 153 seniors perform foot exercises for 30 minutes, three times a week for six months (the exercises included marble pickups and various elastic band exercises). At the end of that study, there was no appreciable change in toe strength. While progressive resistance elastic band exercises can

produce strength gains, these gains are not angle specific because the elastic band's resistance reaches a peak while the ankle and toes are pointing downward; i.e., the calf and arch muscles are shortened. This is in contrast to walking and running, where forces peak while the calf and toe muscles are in lengthened positions.

To produce the best functional outcomes, therefore, the muscles of the foot and ankle should be exercised through ranges that match their real-life movement patterns (55). My favorite way to increase toe strength is with the ToePro exercise platform (Fig. 3.27). This platform was specifically designed to place muscles in their lengthened positions while exercising. The upper surface of the platform tilts down at the sides to target the peroneals, and down from front to back to target the superficial and deep calf muscles. Additionally, an elevated crest is incorporated into the front top edge to place the toe muscles in their lengthened positions.

Strengthening the peroneals is extremely important for improving running performance.

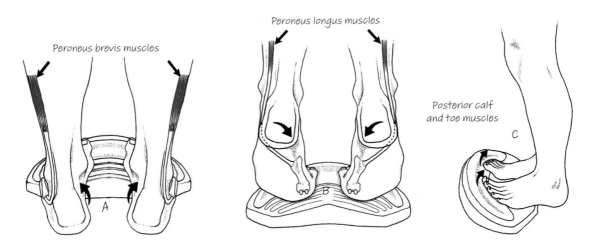

Fig. 3.27. The ToePro exercise platform. *This platform tilts down at the sides to target the peroneals (A and B), and down from front to back to isolate the posterior calf (C). An elevated crest along the top front surface has been added to lengthen the toe muscles.*

In an interesting analysis of muscle activity as athletes transition from slow to fast running, Reber et al. (58) showed that the peroneus brevis experiences a linear increase in activity as running speed increases. Those authors emphasize the importance of strengthening this often-overlooked muscle in order to optimize sprint performance.

A more recent paper, in 2018, confirmed that keeping all of the calf muscles strong is essential for maintaining running speed as we age. In a study comparing running efficiency in young and middle-aged runners, Paquette et al. (59) confirmed that older runners slow down not because of decreased force output from the hips or knees, but because of reduced force output from the calves. In fact, the force output in older runners was 10.5% lower than that of their younger peers. The authors suggest that preserving calf strength could attenuate the decline of speed associated with aging.

The easiest way to tell if your toes are weak is to look at your insoles: A runner with a strong foot should leave clear indents beneath the toes, not just beneath the central metatarsal heads. Another way to identify toe weakness is with the paper grip test. This simple test is performed by placing a standard business card beneath your toes and have someone attempt to slide the card away while you try to prevent the card from moving (Fig. 3.28, A). According to Menz et al. (60), this test is highly reliable, making it a useful screening tool to detect toe weakness. The most accurate way to measure toe strength, however, is with a toe strength dynamometer (Fig. 3.28, B). The inability to generate less than 10% of your body weight beneath your big toe, and less than 7% body weight beneath your little toes, correlates with the development of future injuries.

In a 2019 pilot study of the ToePro exercise platform, researchers from Temple University had 25 subjects perform ToePro exercises for six weeks (61). At the end of the study, in addition to 20% improvements in toe strength during that short period, subjects were also able to balance better and could generate slightly more force beneath their big toe while walking. That latter finding was particularly significant,

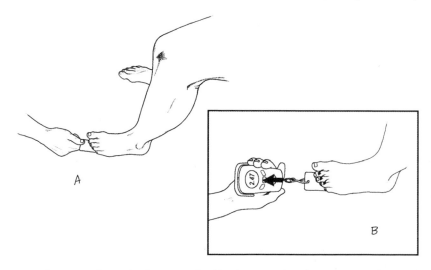

Fig. 3.28. *The paper grip test performed using a standard business card, with someone pulling the card (A) and with a toe strength dynamometer (B).*

as generating pressure beneath the big toe offloads the central metatarsal heads and can protect the plantar fascia from damage. If you don't feel like investing in a ToePro platform, you can do repeat heel raises on an AIREX foam core platform while consciously forcing your toes into the foam platform as you raise your heels. Another option for strengthening the toes is to wear minimalist shoes throughout the day; these have been proven to increase strength and the cross-sectional areas of muscles of the arch (8). Unfortunately, minimalist shoes and heel raises don't target the peroneals as well as the ToePro platform, and so these muscles will need to be exercised separately.

Strength Asymmetries

Because strength asymmetries can be predictors of future injury, it is important to do the exercises on each side and look for subtle differences in strength/endurance. If you notice you are weaker on one side, correct the asymmetry by using the resistance necessary to fatigue your weaker side while exercising both the weak and the strong sides. At first, the strong side won't be getting much of a workout. Over a six to eight-week period of time, however, your strength will gradually become symmetric, and you can begin to increase the resistance on both sides.

Right to left strength differences commonly occur following prolonged injury. For example, runners with chronic Achilles tendinitis and/or tibial stress fractures frequently present with significant weakness of the calf muscles on the injured side. This is especially true if the runner is boot immobilized for more than a few weeks. The weakness is made apparent by performing repeat heel raises on each side until you are fatigued: The injured side will be unable to handle the same number of repetitions as the uninjured side. Surprisingly, the injured runner is almost always unaware of the strength difference.

Another common example, especially in women, is asymmetry in strength of the hip extensors. Asymmetric hip extension strength is strongly correlated with future low back pain. Nadler (62) points out that low back pain patients have a strength imbalance of 15% between the right and left hip extensors, while people without low back pain present with only a 5.3% imbalance. To determine if you're weak in your hip extensors, get on all fours and place a 3-pound weight around each ankle. Perform repeat kickbacks on one side and count the number you can do before you are fatigued, then repeat on the other side. If there is a big difference between the two sides, glute strengthening exercises are recommended until the asymmetry is corrected.

Specific Strengthening Exercises

For whatever reason, most runners dislike strength training. People tend to be drawn to things they're good at, and while most runners are willing to tolerate intensive track workouts and grueling long-distance runs, many of them avoid tedious strengthening exercises. This is unfortunate because, as I pointed out, weak runners are prone to injury.

Maintaining adequate hip strength is not only important in preventing running injuries, but also helpful in preventing the development of osteoarthritis. In an interesting study published in *Arthritis and Rheumatism*, researchers determined that people with strong hip abductors are much less likely to develop osteoarthritis in their knees (63). Apparently, in addition to preventing inward rotation of the thigh, the hip abductors also function to create a compressive force on the outside of the knee that prevents the knee from collapsing inward (Fig. 3.29).

In their 18-month study of the progression of knee arthritis in people with bowed legs, the authors noted that there was a reduced progression of the condition in individuals with strong hips, regardless of age, sex, and, most importantly, the degree to which their legs bowed inward. This research is significant because it demonstrates that strength can protect you from injury even if you are poorly aligned. A range of the most effective home exercises for increasing your strength are reviewed in Fig. 3.30.

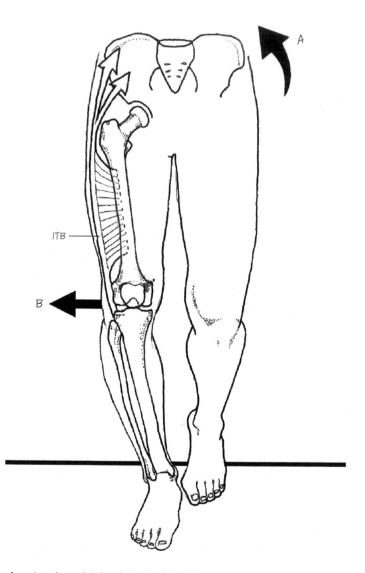

Fig. 3.29. *In addition to keeping the pelvis level (A), the hip abductors pull on the iliotibial band (ITB), creating a compressive force that stops the knee from shifting sideward (B).*

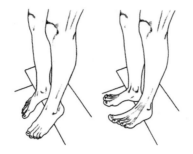

B) Anterior compartment exercises.
Stand with your heels supported on the edge of a stair and alternately raise and lower your forefeet through a full range of motion.

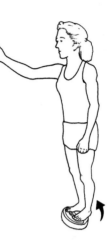

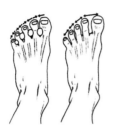

A) Foot intrinsic exercises.
Small corks or rubber tubes are positioned between your toes while you alternate between squeezing and separating the toes.

C) Foot and calf exercises.
Stand on a ToePro platform and gradually raise you heels, rolling in towards your big toe. Finish by forcefully pushing down with your toes. Repeat with knees bent.

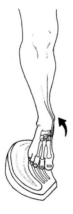

D) Tibialis posterior exercise.
Stand sidewards on a ToePro or AirEx balance pad and raise your heel (arrow). Tilting your upper body slightly towards the opposite side isolates tibialis posterior.

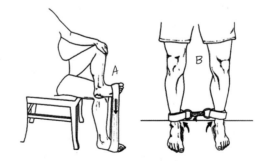

E) Alternate tibialis posterior exercises.
Place the involved foot over the opposite knee with a TheraBand wrapped between the forefeet (A). Tibialis posterior is exercised by raising and lowering the upper forefoot. An alternate tibialis posterior exercise is to wrap a series of elastic tubes between ankle cuffs and alternately raise and lower your arches (B).

Fig. 3.30. *Strengthening exercises.*

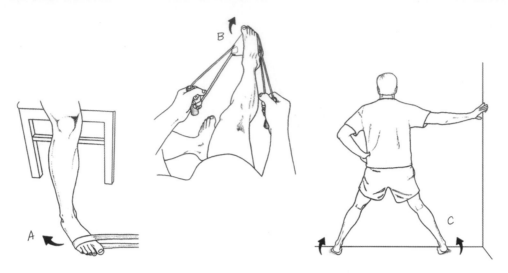

<u>F) Peroneus brevis (A) and longus (B and C) exercises.</u>

Peroneus brevis is exercised by pulling your forefoot outward against resistance provided by an anchored piece of TheraBand (A). Peroneus longus is exercised by pushing down with the inner side of your forefoot against resistance provided by an elastic band (B). A more advanced peroneus longus exercise is to stand with your hips separated and knees slightly bent, while alternately raising and lowering your heels (arrows in C). You can perform this exercise with a weighted backpack to increase resistance.

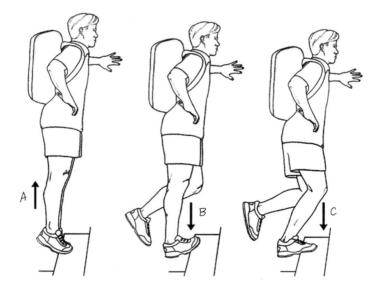

<u>G) Gastrocnemius and soleus eccentric exercises.</u>

Because these muscles are so strong, these exercises are performed wearing a weighted backpack while standing on the edge of a stair with your heels unsupported. To strengthen the gastrocnemius, lift upward with both legs simultaneously (A), and then slowly lower yourself on one leg (B). Three sets of 15 repetitions are performed on each side. To strengthen the soleus muscle, this exercise is repeated with the knee flexed (C). Redrawn from Alfredson (85).

Fig. 3.30. *Strengthening exercises.* *(continued)*

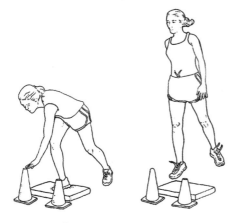

<u>H) Single-leg cone-touch.</u>
While standing on one leg on an unstable surface (such as the AirEx Balance Pad), pivot forward at the hip so you touch the top of a cone placed in front of you. Immediately jump up and repeat the cone-touch on a neighboring cone.

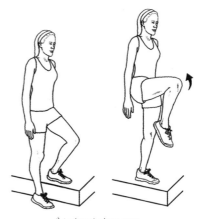

<u>I) Lateral step-ups.</u>
To strengthen the inner quad, stand next to a 4-inch (10-cm) platform and raise the opposite knee (arrow). You can do this exercise with a weighted backpack to increase resistance.

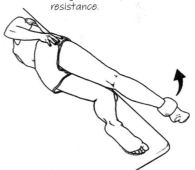

<u>L) Sidelying hip abduction.</u>
Lie on your side near the edge of a workout bench. With a weight placed around your ankle, alternately raise and lower the straight upper leg. This exercise can be performed by repeating the straight leg raises with the hip first in front, and then behind you. Performing the exercise behind you lets you isolate the gluteus minimus muscle.

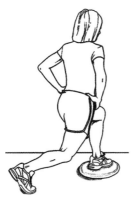

<u>J) DynaDisc lunge.</u>
A conventional lunge can be performed on an unstable surface to enhance coordination. Be very careful while performing this exercise. At first, make sure you have something to grab onto, should you lose your balance.

<u>K) Standing gluteus medius exercise.</u>
Stand with your knee slightly flexed and your hips slightly abducted with a TheraBand placed just above your knees. While keeping your feet in place, alternately move your knees in and our (arrows).

Fig. 3.30. _Strengthening exercises._ (continued)

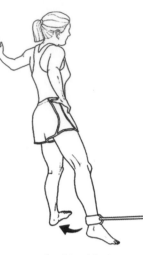

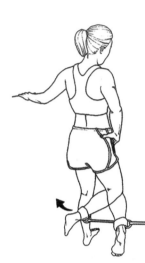

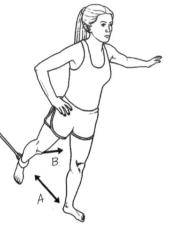

<u>N) Cable adductor exercise.</u>
Pull leg inward against resistance
provided by the cable.

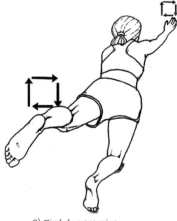

<u>O) Cable hip flexor exercise.</u>
Move the straight leg forward against resistance
provided by a cable machine. This exercise should
be repeated with the knee straight (A)
and flexed (B).

<u>M) Cable piriformis exercise.</u>
Stand with your hip and knee slightly flexed with
an ankle cuff attached to a cable machine. While
keeping your thigh in a fixed position, pull the ankle
inward (arrow).

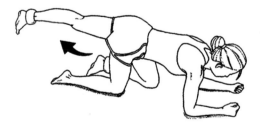

<u>P) Glute max kickbacks.</u>
To strengthen the gluteus maximus, get on all fours
and kick the involved leg out against
resistance provided by an ankle weight.

<u>Q) Bird dog exercise.</u>
Get on all fours and extend opposite arm and leg.
In this position, move each extremity through
4-in. (10 cm) squares.

Fig. 3.30. **Strengthening exercises.** (continued)

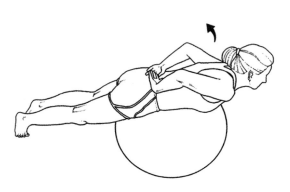

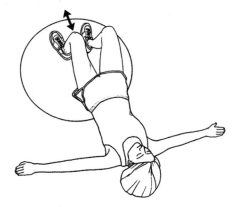

S) Hamstring rollout.

With your arms positioned at your side, place your feet on a 25½-inch (65-cm) physioball with your knees bent and your spine straight. While maintaining a straight spine and pelvis, push and pull the physioball by alternately straightening and flexing your knees. The stronger you become, the farther you can push and pull the physioball.

R) Back extension exercise.

With feet slightly separated for stability, lie facedown on a 2-inch (5-cm) physioball and gently arch your back upward (arrow). Hold this position for five seconds and repeat 10 times. If you feel even slightly unstable while performing this exercise, you can use a workout bench instead of a physioball.

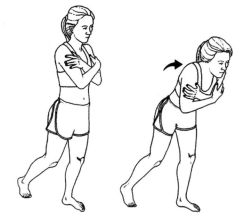

T) Upper hamstring exercise.

Stand with your weight on the leg to be exercised while the toes of the opposite foot lightly touch the ground. While maintaining a slight arch in your low back, bend forward, pivoting at the hip. It is important to maintain a slight curve in your back while performing this exercise. In order to isolate the outer hamstring, tilt slightly away from the involved leg (e.g., the left outer hamstring is isolated by tilting slightly to the right).

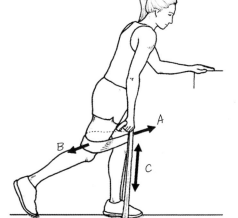

U) Isometric multi-hip exercise.

Place an elastic band or triple-stick strap around your knees and separate your knees in the directions of arrows A and B. Next, place an elastic band beneath your foot and pull up using your hips and hamstring (C). There should be enough tension to produce fatigue after 30 seconds. Repeat this 4 times on each side.

Fig. 3.30. *Strengthening exercises.* (continued)

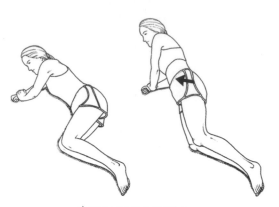

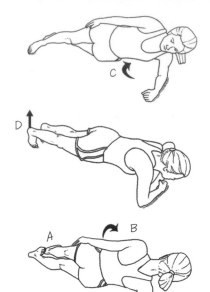

V) Beginner core exercise.

Because conventional core exercises require a fair amount of strength, an alternate method for strengthening the core is to rest on the floor with your hips and knees flexed while your upper body is supported on your flexed elbow. While maintaining ground contact with the legs and the down knee, the pelvis is lifted up and forward as if rising from a chair (arrow).

W) Advanced core exercise.

With the upper heel touching the toes of the downside leg (A), a sidelying plank is maintained for 20 seconds. You then rotate 90° (B), placing your forearms side-by-side with your toes touching the ground. This position is held for 2 seconds before rotating another 90° (C), performing a sidelying plank on the opposite side. The cycle is repeated three times. This exercise can be made more difficult by raising one leg at a time while in the plank position (D).

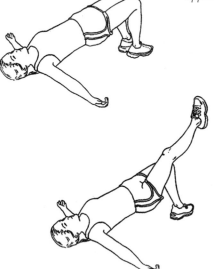

X) Supine bridge with knee extension.

Perform a conventional bridge with knees bent 90° and your pelvis elevated. While maintaining a perfectly level pelvis, alternately raise and lower one leg at a time.

Y) The rollout abdominal exercise.

Kneel beside a physioball with your fists contacting the ball (A). Lean forward, rolling your forearms against the physioball while maintaining a straight spine. Pull yourself back and repeat (B). This exercise was proven to be one of the best ways to recruit the rectus abdominis.

Fig. 3.30. *Strengthening exercises.* (continued)

The Ideal Number of Repetitions and Sets

To strengthen a muscle as quickly as possible, various authors recommend different exercise intensities, sets, repetitions, and weekly frequencies. According to the American College of Sports Medicine, the only way to effectively build muscle is to perform sets of 8 to 12 repetitions using heavy weights (64). The theory is that muscle must be pushed to the limit of its capacity to stimulate repair. The problem with using heavy weights is that unless you have been bulking up for several years, heavy weight training often produces injuries, especially in runners.

Fortunately, research in 2010 proved that the above theory is wrong: Exercising with light weights, when done properly, can rebuild muscles just as effectively as (if not better than) heavy weight training protocols (65). To prove light resistance can build muscle mass, researchers from McMaster University measured the rate of muscle protein synthesis before and after young subjects completed a conventional heavy resistance exercise program (performed at 90% of full effort), or a less intense protocol in which subjects performed 4 sets of 24 repetitions to volitional fatigue (approximately one-third of full effort) (65). Surprisingly, the authors noted significantly more muscle fiber production in the lower resistance group.

More recent research shows it is possible to build muscle mass using resistance provided by body weight alone (66). In this 2018 study, researchers from Japan had 158 senior citizens participate in a weight training program in which they performed 2 sets of 10 to 14 repetitions daily for 12 weeks. The subjects used just body weight and performed the movements very slowly (four seconds up, four seconds down). At the end of the 12-week training program, in addition to significant increases in muscle mass, participants also had decreased hip and waist circumference and decreased abdominal fat. The authors claim their success was related to the total time the muscles were contracting during the protocol. Even though the loads were light, the four-second up and four-second down times resulted in a total of 1,344 seconds of muscle contraction per week (12 repetitions × 8 seconds × 2 sets × 7 times per week). The authors suggest that the long total contraction time is what created muscle mass, not the amount of resistance.

The most important component of all of these exercise protocols is that the light weight is repeatedly lifted until the involved muscle is fatigued. In some cases, the muscle in question fatigued after 60 repetitions performed at 15% full effort. In other situations, the involved muscle fatigued after 24 repetitions performed at about 30% full effort. Regardless of which fatigue protocol is chosen, the rest periods between sets should be short (less than 30 seconds), as this may increase the number of muscle fibers recruited in subsequent sets (67). The more muscle fibers recruited in each set, the more satellite cells work to stimulate remodeling. A growing body of research has proven that the safest way to build muscle mass is to lift light weights with prolonged contraction times (68–70).

Increased muscle remodeling with prolonged contraction times explains why isometric contractions are so effective at building muscle mass (71). For unknown reasons, muscle remodeling occurs more quickly when muscles are isometrically contracted in their lengthened positions. In an extensive review of the literature, researchers from Australia (36) determined that when muscles are isometrically contracted in their lengthened positions, they develop muscle mass more rapidly than muscles exercised in their shortened positions. The authors also point out that "long muscle length training" results in a greater transfer of strength to dynamic activity. This statement is significant for runners wishing to improve performance.

In another important study evaluating the effect of long muscle length training, Goldman et al. (53) measured muscle strength in people who isometrically contracted their toes while they were straight or stretched. The subjects performed 15 repetitions for six weeks. At the end of that time, the subjects strengthening their toe muscles while they were stretched became four times stronger. This information explains why Therabands should rarely be used in strengthening protocols because force output typically peaks while the muscle is in a shortened position. This is in contrast to running, where forces on a muscle almost always peak while it's in a lengthened position.

Concentric versus Eccentric Contractions

Besides altering the number of repetitions and sets, strength training can also be modified by emphasizing either concentric or eccentric muscle contractions. Concentric contractions occur when a muscle is shortening while producing force. In contrast, eccentric contractions occur when the muscle is lengthening while producing force. For example, when you are lifting yourself up while performing a pull-up, the biceps are shortening and are therefore concentrically contracting. When you lower yourself, the biceps are eccentrically contracting, since they are lengthening while producing force.

Differentiating eccentric and concentric contractions is important because exercises are 100% mode specific: If you exercise a muscle only concentrically, it will become strong only when contracting concentrically. Conversely, if you exercise a muscle eccentrically, it is strengthened only during the eccentric component of a contraction. There is no overflow from one type of contraction to the other. This is essential for runners, since many exercises emphasize only one type of contraction. The best example of this occurs while wet vest running in a pool to recover from injuries. Although effective for staying fit while rehabilitating injuries such as stress fractures, pool running almost always results in hamstring injury because resistance from the water forces the hamstrings to fire concentrically only: When you're pulling your leg forward, your quadriceps and hip flexors concentrically contract to overcome resistance provided by the water, and when you pull your leg back, your hamstrings also contract concentrically, again to overcome resistance from the water. Rehabilitating the hamstrings with concentric contractions alone is dangerous because the hamstrings work eccentrically while running to decelerate the forward motion of the swinging leg. When you only tense the muscle concentrically in a pool, the hamstrings become eccentrically weak during your rehabilitation, and as soon as you go back to running fast, the hamstrings are easily strained, since they are no longer able to control the forward swinging leg.

To reduce your potential for injury, muscles therefore should be exercised in the same manner they are used while running. Almost always, both eccentric and concentric components of an exercise should be included.

NEUROMOTOR COORDINATION

This is one of the most important criteria for injury-free running because runners with well-coordinated muscles can tolerate high-mileage training whether they are flat-footed, bowlegged, knock kneed, or hypermobile. In addition to smoothly absorbing impact forces, coordinated muscles work in unison to level your pelvis while keeping your hips and knees moving in a straight line. Coordinated muscles are capable of smoothly decelerating joint motions even if the muscles themselves are relatively weak. In contrast, uncoordinated muscles allow your joints to move rapidly through large ranges of motion, which almost always results in injury and/or altered form.

Motor Engrams

The most common cause of impaired neuromotor coordination is prior injury. To protect you from further injury, the central nervous system essentially rewires itself by creating an alternate pattern of muscle recruitment to avoid stressing the damaged soft tissues. Referred to as a "motor engram," the altered pattern of muscle recruitment persists long after the injury has healed. The perfect example of a faulty motor engram occurs following an ankle sprain. Laboratory evaluation of muscle activity confirms that immediately following an ankle sprain, the peroneal muscles on the outside of the leg pre-tense with greater force just before your foot hits the ground (72). Pre-tensing the peroneals protects the damaged ligament by keeping the rearfoot in a stable position during initial ground contact.

Although usually helpful, all too often the motor engrams created are damaging. For example,

while increased activity in the peroneals following an ankle sprain is protective, ankle sprains have also been shown to impair recruitment of the gluteus maximus on the side of the sprain. While the exact mechanism responsible for producing inhibition is unclear, the decreased activation of the gluteus maximus results in impaired stabilization of the hip and knee. The resultant hip weakness frequently produces a gait pattern in which the knee is allowed to twist inward excessively. As previously mentioned, inward collapse of the knee is associated with the development of a wide range of running injuries.

Faulty motor engrams also occur following knee injury. Even minor knee injuries produce inhibition of the inner quadriceps muscle (the vastus medialis obliquus, or "VMO") that persists after the knee itself has healed. Without proper stabilization from the inner quadriceps muscle, the patella drifts toward the outside of the knee, often resulting in chronic pain.

In one of the more interesting motor engrams I've seen, an Olympic Trials Marathon runner compensated for an outer hamstring muscle injury by switching from a heel to a forefoot strike pattern on the injured side. She also began running with the injured leg turned out almost 35°. Until her uneven shoe wear was pointed out, the runner had no idea that she was striking on her forefoot on one side and her heel on the other. This specific motor engram developed because the forefoot contact point reduced her stride length on the injured side. The reduced stride length lessens strain on the hamstrings because these muscles decelerate forward motion of the swing phase leg: The shorter the stride, the less the hamstring strain. The toe-out gait pattern also reduced strain on the hamstrings because it allowed her to use her hip abductors to decelerate forward motion of the swinging leg. Long after the muscles healed, she continued to run with this faulty running style.

Identifying Faulty Motor Engrams

To help identify faulty motor engrams, a series of functional tests have been developed that test your ability to recruit muscles in a smooth and coordinated manner. These tests are easy to perform and can be done at home. Note that on some occasions, faulty movement patterns are the result of compensating for arthritic joints. Hip and knee arthritis are notorious for producing faulty motor engrams in older runners. Unfortunately, it is often not possible to fully correct a faulty movement pattern associated with arthritis, and runners with arthritis should develop a running form that lessens stress on the arthritic joint; e.g., switching

to a midfoot strike pattern and/or shortening the length of stride. In all situations, the joint responsible for causing the faulty movement pattern should be stretched and strengthened. While this occasionally requires a visit to your local sports chiropractor or physical therapist, it is possible to maintain symmetric strength and flexibility with the previously described stretches and exercises. In the following sections, the more common functional tests used to identify faulty motor engrams are discussed.

Vleeming's Test and the Multifidus Lift Test

Vleeming's test and the multifidus list test are illustrated in Fig. 3.31. Vleeming's test evaluates the ability of the core muscles to lock your ribs against your pelvis while your hip flexors fire. The core exercises on page 223 in Chapter 6

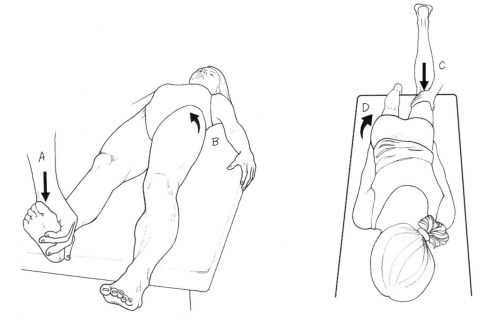

Fig. 3.31. *Vleeming's test and the multifidus lift test.* *As previously described (see Fig. 3.23), Vleeming's test is performed by pushing down on one leg (**A**) and observing if the opposite pelvis lifts off the table (**B**). The multifidus lift test is done with the person face down with the knee bent. The person then resists as you push down just above the knee (**C**). The test is positive if the opposite pelvis lifts off the table (**D**). In both of these tests, a strong core will lock the torso against the pelvis, keeping the hips and spine immobile.*

(Fig. 6.60) illustrate the most effective ways to correct a positive Vleeming's test.

The multifidus lift test evaluates the ability of the back-extensor muscles to lock your spine while your glutes and hamstrings are activated. Research reported in 2019 showed that people with low back pain inappropriately tense their glutes and hamstrings before their low back stabilizers fire (73). As a result, the spine is susceptible to injury because of inadequate muscular stabilization. Prone isometric extensions (Fig. 3.30, R) and bird dogs (Fig. 3.30, Q) are my favorite exercises for strengthening the back extensors. I typically have people perform 30, ten-second prone isometric extension exercises five times per week.

The Modified Romberg's Test

Developed in the 1960s to assess balance after an ankle sprain, the inability to perform this test is a better predictor of future ankle injury than the degree of ligament damage present on MRIs. Because there is a risk of falling during this test, make sure you are standing near a wall or in a corner so you can catch yourself if you start to lose balance. To begin with, stand on one foot with your eyes open and spend about 30 seconds getting your balance. Once you feel secure, close your eyes and count in seconds how long it takes before you feel unstable. The first time you try this, you may lose your balance pretty quickly but after a few attempts, you should be able to maintain your balance for at least 20 seconds. If you are unable to balance with eyes closed despite several attempts, you have impaired muscular stabilization.

The reason closing your eyes affects balance is that when your eyes are open, you are relying on visual cues to maintain balance, but as soon as you close your eyes, you are forced to rely on sensory information provided by the muscles, ligaments, and even the skin on the bottom of your weight-bearing foot. When everything is working properly, the sensory cues from your foot and ankle cause your muscles to immediately tense to stop you from swaying too far in any one direction.

The ability to balance with eyes closed is essential while running because you're not looking down as you run. When your foot hits the ground, subtle changes in terrain cause the foot and ankle to tilt rapidly in a variety of angles, and sensory fibers in the muscles, ligaments, and skin provide immediate information that allow you to adjust. The inability to maintain your balance while standing on one foot with your eyes closed confirms that there is a glitch in the sensory/motor system. The culprit may be a damaged ligament that is failing to provide your central nervous system with information regarding changes in length and/or an injured muscle that fails to react to the sensory information by tensing rapidly. Either way, the impaired balance needs to be corrected.

The easiest way to improve balance is to routinely practice standing on one leg with your eyes closed. After a week or two, you can usually balance for more than 20 seconds. Once your balance has improved, you can practice shifting your weight slightly forward, sideward, and backward until you feel stable in all positions. An alternate method to improve balance is with an ankle rock board device (see Fig. 3.4). Because it forces your ankle to move through a full range of motion, the rock board essentially duplicates the position of a potential sprain and forces you to move out of the high-risk position. The resultant movement pattern eventually becomes wired into your system, and a faulty motor engram associated with your prior injury is replaced with a safer movement pattern. While performing ankle rock board exercises, always make sure you have something to catch on to just in case you lose your balance.

Training on unstable surfaces has been proven to improve coordination and reduce injury rates. In a study of high school football players considered high risk for future ankle sprains (they had a history of prior ankle sprains), researchers from the Nicholas Institute of Sports Medicine (74) confirmed that five minutes of balance board training, performed five times a week for four weeks, resulted in a 77% reduction in the frequency of subsequent ankle sprains.

To improve balance as quickly as possible, consider placing a strip of Kinesiotape along your outer leg and heel prior to performing your rock board exercises. While the rock board is forcing you to move through a full range of motion, the tape gently pulls on your skin providing your nervous system with additional information regarding the position and movement of your ankle. This improved awareness allows for a more effective muscular response. In a study evaluating the length of time necessary to restore balance using ankle rock boards, taped subjects returned to baseline values of balance within six weeks of training, compared to eight weeks with balance board training alone (75).

The Sidelying Hip Abduction Test

Designed to evaluate the coordination of your hip abductors and core muscles, this test is performed by lying on your side with your pelvis vertical and your legs straight. With one arm folded beneath your head and the other resting comfortably at your side, try raising your upper leg toward the ceiling while keeping your knee straight and your pelvis perpendicular to the table (Fig. 3.32, A). When the core and

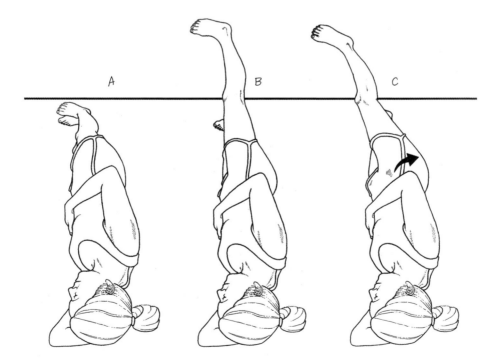

Fig. 3.32. ***The sidelying hip abduction test.*** *Lie on your side (**A**) and raise your upper leg straight toward the ceiling (**B**). When your hip abductors are working properly, the pelvis remains vertical while you raise your leg. When your core and hip abductors are not working properly, the pelvis rotates forward or backward (**C**).*

hip abductor muscles are working properly, it's relatively easy to lift your leg while maintaining alignment between your torso and leg (Fig. 3.32, B). However, when your hip abductors and core muscles are not working in synchrony, your pelvis rotates out of alignment when you raise your leg (Fig. 3.32, C). A study from 2009 confirmed that if you are unable to smoothly raise your leg in a straight line while maintaining your pelvis in a vertical position, you are six times more likely to suffer low back pain while standing for long periods of time (76). I've been using this test for several years and have noticed that it also a predictor of low back and hip problems in runners.

If you fail this test and your hip tilts forward or backward while raising your leg, the first step is to practice performing the test itself while maintaining a vertical pelvis. If necessary, raise your top leg only a few inches until you feel stable. Over time, you should be able to move that leg through a full range of motion without twisting the pelvis. Once you can do 3 sets of 15 repetitions with a stable pelvis, you can progress to a sidelying plank performed while alternately raising and lowering the top leg. Rotating from side plank to full plank and back to opposite side plank while raising the upper leg is a very effective exercise to improve coordination between your core and hip abductors (Fig. 3.30, L). In all cases, the pelvis must always be vertical. If you continue to rotate your pelvis out of alignment, go back to the simpler version of the exercise in which you just lie on your side and practice raising your straight leg toward the ceiling while keeping your pelvis perpendicular to the table. Remember, your goal is to correct a faulty motor engram, and failure to maintain perfect form will reinforce the faulty movement pattern.

The Star Excursion Balance Test

This test is performed by placing a tape measure on the floor, angled 45° backward away from your weight-bearing foot. While balancing on one leg, reach back with your toe and touch the farthest point on the ruler you can without losing your balance (Fig. 3.33). Repeat this measurement on both sides and compare the difference. According to a 2006 study, runners with reach differences greater than 1½ inches (4 cm) are 2.5 times more likely to sustain an injury (77).

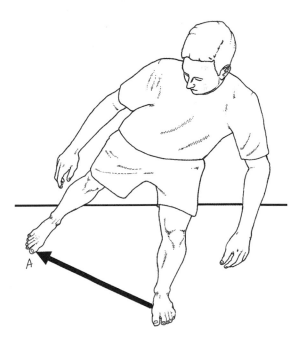

Fig. 3.33. *The star excursion balance test. Place a cloth tape measure on the floor angled 45° backward. While standing on one foot, reach back as far as you can without touching the ground. Note the farthest distance you can reach on the tape measure without losing balance and compare right and left sides. You may need a friend to spot the contact point on the tape measure, or you can place a small box on top of the tape and push it back while maintaining balance.*

The best way to improve your reach distance is to strengthen your knees and hips with the single-leg cone-touch exercise (see Fig. 3.30, H).

Once you feel stable, you can perform the cone-touches while standing on an unstable surface, such as the AIREX balance pad. Research in 2002 suggested that balancing on unstable surfaces allows you to rewire your movements without conscious thought, and the reflexive corrections are more permanently engrained (78).

An alternate way to improve your reach distance is to perform lunges on a DynaDisc (Fig. 3.34). To perform this exercise, place the DynaDisc close to you and do a small range of motion lunge. Until you are confident in your ability to balance, DynaDisc lunges should only be performed while standing near a wall or some stable structure that you can quickly take hold of if necessary. When you initially perform this exercise, even a slight

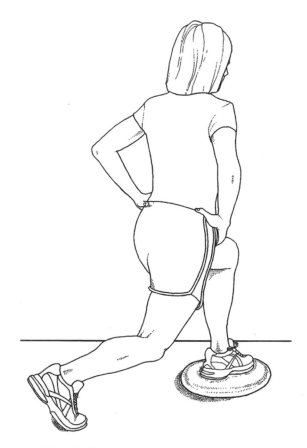

Fig. 3.34. *The DynaDisc lunge exercise.*

problem with coordination will cause your knee and hip to shift rapidly back and forth. Because the supporting disk is unstable, you quickly learn to tense your hip abductors and rotators in order to stabilize yourself. Over time, this movement pattern becomes more natural and the improved muscle function allows you to run with a more stable running form.

The Triple Hop Test

This is my favorite test because it's so simple. Find a clear hallway and stand on one leg with your arms out for balance. Lean forward and hop three times on one leg, making sure you land in a stable position (if you lose balance, the test doesn't count). Mark the spot where you land with a coin or other small object. Repeat this test three times on each side and measure the longest distance you were able to hop on each leg with a metal tape measure (it should be able to measure at least 25 feet (7.6 m)). Your jump distance should be within 10% between the two sides. If you can only jump 80% as far on your right as you can on your left, you need to fix your right side. Runners with prior hamstring injuries are especially prone to failing this test. My favorite exercises to improve hop distance are illustrated in Figs. 3.30, H, I, J, and U.

The Forward Step-Down Test

This test is my preference for evaluating coordination in runners. Besides identifying very specific altered movement patterns, laboratory studies have proven that this test is a reliable predictor of delayed recruitment times in the hip abductor muscles (79). Identifying delayed recruitment times is necessary for injury prevention because muscles need to tense rapidly in order to provide stability while running. Even a slight delay in the time when a muscle begins to contract will allow for potentially dangerous movement patterns. A delayed recruitment time is the muscular equivalent of closing the barn door after the horse is already out: The muscle tenses too late to provide adequate protection.

To perform this test, stand on a 4-inch-high (10 cm) platform positioned in front of a mirror and slowly step down. When the hip abductors are working properly, the pelvis, spine, and weight-bearing leg remain aligned while you are stepping down (Fig. 3.35, A). When the hip abductors are weak and uncoordinated, the step-down occurs with the opposite hip dropping toward the floor excessively or with the weight-bearing knee rotating inward. The faulty form associated with a positive

test often carries over into running: Runners who step down with the recruitment patterns illustrated in Fig. 3.35, C often run with an uneven pelvis, while the movement pattern illustrated in Fig. 3.35, D is almost always associated with an excessive inward collapse of the knee while running. Regardless of how you compensate for your weak hips, the faulty movement pattern should be corrected.

As with the star excursion balance test, the first step in fixing the inappropriate movement is to strengthen the involved muscles. The exercises illustrated in Fig. 3.36 target the hip abductors, extensors, and rotators. Balance exercises on unstable surfaces are helpful to improve coordination. (See also the agility drills listed in Fig. 4.5, which have been proven to improve muscular reaction times.)

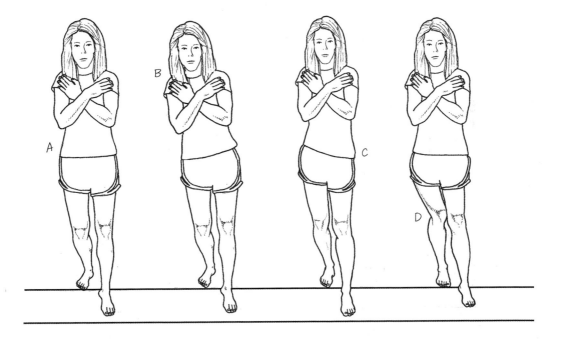

Fig. 3.35. *The forward step-down test.* When the hip abductors are working properly, the leg, pelvis, and spine remain well-aligned while stepping off a 4-inch-high (10 cm) platform (**A**). When the core muscles are weak, the runner performs the step-down by tilting his or her upper body to the side (**B**). When the hip abductors are weak, the runner lowers the opposite hip excessively (**C**). When the hip external rotators are weak, the knee twists in excessively (**D**).

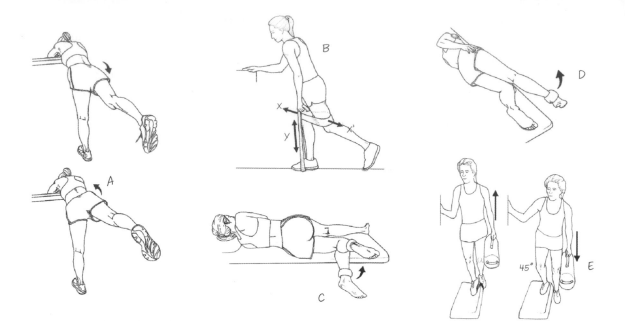

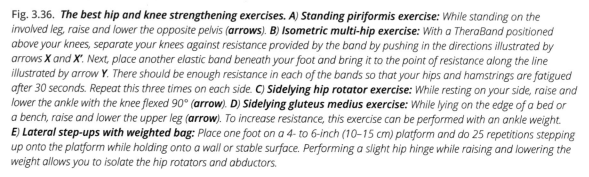

Fig. 3.36. *The best hip and knee strengthening exercises. A) Standing piriformis exercise: While standing on the involved leg, raise and lower the opposite pelvis (arrows). B) Isometric multi-hip exercise: With a TheraBand positioned above your knees, separate your knees against resistance provided by the band by pushing in the directions illustrated by arrows X and X'. Next, place another elastic band beneath your foot and bring it to the point of resistance along the line illustrated by arrow Y. There should be enough resistance in each of the bands so that your hips and hamstrings are fatigued after 30 seconds. Repeat this three times on each side. C) Sidelying hip rotator exercise: While resting on your side, raise and lower the ankle with the knee flexed 90° (arrow). D) Sidelying gluteus medius exercise: While lying on the edge of a bed or a bench, raise and lower the upper leg (arrow). To increase resistance, this exercise can be performed with an ankle weight. E) Lateral step-ups with weighted bag: Place one foot on a 4- to 6-inch (10–15 cm) platform and do 25 repetitions stepping up onto the platform while holding onto a wall or stable surface. Performing a slight hip hinge while raising and lowering the weight allows you to isolate the hip rotators and abductors.*

Because strengthening exercises alone do not correct faulty movement patterns, it is important to modify form consciously, both while performing your exercises and while running. Focusing on form is essential for injury prevention because a strong muscle can still fire inappropriately. In order to change the movement pattern, you have to consciously rewire how the newly strengthened muscles fire. The inability of strengthening exercises alone to correct faulty running form was demonstrated in a study in which researchers measured strength and performed three-dimensional gait evaluations on 10 runners with excessive inward collapse of the knees (80). The runners were all prescribed specific strengthening exercises targeting the hip abductors and external rotator muscles. Six weeks later, the strength and gait evaluations were repeated, and while hip strength increased by almost 50%, there was absolutely no change in the faulty running style. The runners' knees continued to collapse inward in spite of the significant strength gains.

The inability of strengthening exercises to alter movement emphasizes an important point in rehabilitation: You can't just make a muscle stronger—you have to retrain the muscle to interact in synchrony with other muscles. To that end, the next chapter reviews the latest research on gait analysis and goes over specific gait retraining techniques that can be used to reduce your injury risk and correct faulty motor engrams.

REFERENCES

1. Sherry M, Best T. A comparison of 2 rehabilitation programs in the treatment of acute hamstring strains. *J Orthop Sports Phys Ther*. 2004;34:116.

2. DiGiovani C, Kuo R, Tejwani N, et al. Isolated gastrocnemius tightness. *J Bone Joint Surg*. 2002;(84A):962–971.

3. Nigg B, Cole G, Nachbauer W. Effects of arch height of the foot on angular motion of the lower extremities in running. *J Biomech*. 1993;26:909–916.

4. Kolata G. Close look at orthotics raises a welter of doubts. *The New York Times*. January 17, 2011.

5. Williams D, McClay I. Measurements used to characterize the foot and the medial longitudinal arch: reliability and validity. *Phys Ther*. 2000;80:864–871.

6. Williams D, McClay I, Hamill J. Arch structure and injury patterns in runners. *Clin Biomech*. 2001;16:341–347.

7. Nielsen R, Buist I, Parner E, et al. Foot pronation is not associated with increased injury risk in novice runners wearing a neutral shoe: a 1-year prospective cohort study. *Br J Sports Med*. 2014;48(6):440–447.

8. Ridge S, Olsen M, Bruening A, et al. Walking in minimalist shoes is effective for strengthening foot muscles. *Med Sci Sports Exerc*. 2019;51:104–113.

9. Zhang X, Pauel R, Deschamps K, et al. Differences in foot muscle morphology and foot kinematics between symptomatic and asymptomatic pronated feet. *Scand J Med Sci Sports*. 2019;29(11):1766–1773.

10. Sulowska I, Milka A, Olesky Ł, et al. The influence of plantar short foot muscle exercises on the lower extremity muscle strength and power and proximal segments of the kinetic chain in long-distance runners. *Biomed Res Int*. 2019:1–11.

11. Franklyn-Miller A, Wilson C, Bilzon J, McCrory P. Foot orthoses in the prevention of injury in initial military training: a randomized controlled trial. *Am J Sports Med*. 2011;39:30.

12. MacLean C, McClay I, Hamill J. Influence of custom foot orthotic intervention on lower extremity dynamics in healthy runners. *Clin Biomech*. 2006;21:623–630.

13. Verhagen E, van der Beek A, Twisk J, et al. The effect of proprioceptive balance board training for the prevention of ankle sprains. *Am J Sports Med*. 2004;32:1385–1393.

14. Tsai L, Yu B, Mercer V, Gross M. Comparison of different structural foot types for measures of standing postural control. *J Orthop Sports Phys Ther*. 2006;36:942–953.

15. Brantingham J, Adams K, Cooley J, et al. A single-blind pilot study to determine risk and association between navicular drop, calcaneal eversion, and low back pain. *J Manip Physiol Ther*. 2007;30:380–385.

16. Williams D, McClay I, Hamill J, Buchanan T. Lower extremity kinematic and kinetic differences in runners with high and low arches. *J Appl Biomech*. 2001;17:153–163.

17. Landorf K, Keenan AM, Herbert R. The effectiveness of foot orthoses to treat plantar fasciitis: a randomized trial. *Arch Intern Med*. 2006;166:1305–1310.

18. Braga U, Mendonca L, Mascarenhas R, et al. Effects of medially wedged insoles on the biomechanics of the lower limbs of runners

with excessive foot pronation and foot varus alignment. *Gait Posture*. 2019;74:242–249.

19. Trivers R, Manning J, Thornhill R, et al. Jamaican symmetry project: long-term study of fluctuating asymmetry in rural Jamaican children. *Hum Biol*. 1999;71:417–430.

20. Perttunen J, Antilla E, Sodergard J, et al. Gait asymmetry in patients with limb length discrepancy. *Scand J Med Sci Sports*. 2004;14:49–56.

21. Friberg O. Leg length asymmetry in stress fractures: a clinical and radiographic study. *J Sports Med Phys Fitness*. 1982;22:485–488.

22. Tallroth K, Ylikoski M, et al. Preoperative leg-length inequality and hip osteoarthritis: a radiographic study of 100 consecutive arthroplasty patients. *Skeletal Radiol*. 2005;34:136–139.

23. Wang Q, Whittle M, Cunningham J, et al. Fibula and its ligaments in load transmission and ankle joint stability. *Clin Orthop Relat Res*. 1996;330:261–270.

24. Giles L., Taylor J. The effect of postural scoliosis on lumbar apophyseal joints. *Scand J Rheumatol*. 1984;13:209–220.

25. Neely K, Wallmann H, Backus C. Validity of measuring leg length with tape measure compared to CT scan. *J Orthop Sports Phys Ther*. 2013;43:A113.

26. Cummings G, Scholz J, Barnes K. The effect of imposed leg length difference on pelvic bone symmetry. *Spine*. 1993;18:368–373.

27. Malachy P, McHugh M, Connolly D, et al. The role of passive muscle stiffness in symptoms of exercise-induced muscle damage. *Am J Sports Med*. 1999;27:594.

28. Jones B, Knapik J. Physical training and exercise-related injuries: surveillance, research and injury prevention in military populations. *Sports Med*. 1999;27:111–125.

29. La Roche D, Connolly D. Effects of stretching on passive muscle tension and response to eccentric exercise. *Am J Sports Med*. 2006;34:1000–1007.

30. Kubo K, Kanehisa H, Kawakami Y, Fukunaga T. Influence of static stretching on viscoelastic properties of human tendon structures in vivo. *J Appl Physiol*. 2001;90:520–527.

31. Radwan A, Buonomo H, Tataevic E, et al. Evaluation of intrasubject difference in hamstring flexibility in patients with low back pain: an exploratory study. *J Orthop Sports Phys Ther*. 2013;43:A85.

32. Taylor D, Dalton J, Seaber A, et al. Viscoelastic properties of muscle-tendon units: the biomechanical effects of stretching. *Am J Sports Med*. 1990;18:300–309.

33. Bandy WD, Irion JM, Briggler M. The effect of time and frequency of static stretching on flexibility of the hamstring muscles. *Phys Ther*. 1997;77:1090–1096.

34. Stecco C. *Functional Atlas of the Human Fascial System*. London: Churchill Livingstone, 2015.

35. Kay A, Husbands-Beasley J, Blazevich A. Effects of PNF, static stretch, and isometric contractions on muscle-tendon mechanics. *Med Sci Sports Exerc*. 2015;47:2181–2190.

36. Oranchuk D, Storey A, Nelson A, Cronin J. Isometric training and long-term adaptations: effects of muscle length, intensity, and intent: a systematic review. *Scand J Med Sci Sports*. 2018;29(4):484–503.

37. Kubo K, Kanehisa H, Fukunaga T. Effects of different duration isometric contractions on tendon elasticity in human quadriceps muscles. *J Physiol*. 2001;536(2):649–655.

38. Turki O, Chaouachi D, Behm D, et al. The effect of warm-ups incorporating different volumes of dynamic stretching on 10-and 20-m sprint performance in highly trained male athletes. *J Strength Cond Res*. 2012;26:63–72.

39. Pereles D, Roth A, Thompson D. A large, randomized, prospective study of the impact of a pre-run stretch on the risk of injury on teenage and older runners. USATF Press Release 2012.

40. Fritz JM, Cleland JA, Childs JD. Subgrouping patients with low back pain: evolution of a classification approach to physical therapy. *J Orthop Sports Phys Ther*. 2007;37:290–302.

41. Janssens L, Brumagne S, McConnell AK, et al. Greater diaphragm fatigability in patients with recurrent low back pain. *Respir Physiol Neurobiol*. 2013;188(2):119–123.

42. Harms CA, Babcock MA, McClaran SR, et al. Respiratory muscle work compromises leg blood flow during maximal exercise. *J Appl Physiol*. 1997;82:1573–1583.

43. Borghi-Silva A, Oliveira C, Carrascosa C, et al. A respiratory muscle unloading improves leg muscle oxygenation during exercise in patients with COPD. *Thorax*. 2008;63:910–915.

44. Janssens L, McConnell AK, Pijnenburg K, et al. Inspiratory muscle training affects proprioceptive use and low back pain. *Med Sci Sports Exerc*. 2014;47:12–19.

45. Edwards A, Wells C, Butterly R. Concurrent inspiratory muscle and cardiovascular training differentially improves both perceptions of effort and 5000 m running performance compared with cardiovascular training alone. *Br J Sports Med*. 2008; 42:823–827.

46. Johnson M, Sharp G, Brown P. Inspiratory muscle training improved cycling time-trial performance and anaerobic work capacity but not critical power. *Eur J Appl Physiol*. 2007;101:761–770.

47. Kilding AE, Brown S, McConnell AK. Inspiratory muscle training improves 100 and 200 m swimming performance. *Eur J Appl Physiol*. 2010;108:505–511.

48. Leetun D, Ireland M, Willson J, et al. Core stability measures as risk factors for lower extremity injury in athletes. *Med Sci Sports Exerc*. 2004;36:926–934.

49. Khayambashi K, Ghoddosi N, Straub R, et al. Hip muscle strength predicts noncontact anterior cruciate ligament injury in male and female athletes: a prospective study. *Am J Sports Med*. 2015;44(2):355–361.

50. Moon D, Kim K, Lee S. Immediate effect of short-foot exercise on dynamic balance of subjects with excessively pronated feet. *J Phys Ther Sci*. 2014;26:1.

51. Sulowska I, Oleksy Ł, Mika A, et al. The influence of plantar short foot muscle exercises on foot posture and fundamental movement patterns in long-distance runners, a non-randomized, non-blinded clinical trial. *PLoS One*. 2016;11(6):1–12.

52. Kokkonen J, et al. Improved performance through digit strength gains. *Res Q Exercise Sport*. 1988;59:57–63.

53. Goldmann J, Sanno M, Willwacher S, et al. The potential of toe flexor muscles to enhance performance. *J Sports Sci*. 2012;31:424–433.

54. Yuasa Y, Kurihara T, Isaka T. Relationship between toe muscular strength and the ability to change direction in athletes. *J Hum Kinet*. 2018;64:47–55.

55. Kitai T, Sale D. Specificity of joint angle in isometric training. *Eur J Appl Physiol Occup Physiol*. 1989;58(7):744–748.

56. Houck J, Seidl L, Montgomery A. Can foot exercises alter foot posture, strength, and walking foot pressure patterns in people with severe flat foot? *Foot Ankle Orthop*. September 2017.

57. Spink MJ, et al. Effectiveness of a multifaceted podiatry intervention to prevent falls in community dwelling older people with disabling foot pain: randomized controlled trial. *BMJ*. 2011;342:d3411.

58. Reber L, Perry J, Pink M. Muscular control of the ankle in running. *Am J Sports Med.* 1993;21:805–810.

59. Paquette M, DeVita P, Williams D. Biomechanical implications of training volume and intensity in aging runners. *Med Sci Sports Exerc.* 2018;50(3):510–515.

60. Menz H, Zammit G, Munteanu S, Scott G. Plantar flexion strength of the toes: age and gender differences and evaluation of a clinical screening test. *Foot Ankle Int.* 2006;27:1103–1108.

61. Song J, Gorelik S, Husang D, Morgan T. Effects of eccentric exercises on foot structure, balance, and dynamic plantar loading. Gait Study Center, Temple University School of Podiatric Medicine. 2019, in press.

62. Nagler S, Malanga G, Fienberg J, et al. Relationship between hip muscle imbalance and occurrence of low back pain in collegiate athletes: a prospective study. *Am J Phys Med Rehabil.* 2001;80:572–577.

63. Chang A, Hayes K, et al. Hip abduction moments and protection against medial tibiofemoral osteoarthritis progression. *Arth Rheum.* 2005;52:3515–3519.

64. American College of Sports Medicine. *ACSM'S Guidelines for Exercise Testing and Prescription.* Philadelphia, PA: Lippincott Williams & Wilkins, 2006.

65. Burd N, West D, Staples AW, et al. Low-load high-volume resistance exercise stimulates muscle protein synthesis more than high-load low-volume resistance exercise in young men. *PLoS One.* 2010;5(8):e12033.

66. Tsuzuku S, Kajioka T, Sakakibara H, Shimaoka K. Slow movement resistance training using body weight improves muscle mass in the elderly: a randomized controlled trial. *Scand J Med Sci Sports.* 2018;28:1339–1344.

67. Takarada Y, Ishii N. Effects of low-intensity resistance exercise with short interset rest period on muscular function in middle-aged women. *J Strength Cond Res.* 2002;16:123–128.

68. Holm L, Reitelseder S, Pedersen T, et al. Changes in muscle size and MHC composition in response to resistance exercise with heavy and light loading intensity. *J Appl Physiol.* 2008;105(5):1454–1461.

69. Mitchell C, Churchward-Venne T, West D, et al. Resistance exercise load does not determine training-mediated hypertrophic gains in young men. *J Appl Physiol.* 2012;113(1):71–77.

70. Van Roie E, Delecluse C, Coudzer W, et al. Strength training at high versus low external resistance in older adults: effects on muscle volume, muscle strength, and force-velocity characteristics. *Exp Gerontol.* 2013;48(11):1351–1361.

71. Danneels LA, Vanderstraeten GG, Cambier DC, et al. Effects of three different training modalities on the cross-sectional area of the lumbar multifidus muscle in patients with chronic low back pain. *Br J Sports Med.* 2001;35(3):186–191.

72. Delahunt E, Monaghan K, Caulfield B. Altered neuromuscular control and ankle joint kinematics during walking in subjects with functional instability of the ankle joint. *Am J Sports Med.* 2006;34:1970–1976.

73. Sung W, Hicks G, Ebaugh D, et al. Individuals with and without low back pain use different motor control strategies to achieve spinal stiffness during the pro instability test. *J Orthop Sports Phys Ther.* 2019;49:899.

74. McHugh M, Tyler T, Mirabella M, et al. The effectiveness of balance training intervention in reducing the incidence of noncontact ankle sprains in high

school football players. *Am J Sports Med*. 2007;35:1289.

75. Matsusaka N, Yokoyama S, Tsurusaki T, et al. Effect of ankle disk training combined with tactile stimulation to the leg and foot on functional instability of the ankle. *Am J Sports Med*. 2001;29:25.

76. Nelson-Wong E, Flynn T, Callaghan J. Development of active hip abduction as a screening test for identifying occupational low back pain. *J Orthop Sports Phys Ther*. 2009;39:649.

77. Hertel J, Braham R, Hale S, Olmsted-Kramer L. Simplifying the star excursion balance test: analysis of subjects with and without chronic ankle instability. *J Orthop Sports Phys Ther*. 2006;36:131–137.

78. McNevin NH, Wulf G. Attentional focus on suprapostural tasks affects postural control. *Hum Mov Sci*. 2002;21:187–202.

79. Crossley K, Zhang W, Schache A, et al. Performance on the single-leg squat task indicates hip abductor muscle function. *Am J Sports Med*. 2011;39:866.

80. Noehren B, Scholz J, Davis I. The effect of real-time gait retraining on hip kinematics, pain and function in subjects with patellofemoral pain syndrome. *Br J Sports Med*. 2011;45:691–696.

CHAPTER 4

HOW TO DEVELOP THE IDEAL RUNNING FORM FOR ENDURANCE, SPRINTING, AND/OR INJURY PREVENTION

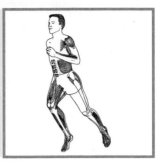

From a biomechanical perspective, it makes sense that nearly every runner has some slight anatomical imperfection that can detract from optimal performance. Think of how automakers have to blow streams of smoke over a car's exterior in a wind tunnel to identify subtle design flaws that could affect gas mileage and/or speed. In regard to running, by far the most common factor that can result in less than optimal performance is prior injury. A perfect example of this is how a damaged Achilles tendon fails to store and return free energy, thereby significantly decreasing efficiency. Muscle weakness is also notorious for causing problems with performance. This is especially true for weakness of the external hip rotators, which may allow the entire lower extremity to rotate inward too far. This inward rotation not only detracts from performance but also greatly increases the risk of injury.

It's not just prior injuries that can create problems. The routine use of heavy motion control sneakers reduces the range that your toes bend during push-off, gradually weakening the intrinsic muscles of the arch. Arch weakness correlates with the development of plantar fasciitis and impaired athletic performance, particularly as we age. Given the potential for creating movement patterns associated with

less than optimal performance, it's essential you identify each and every risk factor potentially affecting performance.

Assuming you've read Chapters 1–3 and you're working on correcting your specific biomechanical glitches, the next step is to develop the ideal running form to maximize efficiency and reduce your overall risk of injury. The specific running form you choose depends upon how fast you plan on running. Because the running form of sprinters is different to that of endurance runners, which in turn is different to that of recreational runners, you'll need to select the running form that matches your desired speed. For example, the world's fastest sprinters require larger ranges of hip motion than distance runners in order to achieve the 16-foot stride lengths necessary for top performance. The neuromotor coordination necessary to attain a sprinting cadence of 250 foot strikes per minute is nearly unimaginable and needs to be addressed with specific running drills. Conversely, elite marathon runners require less overall mobility than sprinters, but their tendons need to be extremely resilient to store and return the free energy needed to run 26.2 miles at a sub-five-minute mile pace. Over the course of a marathon, elite runners must absorb and attempt to return over 6,500 tons of impact force, and so they need to focus on maximizing their shock absorption systems. Finally, the movement patterns of elite sprinters and distance runners are very different from those of slower recreational runners, who have stride lengths of about 5 feet (1.5 m), cadences of 150 foot strikes per minute, and often avoid the airborne phase of running altogether by ground running with one foot or the other constantly on the ground. Avoiding an airborne phase won't allow you to run fast, but it will greatly decrease your risk of injury.

The following section reviews the biomechanical differences between elite long-distance runners and sprinters, and applies this information to ways in which you can improve performance and efficiency yourself. The chapter concludes by explaining how to perform a detailed video gait analysis, with recommendations for visual and auditory gait retraining. Lastly, you will find a list of specific exercises and agility drills that can help you run faster and more efficiently regardless of your running level.

THE MAKING OF A GREAT ENDURANCE RUNNER

According to the exercise physiologist Tim Anderson (1), the best male long-distance runners tend to be slightly shorter than average, while females tend to be slightly taller than average. Male or female, the best long-distance runners possess muscular hips, thin legs, and small feet. Distance runners with muscular hips and relatively thin lower legs are more efficient because accelerating and decelerating heavy legs contributes greatly to the metabolic cost of locomotion. Since the feet and legs have long levers to the hips, even a slight increase in weight applied to the foot will greatly reduce efficiency. To prove this, researchers measured oxygen

consumption before and after adding weights to either the foot or thigh of recreational runners, and determined that while adding weight to the thighs had little effect on efficiency, the same weight added to the feet more than doubled the metabolic costs of locomotion. Other studies have confirmed that every 100 grams (3.5 oz.) of weight you add to a running shoe increases the metabolic cost of running by 1%. These findings explain why endurance runners with small feet are more efficient than their large-footed rivals (2).

One of the most important factors that separates the world's best distance runners from their less successful peers is that successful distance runners plantar flex their ankles 10° less during propulsion, and this reduced movement occurs at a faster velocity (Fig. 4.1) (3, 4). The decreased range and increased speed of ankle plantar flexion

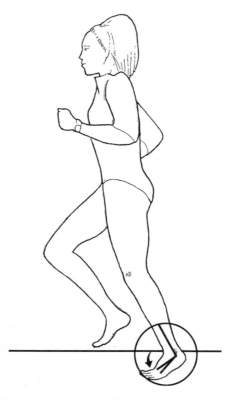

Fig. 4.1. *The best runners plantar flex their ankles more rapidly, through a smaller range of motion.*

is most likely the result of the Achilles tendon rapidly snapping back during early propulsion when it shortens to return stored energy.

In a paper published in the *European Journal of Applied Physiology*, world-class Kenyan endurance runners were found to have longer Achilles tendons that more effectively stored and returned energy compared to height-matched control subjects (5). According to the authors, the longer, more resilient, Achilles tendons present in the Kenyan runners were "optimized to favor efficient storage and recoil of elastic energy." The only flaw with this paper is that the authors compared world-class Kenyans to non-world-class controls. It is likely that all world-class endurance runners have longer, more resilient, Achilles tendons compared to controls. As mentioned in the previous chapter, you can improve the ability of your Achilles tendon to store and return energy by performing isometric contractions with the tendon maintained in a lengthened position. While you can't make your Achilles tendon longer, you can easily make it more resilient.

In an interesting study of efficiency in middle- and long-distance runners competing in a 5K race, researchers from Japan determined that the center of mass in the best runners moved with a vertical displacement of only 2½ inches (6 cm), while the less efficient runners averaged vertical displacements of 4 inches (10 cm) (6). The authors also noted that the good runners ran 5K in 2,825 steps, while the poor runners required 3,125 steps. The added work associated with lifting the center of mass the additional 1½ inches (4 cm) with each stride produced an increased workload roughly the equivalent to the cost of running up a 50-story building.

In what is without doubt the most thorough paper on running economy and performance to date, researchers from the United Kingdom evaluated 97 experienced distance runners (47 females) to determine exactly which biomechanical factors were associated with improved running economy and which factors were related to performance (7). To evaluate economy, the authors analyzed a range of respiratory gases and the velocity of lactate turn point (a marker of fatigue). The correlation between running performance and running form was determined by measuring three-dimensional motion of the spine, pelvis, and lower extremity during all phases of gait, and then analyzing which specific movement patterns correlated with each runner's season's best running time. The authors looked at stride length normalized to height, cadence, vertical oscillation of the pelvis, braking forces, posture, and the position of the hip, knee, and foot during different phases of the running cycle.

Surprisingly, even though all participants were experienced distance runners, including 29 elite runners, there were huge variations in all aspects of running form. For example, vertical oscillation of the pelvis varied twofold and braking forces differed by 280%. Cadence ranged from 144 to 222 foot strikes per minute, while stride length normalized to height was between 1.04 and 1.49 times the runner's height. Runners also showed significant differences in the positions of their feet, legs, and hips at touchdown. Some runners made initial ground contact with their foot plantar flexed 11°, while others hit the ground with their foot dorsiflexed 24°. The position of their lower legs varied from 1 to 16° relative to vertical, and the forward lean of the trunk varied by 20°.

After analyzing all the data, the authors found that the most economical runners had reduced vertical oscillation of the pelvis, lower braking force, stiffer knees, shorter stride lengths, and a more vertical leg during initial ground contact. Running performance was predicted by lower braking forces, a more vertical leg during contact, reduced spinal motion, and reduced ground contact times. The best part of this study was the conclusion that simply positioning your leg in a near vertical position at initial touchdown could improve both economy and performance. In fact, having a nearly vertical leg at touchdown explained 10% of a runner's performance, and this is one of the easiest changes in running form you can make. Fig. 4.2 summarizes the various

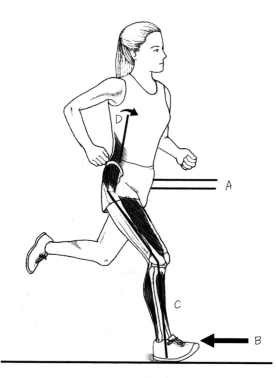

Fig. 4.2. *Biomechanical measurements associated with improved performance and efficiency.* *Folland et al. (7) proved that the most economical runners presented with reduced vertical oscillation of the pelvis (**A**), lower braking forces (**B**), shorter stride lengths, and a more vertical leg during initial ground contact (**C**). Runners with the fastest running times presented with decreased braking forces, shorter ground contact times, a more vertical leg at initial contact (**C**), and a reduced range of spinal motion (**D**). Reduced vertical oscillation of the pelvis and a more vertical leg at touchdown most strongly correlated with both improved economy and faster running times.*

joint interactions associated with improved performance and efficiency. The authors point out that their study provides "novel and robust evidence" that running form strongly influences running economy and performance.

FACTORS RESPONSIBLE FOR SUCCESSFUL SPRINTING

In a classic study published in the *Journal of Applied Physiology*, Peter Weyand and colleagues proved that the fastest sprinters spend less time on the ground and generate significantly more force while they are making ground contact (8). Interestingly, fast and slow sprinters spend about the same amount of time in the air and reposition their swinging limbs at about the same rate. These authors demonstrate that increasing the force applied to the ground by $\frac{1}{10}$ body weight will increase the top speed of running by 1 m/s. While stride length increases significantly with faster running, each runner has an upper limit to the length of his/her stride, after which continued increases will actually lessen speed. For the 30 sprinters in their study, stride length was maximized at 8 m/s (a 3:20 mile pace), while cadence gradually increased to the maximum speed of 9 m/s (3:00 mile pace). In all of the sprinters, the aerial phase of running continued to increase until the 4:30 mile pace, at which time it decreased slightly until the maximum sprint speed was achieved.

To understand stride mechanics, researchers from the United Kingdom (9) studied stride lengths in different sprinters and noted that some sprinters self-selected excessively long strides with low cadences, while others ran with short strides and high cadences. The authors suggest that the sprinters with the longest strides may have chosen long stride lengths because of an inability to rapidly turn their legs over. Conversely, the sprinters that self-selected high cadences may have done so because of an inability to lengthen their stride. These researchers propose that athletes who are overly reliant on long strides should do drills to increase their leg turnover (such as pool running with a high cadence), while athletes dependent upon high cadences should focus on improving flexibility and strength in order to achieve longer strides. By giving the athlete the option of increasing cadence and/or stride length, faster running times may be possible.

Anatomical studies have shown that sprinters have significantly longer muscle fibers in their gastrocnemius muscles compared with non-sprinters (10, 11). The longer fibers might allow these muscles to behave like large rubber bands that store and return energy more effectively than short fibers. The longer fibers can be inherited but more likely result from training, since muscles rapidly adapt to high-intensity training by increasing muscle fiber length. Research in 2006 showed that muscle fiber length can be increased by exercising muscles in their lengthened positions (12).

Unlike distance runners, sprinters flex their hips and knees through larger ranges during swing phase, and these motions occur at faster velocities. As a result, the trailing knee of the fastest sprinters is farther forward when the lead foot touches the ground (Fig. 4.3).

According to some experts, recovering the back leg more quickly allows sprinters to immediately pull the lead foot backward upon impact. Excessive knee flexion during swing phase is essential to sprint rapidly because flexion of the knee shortens the relative length

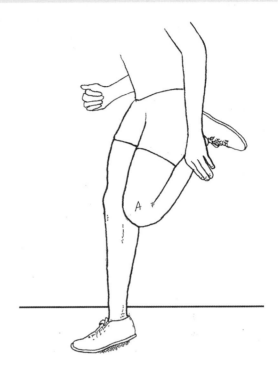

Fig. 4.3. *The best sprinters flex their knees and hips through large ranges of motion, and the trail knee is farther forward (A) when the lead foot contacts the ground.*

of the lower extremity, which decreases muscular strain on the hip flexors (the lever arm to the hip is shorter when the knee is flexed). You can demonstrate this on yourself by placing an exercise band around your ankle and pulling forward: When your leg is straight you can feel the hip flexors strain, but when you bend your knee, there's a significant decrease in stress placed on the hip flexors. The world's fastest sprinters take advantage of the reduced lower extremity lever arm associated with knee flexion by pulling their heels up toward their hips as they pull their knees forward. Since marathon runners occasionally need to sprint toward the finish line, the best coaches suggest that endurance runners learn to move their hips and knees like sprinters. Watch a few slow-motion videos of elite marathon runners and you'll notice that during swing phase, the best

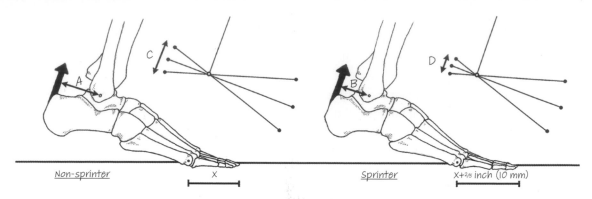

Fig. 4.4. *Because the distance from the Achilles tendon is 25% longer in non-sprinters (compare A and B), the gastrocnemius and soleus muscles must move through larger ranges of motion to plantar flex the ankle (compare C and D).* Notice that the toes of sprinters are ⅖ inch (10 mm) longer than those of non-sprinters.

elites move their hips and knees similarly to sprinters.

In an interesting study of foot shape in sprinters, Lee and Piazza (13) determined the distance from the back of the heel to the center of the ankle is 25% shorter in elite sprinters than in the non-sprinter controls. Conversely, sprinters possess toes that are almost ⅖ inch (10 mm) longer than the toes of the non-sprinter controls. While counterintuitive, the 25% shorter lever arm allows the Achilles to plantar flex the ankle effectively, with little change in length occurring in the gastrocnemius and soleus muscles (Fig. 4.4). The reduced lever arm may decrease mechanical efficiency of the Achilles tendon, but it allows the gastrocnemius and soleus muscles to move the ankle with a nearly isometric contraction.

On the opposite side of the fulcrum, the longer toes result in greater force production in the forefoot because the increased toe lengths provide the toe muscles with significantly longer lever arms that allow a more powerful push-off. Even though the added metabolic cost of accelerating and decelerating the longer, heavier toes would lessen efficiency while walking and running long distances (which is why

evolution has favored shorter toe lengths), the longer toes provide increased force production during propulsion, thereby allowing the elite sprinter to run at the fastest speed possible. The combination of a short Achilles lever arm coupled with long toes is also found in nature; e.g., cheetahs, which are capable of sprint speeds exceeding 70 mph, have shorter heels and longer toes than lions. While you can't change your toe length, you can significantly improve sprinting speed by increasing toe strength.

THE BEST DRILLS AND EXERCISES FOR IMPROVED PERFORMANCE

Whether you're a sprinter, distance runner, or recreational runner trying to get faster, you should consider incorporating specific plyometric drills designed to improve the storage and return of energy. My favorite plyometric drills are illustrated in Fig. 4.5.

One particular study showed a 5% improvement in VO$_2$ and a 3% improvement in 3K race performance after just six weeks of plyometric training (14). The authors attributed the improved performance and speed to an

Glutes	While walking, lift knee toward chest, raising the body on the toes of the opposite leg.	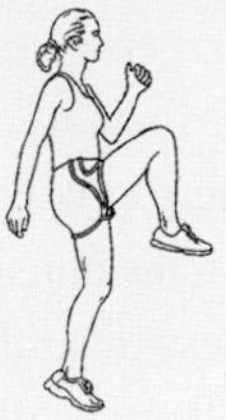
Hamstrings	Walk while swinging your leg forward until a stretch is felt in your hamstrings. Keep your toes pointing toward your knee.	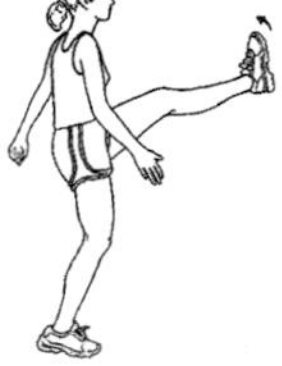
Adductors	While moving forward, raise the trail leg by abducting the hip 90°, while keeping the knee flexed. Move as though you were stepping over an object just below waist height.	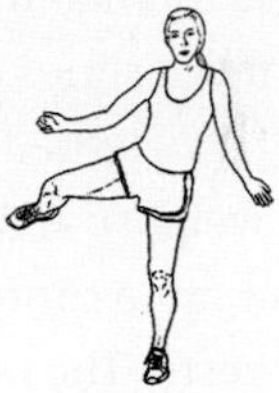
Gastrocnemius	Tip-toe walking. Move forward while alternating walking on your tiptoes. The aim is to raise your body as high as possible with each step.	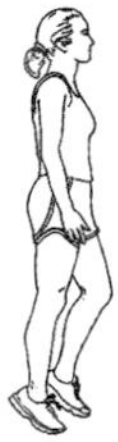
Quadriceps	Rapidly kick heels toward buttocks while moving forward.	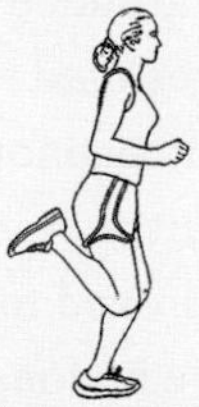
Abductors	Quickly move sideward alternating one leg in front of the other. Go 15 yards (13.5 m) and repeat in opposite direction.	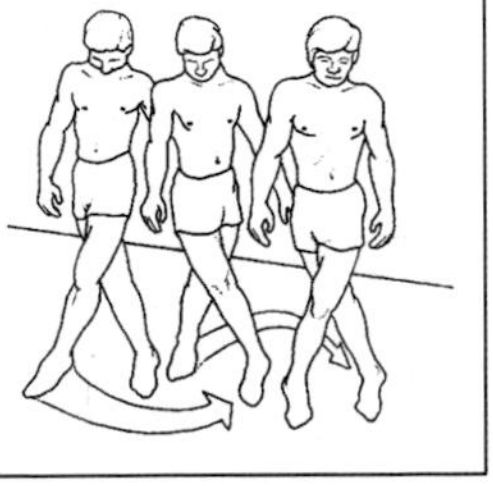

Fig. 4.5. **Dynamic stretching drills.** (Modified from Turki et al. [15].)

enhanced ability of the muscles and tendons to store and return energy following the completion of the plyometric drills. By increasing the speed of force production without increasing muscle size (large muscles consume more calories and are therefore less desirable for distance running), plyometric drills may allow athletes to spend less time on the ground while simultaneously producing greater force. Bounding drills that encourage rapid ankle plantar flexion during propulsion are especially helpful when trying to improve efficiency.

In another interesting paper (16), researchers from New Zealand had high-level distance runners perform a series of six ten-second strides while wearing a weighted vest (loaded with 20% of their body weight). A control group of runners performed the same running drills without the weighted vests. The researchers noted that shortly after performing the drills, the runners with the weighted vests had huge improvements in peak running speed and economy. Apparently, the weighted vests allowed for faster running times and improved efficiency because the runners were forced to stiffen their knees and hips in order to absorb the forces associated with carrying the added weight. The increase in leg stiffness resulted in big improvements in performance and economy because stiff muscles are more efficient at storing and returning energy. The improved form persisted even after the weights were no longer worn.

I really like that study, as the added weight allows your central nervous system to analyze impact forces at contact and modify limb position and stiffness accordingly. For example, if you had excessive up-and-down oscillation of the center of mass and/or were overstriding, you might not notice this if you're strong and healthy, but the amplified impact force associated with wearing the weighted vest would make it more obvious. My only concern is that the weighted vests used in this study were pretty heavy, which could increase the risk of injury. Less fit or inexperienced runners should definitely start out with lighter weights and gradually increase the load based on comfort. Runners who don't want to experiment with weighted vests can also increase their efficiency and performance with plyometric training and/or high-intensity uphill interval training. As with weighted vests, plyometrics and high-intensity training can increase the risk of injury so these drills should be initiated cautiously.

Lastly, because isometric contractions performed with muscles maintained in their lengthened positions have been proven to enhance tendon resiliency, I've outlined a few simple exercises that you can do in five minutes or less to keep your muscles and tendons strong and supple (Fig. 4.6). Whether you run a marathon in two hours or six hours, these exercises can help improve performance and reduce your risk of injury.

To improve resiliency in your glutes and quadriceps tendons, warm up with 25 lateral step-ups (Fig. 4.6, A). Next, move into a long-step forward lunge position and hold this position with your back knee held slightly off the ground (Fig. 4.6, B). This exercise places less stress on your knee than conventional lunges (17), and in addition to placing the glutes and quads in the forward leg in their lengthened positions, the rectus femoris in the back leg is isometrically tensed in a lengthened position. Maintain this position for 20 seconds and repeat four times. A resilient rectus femoris tendon is essential for fast running, as it snaps the trail leg forward to initiate swing phase.

Your Achilles and calf tendons can be made more resilient using the ToePro platform. Warm up by

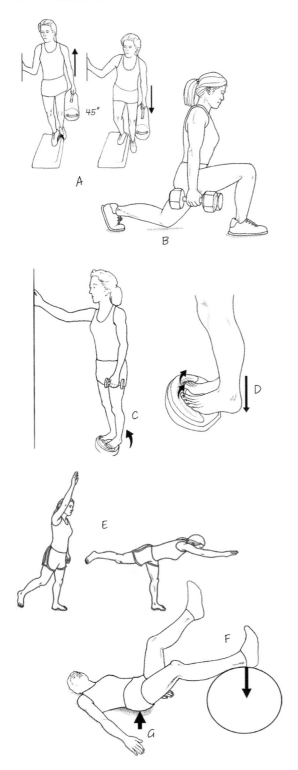

Fig. 4.6. *The best exercises to improve tendon resiliency.*

doing 25 repetitions on the ToePro (Fig. 4.6, C) and then slowly lower your heels so they are ½" from the ground (Fig. 4.6, D). Hold this position isometrically for 20 seconds and repeat that routine four times. With each set, alternate between raising and lowering your arch to isolate different tendons: Your peroneals are lengthened when your weight is on the outside of your foot, while your tibialis posterior tendon is lengthened when your foot is rolled inward. If you don't want to use a ToePro, you can do this exercise by leaning forward into a wall while standing on an AIREX balance pad. With all of these exercises, you need to be fatigued when you finish, and so stronger runners may need to wear a weighted backpack or hold a dumbbell.

The most effective exercise to improve resilience in the glutes and hamstrings is the single-leg push-down. Before performing this exercise, warm up with a standing windmill exercise, illustrated in Fig. 4.6, E. After you're warmed up, lie face up on the floor with your arms out for stability, then place your foot on a physioball or workout bench and push-down with your heel (Fig. 4.6, F) with enough force to raise your pelvis off the ground (Fig. 4.6, G). Try to duplicate the position your hip is in during initial contact, which is typically between 20 and 30° of flexion. Hold this position for 20 seconds and repeat four times on each leg. If this exercise is too difficult, bring the opposite knee toward the chest. Conversely, if you're not fatigued after 20 seconds, straighten the opposite leg so it is closer to the leg that is pushing down, which makes the exercise significantly more difficult. This exercise duplicates the position your foot is in just before initial ground contact and markedly strengthens the hamstring tendons, which are important for both shock absorption and storing and returning energy.

MODIFY YOUR RUNNING FORM TO AVOID INJURY

Because the best predictor of future injury is prior injury, the most effective way to avoid future running injuries is to accommodate your prior running injuries. The easiest way to do this is to select either a heel or forefoot contact point depending upon your prior injuries. While studies comparing impact forces associated with different contact points consistently show that the same force is absorbed by your body, regardless of how your foot strikes the ground, it is possible to shift the location of the impact force simply by changing your contact position. If you have been plagued with chronic knee pain, transitioning to a forefoot strike pattern can reduce load on the back of your knee by 50%. Conversely, if you been struggling with plantar fascial or Achilles injuries, definitely consider switching to a lateral heel strike, as this will significantly reduce stress on the back of your calves and arches. The same is true for runners with a history of recurrent ankle sprains, since forefoot contact points increase the risk of inversion ankle sprains. As a general rule, midfoot and forefoot contact points tend to be more comfortable in runners with neutral arches and wide forefeet, while runners with low arches and narrow forefeet tend to prefer making ground contact along the outer heel.

If you have been dealing with an injured knee and you don't want to switch to a forefoot contact point, an alternate technique to offload your knee is to lean slightly farther forward at the hips during initial contact. This slight forward lean has been shown to redistribute pressure away from the knee and into the hamstrings (Fig. 4.7).

While not an option for fast runners, ground running is absolutely the easiest way to avoid ever being injured. The problem is, you have

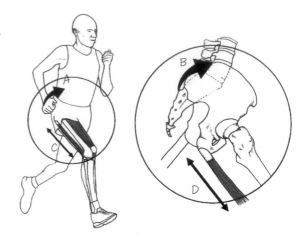

Fig. 4.7. *By leaning slightly forward at the hips (arrows A and B), runners use their upper hamstring muscles (C and D) to absorb force that would normally be absorbed by the knee.* Some great research proves that the world's best runners make initial ground contact with their upper bodies tilted slightly forward, while less efficient runners contact the ground with their spines almost vertical (2).

to run slower than a 13-minute mile pace. If you're a faster runner less concerned with performance and more concerned with staying healthy, the easiest way to avoid injury is to reduce your stride length. In addition to reducing impact forces, slight reductions in stride length cause you to strike the ground with your feet slightly farther apart. Researchers from Iowa State University (18) demonstrated in 2015 that reducing stride length by 5 to 10% caused runners to strike the ground with their feet almost ⅖ inch (10 mm) farther apart. The increased distance between their feet was accompanied by slight decreases in pelvic drop and reduced strain on the iliotibial band. Prior research has shown that increasing the distance between your feet while running may also be an effective way to decrease the risk of developing tibial stress fractures (19).

In an astute study of runners with patellofemoral pain, researchers from the United Kingdom had runners with chronic knee pain increase their cadence by 10% with the aid of an audible metronome (20). The training consisted of a single session of changing cadence to match the metronome and the outcomes were pretty impressive: Metronome training resulted in significantly less pelvic drop, decreased adduction of the thigh, and decreased knee flexion upon contacting the ground. These changes persisted when the runners were reevaluated three months later, and during that time, runners were able to increase their weekly mileage and reported significantly less knee pain. You can download any of a variety of running metronome apps from the iOS App Store for an iPhone or from Google Play for an Android device.

An important fact to remember is that because runners come in all shapes and sizes, there is no one form that is ideal for everyone and each runner should develop a style of running that suits his or her own specific biomechanical needs. A perfect example of this is how some people naturally run with a toe-out running form. While most running experts will tell you that runners should keep their feet straight and aligned, runners with external tibial torsion would be chronically injured if they ran with their feet pointing straight. Given the high impact forces associated with running and the nearly 90% annual injury rate, the best way to remain injury free is to accommodate your specific biomechanical alignment patterns, improve strength, flexibility, and endurance, and analyze your gait to identify subtle problems that might be increasing your risk of injury; e.g., excessive inward rotation of the hip, overstriding, excessive pelvic drop, and/or running with a crossover gait pattern.

PUTTING IT ALL TOGETHER: PERFORMING AN AT-HOME GAIT ANALYSIS

Although gait evaluation is complex and often requires the skilled eye of an expert, there are specific measurements that can be taken with an at-home gait analysis to help you improve performance and prevent injury. While it is usually possible to correct gait asymmetries with specific stretches, exercises, and/or gait retraining, runners with complex movement patterns should consider setting up a time with a local running expert, as there are many variables in neuromotor coordination and/or soft tissue contracture that are difficult to figure out on your own. For most runners, however, a thorough at-home gait evaluation can reveal obvious alignment problems that, when corrected, can make a huge difference in performance and in running longevity.

To perform your gait evaluation, find a treadmill that has enough space around it to place a camera in front, at the side, and behind while you're running. If possible, borrow a friend's camera or phone so you can capture all three angles at once. It's not necessary to use three cameras, but it makes the process quicker. Ideally, each camera should be mounted on a tripod, but you can also have a friend with a steady hand record the videos. The videos should capture your entire body from the back and side cameras, but you'll only need a view from the hips down for the front view. The front and back cameras should be placed along the midline of the treadmill, while the side camera should be placed at 90° to the location where the center of your hips will be while running. If you're using the camera on your phone, go to the settings and select 120 frames per second. Next, get on the treadmill and run at a self-selected pace for

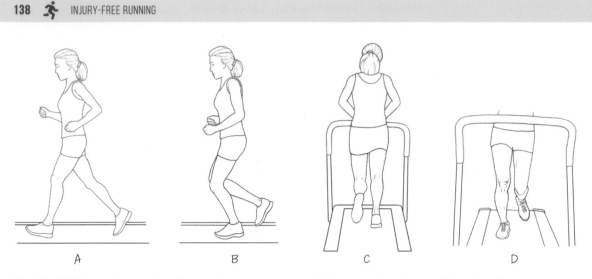

A   B   C   D

Fig. 4.8. *Still frame images taken from each camera, corresponding to precise phases of the gait cycle.* Image **A** represents the position of your body at initial contact, while images **B**, **C**, and **D** are views from the side, back, and front during midstance.

about five minutes. After you're warmed up, you'll only need a few minutes to perform the gait analysis.

Once the cameras are recording, you'll need about two minutes of video from each of the three positions. Again, it's not necessary to have all three cameras going at once, but it does make things simpler. When finished, you'll need to extract specific still frame images from each camera that correspond to precise phases of the gait cycle (Fig. 4.8). You can import the videos into any of a variety of software programs that allow you to mark specific angles on the selected shots.

In the following sections, the clinical significance of each measurement is described, and recommendations are then made for improving your running form by means of specific exercises, stretches, and/or gait retraining. Even though every runner has his or her own unique running style, almost all running styles fall within the parameters of this gait assessment. Information gleaned from completing your gait analysis will hopefully help you run faster and more efficiently as well as greatly reduce your overall risk of injury.

Initial Ground Contact

On the side view of the initial contact image (Fig. 4.8, A), draw a vertical line from the center of your hip to the treadmill (Fig. 4.9). Now measure the distance between the back of your heel and the vertical line (Fig. 4.9, A).

While most running experts tell you to make initial contact with your foot directly beneath your center of mass, this is only possible at extremely slow running speeds. Researchers from the University of Wisconsin proved that the location where your foot makes initial ground contact is dependent upon not just your stride length but also your cadence (21). These researchers took 45 recreational runners and had them vary their cadence from 5–10% above and below their preferred running cadence. The table on the right of Fig. 4.9 summarizes their results. Notice how the heel to center of mass distance decreased from 4½ to 2¾ inches (11.5 to 7 cm) when runners transitioned from their lowest cadence and highest stride length to their highest cadence and lowest stride length. The vertical

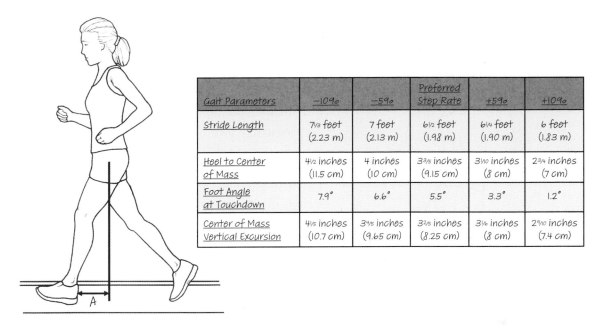

Gait Parameters	−10%	−5%	Preferred Step Rate	+5%	+10%
Stride Length	7⅓ feet (2.23 m)	7 feet (2.13 m)	6½ feet (1.98 m)	6¼ feet (1.90 m)	6 feet (1.83 m)
Heel to Center of Mass	4½ inches (11.5 cm)	4 inches (10 cm)	3⅗ inches (9.15 cm)	3¹⁄₁₀ inches (8 cm)	2¾ inches (7 cm)
Foot Angle at Touchdown	7.9°	6.6°	5.5°	3.3°	1.2°
Center of Mass Vertical Excursion	4⅕ inches (10.7 cm)	3⅘ inches (9.65 cm)	3⅖ inches (8.25 cm)	3¼ inches (8 cm)	2⁹⁄₁₀ inches (7.4 cm)

Fig. 4.9. *Initial ground contact.* *Measure the distance **A** from the back of your heel to a vertical line drawn from the center of your hip to the treadmill.*

excursion of the center of mass also flattened out as the runners increased their cadence.

One of the most fascinating parts of the study was how drastically and consistently the foot angle at touchdown changed as stride length increased. When initial ground contact was made with the foot 2¾ inches (7 cm) in front of the center of mass, the foot was at a near midline position relative to the ankle. As stride length increased and cadence decreased, the foot angle at touchdown consistently increased until it hit almost 8° when running at 10% below the preferred cadence. I feel the increased touchdown angle represents an attempt by these runners to decrease the braking forces by using their ankles to absorb shock as their stride lengths increased. Remember, extremes of foot position correlate with reduced impact forces while running (22). The forward-most position of 4½ inches (11.5 cm) associated with the longest strides wasn't even that large of a number.

In a study of elite runners participating in a 5K road race (23), both men and women made initial ground contact with the foot 13 inches (33 cm) in front of their center of mass. This extreme forward foot position was necessary in order to achieve the 11- to 12-foot stride lengths present in these athletes.

Sagittal Plane Angle at Initial Contact

From the side view at initial contact image (Fig. 4.8, A), measure the important sagittal plane angles **A**–**D** indicated in Fig. 4.10.

Angle **A** represents the foot touchdown angle. As mentioned in the previous section on initial ground contact, higher angles are often associated with excessively long stride lengths. The fastest most efficient runners typically make ground contact with the ankle in a near midline position. Subtle changes from slightly

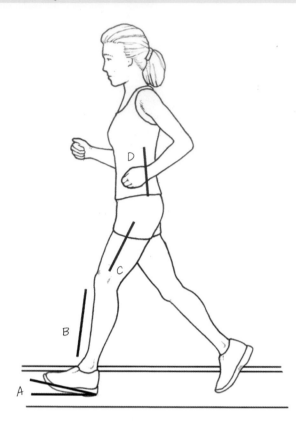

Fig. 4.10. *Important sagittal plane angles taken from the side view at initial contact. Measure the foot touchdown angle (**A**), the tibial inclination angle (**B**), the angle of the thigh relative to the vertical (**C**), and the forward lean of the trunk (**D**).*

plantar flexed to slightly dorsiflexed are a matter of individual preference, although most recreational runners are more efficient with a slight heel strike.

The most important angle in Fig. 4.10 is the tibial inclination angle **B**. This is the angle formed between the vertical and the longitudinal axis of the tibia and should be 7° or less. High angles correlate with inefficiency, decreased performance, and exaggerated braking forces (7). Runners with high tibial inclination angles often make a lot of noise when their lead foot hits the ground. An effective tool for gait retraining is to focus on hitting the ground softly and quietly.

Angle **C** is the angle of the thigh relative to the vertical at initial contact, and recreational runners tend to have between 20 and 25° of hip flexion at initial ground contact, while elite men and women have between 25 and 35°. The more forward position of the hip in elite athletes is related to their incredible stride lengths.

Angle **D** represents the forward lean of the trunk at initial ground contact. A slight forward lean offloads the knee, while a backward lean increases the risk of developing low back pain.

Peak Knee Flexion During Midstance

From the side view at midstance image (Fig. 4.8, B), measure the peak knee flexion angle (Fig. 4.11, A).

Most recreational runners tend to reach a peak knee flexion of around 40° by midstance. Slower hybrid runners tend to keep their knees a little stiffer, and it is not uncommon for a slow runner with a short stride to only flex the knee 25 to 30°. As long as you are keeping your stride length short, the smaller degree of knee flexion is not a problem and, in fact, can improve efficiency.

Because fast runners have such long stride lengths, greater degrees of knee flexion are necessary for adequate shock absorption. As mentioned, recreational runners typically bend their knees about 40° by midstance, but elite male and female distance runners average a little over 50° of knee flexion by midstance, with some runners bending their knees more than 65°. While excessive knee flexion can improve shock absorption, it is metabolically expensive and correlates with decreased efficiency.

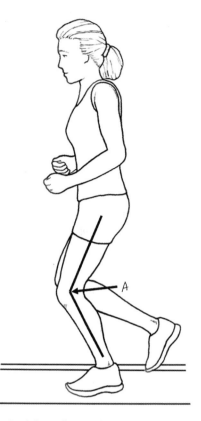

Fig. 4.11. *Peak knee flexion during midstance.* *Measure the angle of peak knee flexion (**A**).*

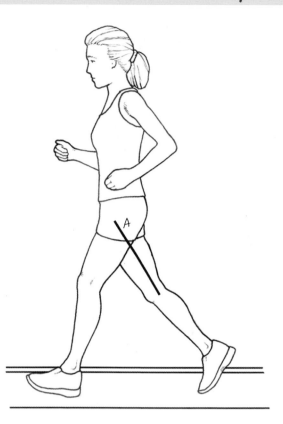

Fig. 4.12. *Thigh extension during toe-off.* *Measure the amount of thigh extension (**A**).*

Thigh Extension During Toe-Off

Measuring thigh extension during toe-off (Fig. 4.12, A). In my opinion, this is one of the most important measurements to take during the gait evaluation.

Slower recreational runners average 15 to 20° of hip extension by toe-off, while faster recreational runners extend their hips 20 to 30°. Because they have to generate so much force during midstance and propulsion, elite distance runners consistently average between 35 and 40° of hip extension by toe-off. This high number is necessary for the glutes and hamstrings to propel the center of mass forward as the hips extend through a larger range of motion.

Greater force generated through a larger range allows these athletes to accomplish the 10- to 12-foot stride lengths necessary to run sub-five-minute miles. While essential for elite marathon runners, almost all runners will benefit from strengthening their glutes and hamstrings and lengthening their hip flexors, which will allow them to generate more force as the leg extends farther behind them.

Knee Flexion of Swing Leg

Because 20% of all energy is spent to bring the swing leg forward while running, bending your knee (Fig. 4.13, A) improves efficiency by effectively shortening the length of the lever

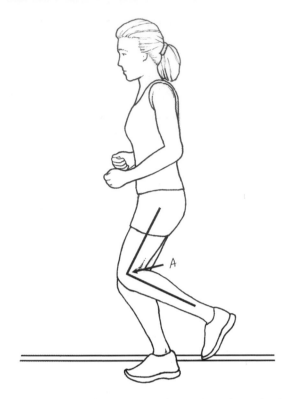

Fig. 4.13. *Knee flexion of swing leg.* Measure the angle of knee flexion (**A**).

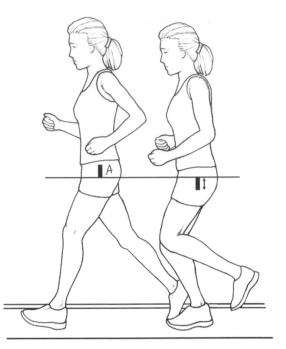

Fig. 4.14. *Vertical excursion of center of mass during stance phase.* Stick a 2-inch (5 cm) strip of duct tape on the side of the hip (**A**). Mark a horizontal line along the top edge of the tape when at the lowest point and compare it to its position at the highest point (**arrow**).

arm that your hip flexors have to work against (refer back to Fig. 4.3).

While recreational runners tend to flex their swing phase knee around 90°, elite male and female distance runners average 135° of knee flexion by midswing. Most recreational runners are fine with approximately 90° of flexion, but faster runners are encouraged to flex their knee a minimum of 130° during swing phase.

Vertical Excursion of Center of Mass During Stance Phase

The vertical excursion of the center of mass during stance phase is one of the most important predictors of speed and efficiency (7). To take this measurement, place a 2-inch (5 cm)

piece of duct tape along the side of your hip, as shown in Fig. 4.14, A. Next, go through the side view video and freeze the frames where your center of mass is at its highest and lowest points. Place a horizontal line along the top edge of the tape when at the lowest point and compare it to its position at the highest point (Fig. 4.14, arrow).

In Fig. 4.14, the vertical excursion of the center of mass is 2 inches (5 cm) (1.0 times the length of the tape). If the upper distance was 1.5 times the length of the tape, the vertical excursion would be 3 inches (7.6 cm). This sounds complicated but it's really easy. Typical values for the vertical excursion of the center of mass vary between $1\frac{9}{10}$ and $4\frac{1}{10}$ inches (5–10 cm), with the average vertical excursion being about 3 inches (7.5 cm) (7).

As mentioned, an excessive vertical excursion correlates with inefficiency and decreased performance. Like runners with an excessive tibial inclination at contact, those with too much vertical movement often make a lot of noise when striking the ground. This is especially apparent with treadmill running. The best way to reduce the vertical excursion of the center of mass is to stiffen your knees during contact, and focus on striking the ground softly. Learning how to run quietly is one of the most important things you can do to avoid injury and improve performance.

Side Bending of the Trunk

From the back view at midstance image (Fig. 4.8, C), measure the side bending of the trunk (Fig. 4.15, A). Ideally this angle will be less than 5°.

Runners with gluteus medius tendon problems and/or early hip arthritis will lean slightly toward the involved hip. Treatment in that situation is to strengthen the hip abductors, improve hip flexibility, and perform core exercises.

Lateral Pelvic Drop

The lateral pelvic drop is represented by the angle between a line drawn through the top of the pelvis and the horizontal (Fig. 4.16, A). Typical ranges of this angle for males are between 3 and 5° and for females, between 4 and 7°.

Excessive pelvic drop correlates with a wide range of injuries, including iliotibial band, anterior knee pain, and lateral hip pain (24). My favorite way to correct excessive pelvic drop is with the exercises illustrated in Fig. 3.36 (the isometric contractions in Fig. 3.36, B are particularly effective).

While excessive drop is almost always blamed on weakness of the hip abductors, new research suggests that some runners compensate for a weak gluteus maximus by firing the adductor magnus excessively during initial ground contact (25). The inappropriate co-contraction of the adductor magnus pulls the pelvis downward (Fig. 4.16, B), creating a pelvic drop that does not respond to conventional exercises. Because the adductor magnus functions as a hip extensor when the hip is flexed (Fig. 4.16, C), exercises to strengthen the glutes are ineffective because the adductor magnus takes over. That being the case,

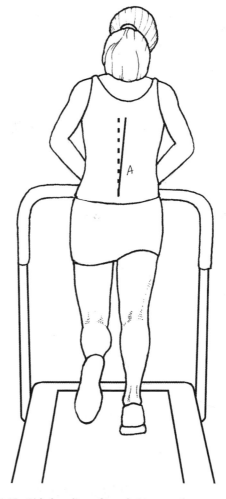

Fig. 4.15. *Side bending of trunk.* Measure the amount of side bending of the trunk (**A**).

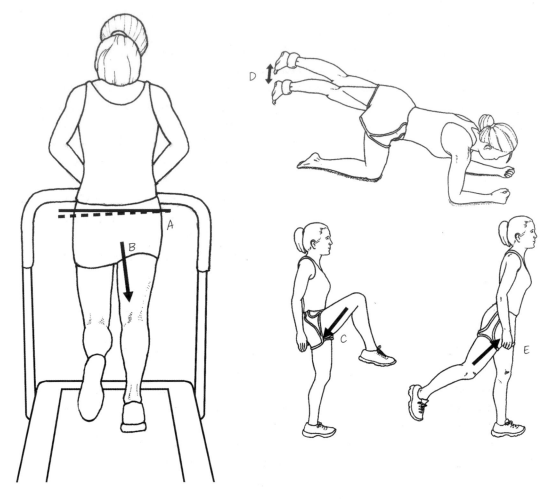

Fig. 4.16. ***Lateral pelvic drop.*** *Measure the angle between a line drawn through the top of the pelvis and the horizontal (**A**). Inappropriate co-contraction of the adductor magnus pulls the pelvis downward (**arrow B**), creating a pelvic drop. When the hip is flexed, the adductor magnus functions as a hip extensor (**C**), so it is recommended to perform glute exercises from neutral to extension only (**D**). When the hip is extended, the adductor is forced to behave as a hip flexor (**E**).*

I recommend runners perform glute exercises from neutral to extension only (Fig. 4.16, D), which forces you to fire just the gluteus maximus. The reason this exercise targets the gluteus maximus is that when the hip is extended, the insertion of the adductor magnus is displaced behind the axis of motion for the hip, forcing the adductor to behave as a hip flexor (Fig. 4.16, E). By exercising the gluteus maximus from neutral to extension, the adductor is unable to participate and the weak gluteus muscle eventually gets stronger. Performing 4 sets of 25 repetitions, four times a week for four weeks, is usually sufficient to strengthen the gluteus maximus so that the adductor magnus no longer takes over.

Arm Motions During Stance Phase

Typically, during stance phase the shoulder is extended 45° (Fig. 4.17, A), while the elbow is flexed about 70° (Fig. 4.17, B).

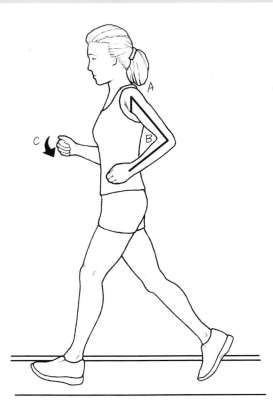

Fig. 4.17. ***Arm motions during stance phase.*** *Note the angles of shoulder extension (**A**) and elbow flexion (**B**). The hand should never cross the midline (**C**).*

There can be significant variation in the degree of elbow flexion, however, as typical ranges vary between 42 and 102° (23). While the degree of shoulder extension and elbow flexion don't correlate that strongly with efficiency, your hand should never cross the midline (Fig. 4.17, C), as excessive rotation of the torso does correlate with inefficiency (7).

Position of Center of Knee

A line drawn between the center of your hip and the center of your Achilles tendon should bisect the middle of the knee (Fig. 4.18, A).

In bowlegged runners, the line will bisect the inner side of the knee, while in knock kneed

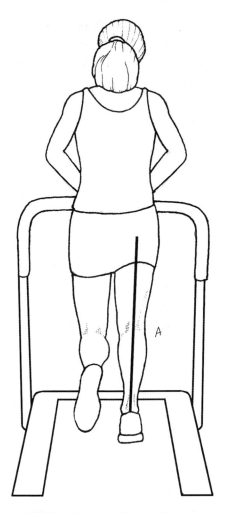

Fig. 4.18. ***Position of center of knee.*** *Observe where the center of the knee lies relative to a line drawn from the center of the hip to the Achilles tendon (**A**).*

runners, the bisection line will traverse the outside of the knee. Bowlegged runners should do everything they can to strengthen the hip abductors, as strong hip abductors correlate with reduced progression of knee arthritis in these individuals (26). Knock kneed runners should strengthen their hip abductors and rotators. My favorite exercises are illustrated in Fig. 3.36. Lateral step-ups are important for both knock kneed and bowlegged runners because these exercises place less stress on the knee than squats and target the hip muscles more effectively.

Knee Separation During Midstance

When viewed from behind, there should be a slight separation of the knees during midstance (Fig. 4.19, A). Excessive narrowing correlates with valgus collapse of the knees, while an increased degree of knee separation is usually seen in bowlegged older males. When viewed from the front, the center of the patella should be in the middle of the knee during midstance (Fig. 4.19, B).

Excessive inward rotation of the knee (Fig. 4.19, C) decreases efficiency and greatly increases the risk of sustaining a running injury. The excessive rotation can be the result of anteverted hips, external tibial torsion, weak hip external rotators, and/or excessive pronation,

and it is important to identify the exact cause of the issue and correct the faulty movement. This can be accomplished with hip strengthening exercises, accommodating external tibial torsion by landing with a slight toe-out running pattern while running, and/or using varus posts or orthotics to control excessive pronation.

Foot to Center of Mass Position

The inner aspect of the foot should always be lateral to a vertical line dropped from the center of mass to the treadmill (Fig. 4.20, A). An alternate way to take this measurement is to use a piece of chalk and place it down the center of the treadmill while it's running. This creates a temporary chalk line down the middle of the

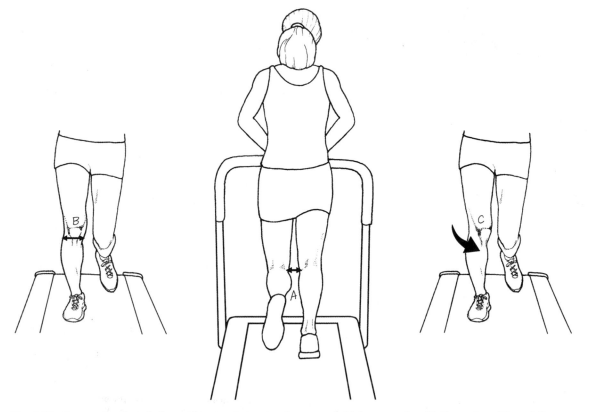

Fig. 4.19. ***Knee separation during midstance.*** *Determine the amount of knee separation (**A**). The center of the patella should be in the middle of the knee (**B**). Excessive inward rotation of the knee (**C**).*

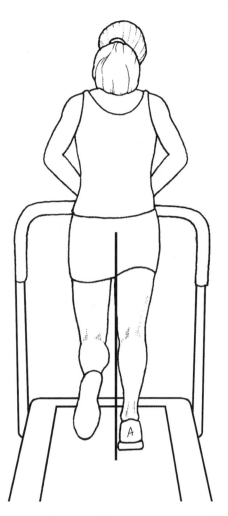

Fig. 4.20. ***Foot to center of mass position.*** *Check the position of the foot relative to a vertical line from the center of mass to the treadmill (**A**).*

between tibial stress fractures and crossover gait patterns (19). Common causes of crossover gait patterns include long stride lengths, low cadences, and/or weakness of the hip abductors.

In addition to reducing your stride length and strengthening your hip abductors, correcting a crossover gait pattern almost always includes gait retraining, which involves the runner focusing on not letting either foot cross the midline while running on a treadmill positioned in front of a mirror. Most gym owners don't mind you putting a chalk mark along the center the treadmill belt, as it gradually disappears over time. Start out by running slowly and make sure each foot consistently lands on the outer side of that centerline. In difficult cases, I have runners place a Triple Stick Strap just below their hips and have them run slowly on a treadmill. The strap forces them to fire their hip abductors constantly during the gait cycle, which allows for rapid resolution of a crossover running pattern. Of course, you have to run slowly as you're getting used to the strap.

Position of Foot During Midswing and Midstance

During midswing, the longitudinal bisection of the foot should be straight. When external tibial torsion is present, this bisection rotates out (Fig. 4.21, A). If you do not have external tibial torsion and the foot rotates out, this could be the result of excessive pronation, a weak tibialis posterior, and/or a tight gastrocnemius.

In addition to stretching your calves and strengthening your hips and feet, outward rotation of the foot almost always requires gait retraining, where you consciously modify the position of your foot during push-off. You should

treadmill, and the inner aspects of your running shoes should never cross this line.

In crossover gait patterns, the foot lands medially to the bisection line, which increases the risk of a wide range of injuries, including medial tibial stress syndrome, Achilles tendinitis, plantar fasciitis, and especially tibial stress fractures. Crossover gait patterns are problematic because the striking of the ground with the tibia at an angle increases the bending strains on the tibial cortex (27), which explains the connection

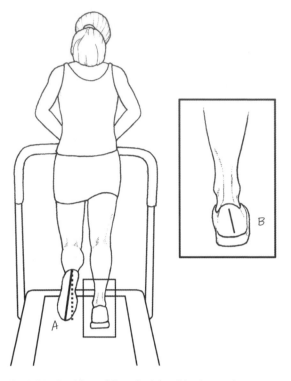

Fig. 4.21. ***Position of foot during midswing and midstance.*** *The longitudinal bisection of the foot should be straight, but rotates out if there is external tibial torsion (**A**). Identifying the rearfoot position during midstance (**B**).*

know your specific degree of tibial torsion on each side and try to match that degree while running. It's fine to land with your feet at angles less than your degree of torsion as long as your knees point straight forward.

Fig. 4.21, B illustrates how to identify the rearfoot position during midstance. Typically, the bisection of the heel should be vertical during midstance, but when excessive pronation is present, the vertical bisection of the heel rolls inward. Excessive pronation correlates with the development of Achilles injuries, medial tibial stress syndromes, and anterior knee pain. In contrast, runners with high arches present with their heels inverted and are more likely to develop stress fractures, lateral knee pain, and outer hip pain.

Overpronators should consider performing foot strengthening exercises and/or wearing minimalist shoes throughout the day, since overpronators who are strong are less likely to be injured (28). Runners who are overpronators almost always prefer stability running shoes, while high-arched runners prefer soft running shoes (see Chapter 5 for details regarding the selection of running shoes). High-arched runners should also consider doing gait retraining, where they try to reduce impact sounds during initial contact. As mentioned in Chapter 3, high-arched runners should work on maintaining adequate range of foot and ankle motion and learn to strike the ground with the tibia nearly vertical in order to reduce braking forces.

REFERENCES

1. Anderson T. Biomechanics and running economy. *Sports Med*. 1996;22:76–89.
2. Williams K, Cavanagh P. Relationship between distance running mechanics, running economy, and performance. *J Appl Physiol*. 1987;63:1236–1246.
3. Cavanagh P, Pollock M, Landa J. A biomechanical comparison of elite and good distance runners. *Ann NY Acad Sci*. 1977;301:328–345.
4. Anderson T, Tseh W. Running economy, anthropometric dimensions and kinematic variables (abstract). *Med Sci Sports Exerc*. 1994;26(5):S170.
5. Sano K, Ishikawa M, Nobue A, et al. Muscle–tendon interaction and EMG profiles of world class endurance runners during hopping. *Eur J Appl Physiol*. 2013;113(6):1395–1403.
6. Miyashita M, Miura M, Murase Y, et al. Running performance from the viewpoint of aerobic power. In: Folinsbe L (ed.)

Environmental Stress. New York: Academic Press, 1978:183–193.

7. Folland J, Allen S, Black M, et al. Running technique is an important component of running economy and performance. *Med Sci Sports Exerc*. 2017;49:1412–1423.

8. Weyand P, Sternlight D, Belizzi J, Wright S. Faster top running speeds are achieved with greater ground forces not more rapid leg movements. *J Appl Physiol*. 2000;89:1991–1999.

9. Salo A, Bezodis I, Batterham, A, et al. Elite sprinting: are athletes individually step-frequency or step-length reliant? *Med Sci Sports Exerc*. 2011;43:1055–1062.

10. Abe T, Fukashiro S, Harada Y, et al. Relationship between sprint performance and muscle fascicle length in female sprinters. *J Physiol Anthropol*. 2001;20:141–147.

11. Kumagai K, Abe T, Brechue W, et al. Sprint performance is related to muscle fascicle length in male 100-meter sprinters. *J Appl Physiol*. 2000;88:811–816.

12. Kubo K, Ohgo K, Takeishi R, et al. Effects of isometric training at different knee angles on the muscle–tendon complex in vivo. *Scand J Med Sci Sports*. 2006;16:159–167.

13. Lee S, Piazza S. Built for speed: musculoskeletal structure and sprinting ability. *J Exper Biol*. 2009;212:3700–3707.

14. Pellegrino J, Ruby B, Dumke C. Effect of plyometrics on the energy cost of running and MHC and titin isoforms. *Med Sci Sports Exerc*. 2016;48(1):49–56.

15. Turki O, Chaouachi D, Behm D, et al. The effect of warm-ups incorporating different volumes of dynamic stretching on 10-and 20-m sprint performance in highly trained male athletes. *J Strength Cond*. 2012;26:63–71.

16. Barnes K, Hopkins W, McGuigan M, et al. Form-up with a weighted vest improves writing performance via leg stiffness and running economy. *J Sci Med Sport*. 2015;18(1):103–108.

17. Escamilla R, Zheng N, Macleod T, et al. Patellofemoral joint force and stress between a short- and long-step forward lunge. *J Orthop Sports Phys Ther*. 2008;38:681–690.

18. Boyer E, Derrick T. Select injury-related variables are affected by stride length and foot strike style during running. *Am J Sports Med*. 2015;43:2310.

19. Creaby M, Dixon S. External frontal plane loads may be associated with tibial stress fracture. *Med Sci Sports Exerc*. 2008;40(9):1669–1674.

20. Bramah C, Preece S, Gill N, et al. A 10% increase in step rate improves running kinematics and clinical outcomes in runners with patellofemoral pain at 4 weeks and 3 months. *Am J Sports Med*. 2019;47:3406–3413.

21. Heiderscheit B, Chumanov E, Michalski M, et al. Effects of step rate manipulation on joint mechanics during running. *Med Sci Sports Exerc*. 2011;43(2):296–302.

22. Stiffler-Joachim M, Wille C, Kliethermes S, et al. Foot angle and loading rate during running demonstrate a nonlinear relationship. *Med Sci Sports Exerc*. 2019;51:2067–2072.

23. Hanley B, Smith L, Bissas A. Kinematic variations due to changes in pace during men's and women's 5 km road running. *Int J Sports Sci Coach*. 2011;6:243–252.

24. Pipkin A, Kotecki K, Hetzel S, et al. Reliability of qualitative video analysis for running. *J Orthop Sports Phys Ther*. 2016;46:556–561.

25. Elsais W. EMG measurement of the adductor muscles during walking and running. PhD dissertation 2019. University of Salford, Salford, UK.

26. Chang A, Hayes K, et al. Hip abduction moments and protection against medial

tibiofemoral osteoarthritis progression. *Arth Rheum*. 2005;52:3515–3519.

27. Turner CH, Wang T, Burr DB. Shear strength and fatigue properties of human cortical bone determined from pure shear tests. *Calc Tiss Res*. 2001;69:373–378.

28. Zhang X, Pauel R, Deschamps K, et al. Differences in foot muscle morphology and foot kinematics between symptomatic and asymptomatic pronated feet. *Scand J Med Sci Sports*. 2019;29(11):1766–1773.

CHAPTER 5

SELECTING THE IDEAL RUNNING SHOE

Given the potential for lacerations, abrasions, and/or thermal injury, it seems odd that for almost all of our seven-million-year history as bipeds, we got around the planet barefoot. Although we perceive our feet as being delicate structures in need of protection, when barefoot from birth, the human foot is remarkably resilient. In a study comparing lifelong shod feet with the feet of people who have never worn shoes, researchers from Belgium confirmed that the unshod forefoot is 16% wider than the shod forefoot (1). The increased width allows for improved distribution of pressure while walking and running. In their analysis of pressure centered beneath the forefoot in lifelong shod versus unshod individuals, the authors confirmed that regular shoe use is associated with significantly more pressure being centered directly beneath the middle of the forefoot. When barefoot from birth, your toes become so strong that they push down with more force, distributing pressure away from the center of the forefoot toward the tips of the toes. This is consistent with an analysis of skeletal remains dating back 100,000 years, confirming that people who are barefoot from birth get less forefoot arthritis because their strong toes distribute pressure more effectively (2). To enhance protection against perforation, the skin of an unshod foot becomes extremely tough and is remarkably similar to leather. These features allowed the feet of our earliest ancestors to effectively manage the stresses associated with moving around sub-Saharan Africa.

Surprisingly, our unshod feet could even handle the extremely cold temperatures and jagged mountainous terrain associated with traversing Eurasia, as evidence suggests that we did not begin routinely using protective footwear until 30,000 years ago. This means that for 80,000 years following our exodus from Africa, we crossed the Swiss and Italian Alps and quickly spread through the cold climates of Europe and Asia without protective shoe wear. Remember, the fat pads beneath our feet contain 4.5 times the amount of polyunsaturated fat as conventional fat, and the reduced viscosity associated with greater amounts of polyunsaturated fats insulates our soft tissues from even subzero temperatures. The skin on the bottom of our feet also developed the peculiar ability to create a variable surface depending on whether we walk on slippery wet rocks or smooth dry terrain. Have you ever wondered why only the skin on the bottom of your hands and feet wrinkles when you get out of a bath or shower? Neurobiologists from a research lab in Idaho (3) claim that these wrinkles act like treads on a tire to improve our ability to grasp wet surfaces. In contrast, we have better traction on dry surfaces when our skin is smooth. Notice how the world's fastest race cars can take turns at 240 mph on dry surfaces by having perfectly smooth tires, while these same tires would be disastrous when driving in the rain, as they would hydroplane.

THE FIRST EVIDENCE OF SHOE USE

Determining the exact date we began routinely using shoes has been difficult, since the early shoes were made of leather, grass, and other biodegradable materials that left no fossil evidence. Although Neanderthals were suspected of occasionally using insulated foot coverings, the first direct evidence of shoe use dates back to only 3,500 years ago (Fig. 5.1). While primitive sandals and moccasins discovered in Oregon and Missouri have been carbon dated to 10,000 years ago, the actual time period that our ancestors first introduced protective shoe wear remains a mystery.

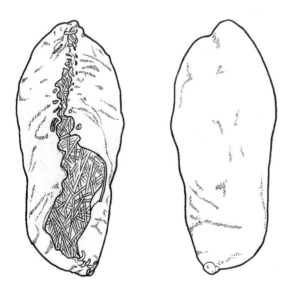

Fig. 5.1. *The earliest shoes resembled stitched leather bags.*

To get around the fact that ancient shoes rapidly decayed, leaving no evidence of use, Trinkaus and Shang (4) decided to date the initiation of shoe wear by searching for changes in the shapes of the toes of our early ancestors. Because regular shoe use lessens strain on the toe muscles, the authors theorized that habitual shoe use would be associated with the sudden appearance of a thinning of the proximal phalanges (the bones at the base of our toes). By precisely measuring all aspects of toe shape and composition, the authors discovered a marked decrease in the robusticity of the toe bones during the late Pleistocene era, approximately 30,000 years ago (Fig. 5.2).

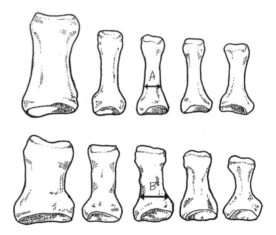

Fig. 5.2. *Compare the width of the toe bones from the early (bottom row) and late (top row) Pleistocene era.* *Trinkaus and Shang (4) claim that the decreased strain on the toes associated with regular shoe use produced bony remodeling with a gradual narrowing of the toe bones (compare **A** and **B**).*

Because there was no change in overall limb robusticity, the anatomical inference is that shoe gear eventually resulted in the development of narrower toes. The authors state that because there is no evidence of a meaningful reduction in biomechanical loads placed on human lower limbs during the late Pleistocene era (e.g., reduced foraging distances), the logical conclusion is that the thinner toes could only have only resulted from the use of shoes. The authors evaluated numerous skeletal remains from different periods and concluded that based on the sudden reduction in toe diameter, the use of footwear became habitual sometime between 28,000 and 32,000 years ago.

The first shoes were most likely similar to the shoes discovered in the Armenian cave; i.e., they were simple leather bags partially filled with grass to insulate the foot from cold surfaces. Because shoe gear varied depending on the region, the earliest shoes worn in tropical environments were most likely similar to the 3,000-year-old sandals recently found in Israel. Once discovered, the use of protective shoe wear quickly spread. The early Egyptians were believed to be the first civilization to create a rigid sandal, which was originally made from woven papyrus leaves molded in wet sand. Affluent citizens even decorated their sandals with expensive jewels.

While wealthy Greeks and Egyptians had separate shoes/sandals made for their right and left feet, the practice of wearing different shoes on each foot was short-lived, and throughout the Dark and Middle Ages, shoes were made to be worn on either foot. Improvements in manufacturing techniques before the American Civil War changed that. By modifying a duplicating lathe used to mass produce wooden gunstocks, a Philadelphia shoemaker was able to manufacture mirror-image lasts that allowed for the production of separate shoes for each foot. (Lasts are three-dimensional foot models used for the manufacturing of shoes.) Using this new technology, the Union Army supplied over 500,000 soldiers with matching pairs of right and left leather shoes.

ATHLETIC SHOES FROM THE EARLY 1900S

Leather continued to be the most popular material used for making shoe gear until the late 1800s, when Charles Goodyear accidentally dropped rubber into heated sulfur, creating vulcanized rubber. Prior to his serendipitous discovery, rubber was a fairly useless material because it melted at relatively low temperatures. The newfound resiliency of this material would have numerous applications, including the production of the first athletic shoe. Although alternative names for the new footwear include tennis shoes, trainers, and runners, the term "sneaker" became the most popular, and its origin can be traced back to an 1887 column in the *New York Times* (5), quoting an article from the Boston *Journal of Education*: "It is only the harassed schoolmaster who can fully appreciate the pertinency of the name boys give to tennis shoes—sneakers." Apparently, the soft rubber soles allowed schoolchildren to sneak up quietly on unsuspecting teachers.

Spalding manufactured one of the earliest athletic shoes: the Converse All-Star. Used by athletes at Springfield College to play the newly invented game of basketball, the All-Star was immediately popular. Since their introduction in 1908, more than 70 million pairs of Converse have been sold worldwide. In 1916, the US Rubber Company introduced Keds, an athletic shoe made with a flexible rubber bottom and canvas upper comparable to the Converse All-Star. The first orthopedic athletic shoe was developed by New Balance shortly before the Great Depression. New Balance continues to be the world's largest manufacturer of athletic shoes available in different widths. The German shoemaker Adi Dassler formed Adidas in the 1930s, while his brother Rudi formed Puma in the 1940s. Adidas was the more popular company and was the dominant manufacturer of sneakers until the 1960s, when Phil Knight and Bill Bowerman created Blue Ribbon Sports. Renamed Nike Inc. in 1978, after the Greek goddess of victory, this company has remained the world's largest producer of athletic shoes and sporting apparel for more than 50 years.

RUNNING SHOES FROM THE 1970S THROUGH 2010

The design of the first sneaker manufactured specifically for running was simple: A thin rubber sole was covered with a canvas upper, providing nominal cushioning and protection. The next generation of running shoes was built with thicker midsoles possessing large medial and lateral heel flares designed to improve stability. Unfortunately, the lateral heel flares were quickly proven to increase the potential for injury, as they provided the ground with a longer lever for pronating the rearfoot during heel strike (6) (Fig. 5.3). While this research was published in the late 1980s by one of the top biomechanists in the world, shoe manufactures were slow to respond and continued to include lateral flares for years to come.

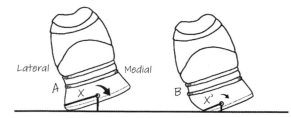

Fig. 5.3. *The first running shoes were made with large lateral flares (A), which provided ground reaction forces with a longer lever arm (X) for pronating the rearfoot at heel strike.* This feature produces significant increases in the initial range and velocity of pronation. Note that a midsole with a negative flare (B) provides ground reaction forces with a shorter lever arm (X') for pronating the rearfoot.

The most significant design change from the flimsy running shoes of the 1960s was that manufacturers began to build sneakers to fit runners with one of three different arch heights: cushion sneakers for high-arched runners,

stability sneakers for neutral-arched runners, and motion control sneakers for flat-footed overpronators (Fig. 5.4).

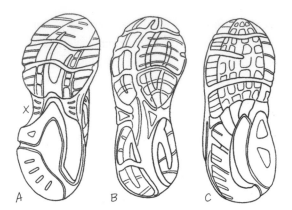

Fig. 5.4. *Bottom view of the three types of running shoe.* Cushion sneakers (A) are made for individuals with high arches. They are slightly curved to match the shape of the typical high-arched foot and possess flexible midsoles with significantly less bulk in the midfoot region (X). The reduced midsole material in the midfoot gives the shoe an hourglass appearance when viewed from below. Stability sneakers (B) are suited to individuals with neutral foot types. They are straighter and have slightly more midsole material reinforced beneath the arch. In contrast, motion control sneakers (C) are very straight and are strongly reinforced throughout the midfoot with extra-thick midsole material. Because of the additional midsole material, motion control sneakers are extremely stiff.

The vast majority of midsoles were made of polyurethane (PU) or ethylene vinyl acetate (EVA). Polyurethane is the most resilient of these materials because it provides maximum resistance against compression without breaking down. It can be identified by its weight (it is the heaviest midsole material), and by its tendency to turn yellow over time. In contrast, EVA is lighter but breaks down quicker, as it rapidly deforms with repeated impacts. As a result, EVA was often used in entry-level sneakers because it's inexpensive to produce.

Other hybrid midsole materials were later incorporated into midsoles, such as Phylon, which is made from EVA pellets heated and cooled in a mold, and Phylite, a combination of Phylon and rubber. Both of these materials could be injection-molded and easily shaped. Because Phylite is durable enough to be used without an outsole, it makes for an extremely light and flexible sneaker.

The density of the different midsole materials varies considerably and this is useful when designing sneakers for runners with high and low arches. High-arched runners need the least dense midsoles to improve shock absorption, while overpronators usually require a blend of midsole materials with soft material incorporated into the lateral midsole and firm material used along the medial midsole. Referred to as a "dual-density midsole," the softer material on the outer side softens the impact forces and decreases the initial velocity of pronation, while the firmer material on the inner side provides protection against excessive pronation (7). The dual-density midsole essentially creates a functional rearfoot varus post that lessens the amount of rearfoot pronation following heel strike.

Despite early thick midsoles providing cushioning and motion control, one main drawback of them was their weight. Because a running shoe is located so far from your hip, it has a very long lever arm to your hip muscles, forcing these muscles to work harder to accelerate and decelerate the added weight. It's comparable to sitting on a seesaw when the person on the other side suddenly moves farther back: Because the person's body weight suddenly has a longer lever arm to the pivot of the seesaw, you get stuck in the air. In regard to running, every 100 grams (3.5 oz.) of midsole material you add to a running shoe increases the metabolic cost of running by 1%. This is known as the "1% rule," and the increased

exertion associated with accelerating and decelerating a heavy midsole can be extremely fatiguing over the course of a marathon.

Until recently, the heels of running shoes were almost universally elevated with an additional ⅜ to ½ inch (10 to 12 mm) of midsole material to support and protect the heel from impact forces. Unlike the flat Converse All-Star and Keds, the forward portions of the early midsoles were also modified by adding different degrees of toe spring (Fig. 5.5).

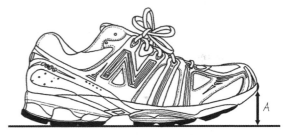

Fig. 5.5. *The typical running shoe is manufactured with a toe spring (A), which allows the foot to move in a more natural manner and reduces strain on the Achilles tendon and plantar fascia.*

The toe spring modification, which represents a superior angulation of the far end of the midsole, effectively shortens the functional length of the shoe while also allowing the toes to move through reduced ranges of motion during propulsion. This midsole design is invaluable in the treatment of Achilles tendinitis, plantar fasciitis, metatarsal stress syndrome, and/or bunion pain, as it allows to the foot to go through push-off with a rolling action.

Running shoe manufacturers were positive that, compared to the flimsy sneakers of the 1960s, running shoes specifically designed to match the biomechanical needs of runners with different arch heights would not only reduce the risk of injury but also improve performance.

Some argue that the long-term use of excessive toe springs would result in weakness of the intrinsic muscles of the arch.

In 2010, several quality studies evaluated whether or not the prescription of running shoes based on arch height had merit. In one of the largest studies done to date, Knapik et al. (8) divided 1,400 male and female Marine Corps recruits into two groups: an experimental group in which running shoe recommendation was based on arch height, and a control group that wore neutral stability running shoes regardless of arch height. After completing an intensive 12-week training regimen, the authors concluded that prescribing running shoes according to arch height was not necessary, since there was no difference in injury rates between the two groups.

In another study evaluating the value of prescribing running shoes according to arch height, Ryan et al. (9) categorized 81 female runners as supinators, neutral, or pronators, and then randomly assigned them to wear neutral, stability, or motion control running shoes. Again, the authors concluded that there was no correlation between foot type, running shoe use, and the frequency of reported pain. One of the more interesting findings of this research was that the individuals classified as pronators reported greater levels of pain when wearing the motion control running shoes, which didn't surprise me, as these shoes are often as stiff as a board.

THE MIDSOLE

Problems Associated with Too Much Midsole Material

Throughout the 1980s and 1990s, researchers from Canada questioned the belief that cushioning the foot by adding more midsole material would protect against injury (10, 11). They claimed that highly cushioned running shoes might increase the potential for injury, as people are unable to feel the ground properly. To prove this, they poked small metal balls into different spots along the bottom of the foot and determined that the skin beneath the first metatarsal head is nearly 10 times more sensitive to pressure than the skin beneath the heel. The increased sensation beneath the first metatarsal allows the sensory receptors to produce a reflex contraction of the toe muscles when these receptors are stimulated while walking and running. As the toes push down to offload the sensitive first metatarsal head, they distribute pressure over a broader area, effectively negating the heavy loads centered beneath the metatarsal heads (Fig. 5.6). This research explains why over 100,000 years ago, our ancestors rarely developed arthritis in the joints of their forefeet, while we regularly get severe arthritis and bunions in those joints now.

In 1997, Robbins and Waked (10) did a simple test to evaluate the effect that soft materials have on our ability to respond to impact. They measured the impact forces as healthy subjects stepped off a perch onto a platform 1⅘ inches (4.5 cm) below. The platform was made from 0, 1, 2, or 3 inches (0, 2.5, 5, or 7.5 cm) of EVA foam. Paradoxically, the subjects landing on the thickest foams had the highest impact forces. The authors claim that because soft surfaces make it difficult to feel the ground properly, the subjects hit the softer surface harder by reducing their knee and hip flexion so they could compress the foam and thereby feel the surface better. They reference another interesting study showing that gymnasts landing on soft 4-inch (10 cm)-thick mats generate 20% more impact force than when they land on a hard floor (12). The only problem

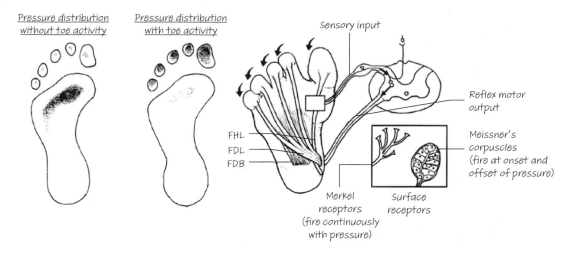

Fig. 5.6. *When stimulated, the skin receptors located beneath the first metatarsal head produce a reflex contraction of the toe muscles, which transfers pressure away from the central forefoot to the tips of the toes.* *This reflex contraction protects our forefeet from injury. (**FDB** = flexor digitorum brevis; **FDL** = flexor digitorum longus; **FHL** = flexor hallucis longus.)*

with Robbins and Waked's research is that the subjects were landing on 1–3 inches (2.5–7.5 cm) of EVA foam, which at the time was way more foam than you could fit into a running shoe.

Problems Associated with Too Little Midsole Material

Given the fact that excessive midsole cushioning can increase impact force and reduce efficiency (remember the 1% rule), it might seem that the best midsole would be no midsole at all. While this is often suggested by advocates of barefoot running, the complete removal of a midsole may result in chronic injury because some degree of midsole cushioning is necessary to protect the heel and forefoot fat pads from trauma. Researchers from the Netherlands have proven that barefoot running results in a 60% deformation of the protective fat pad beneath the heel, while running with running shoes with conventional midsoles results in only a 35% deformation of the fat pad (13). When repeated tens of thousands of times over your running

career, the 60% deformation may permanently damage the walls of your protective fat pads, resulting in chronic heel and/or forefoot pain.

In addition to extending the lifespan of your heel pads, research proves that the softer running shoe midsoles are capable of storing and returning energy, offsetting the reduced efficiency associated with its added weight. By studying oxygen consumption while runners ran either barefoot or with running shoes having 10-mm-thick midsoles, researchers from the University of Colorado proved that despite the added midsole weight associated with wearing running shoes, there is no difference in efficiency when running barefoot and running with cushioned midsoles (14). The authors state: "The positive effects of shoe cushioning counteract the negative effects of added mass, resulting in the metabolic cost for shod running approximately equal to that of barefoot running."

One of the more intriguing results of this study was that the researchers also evaluated efficiency as the runners ran on specially designed treadmills fitted with ⅖ and ⅘ inch (10 and 20 mm) of midsole material attached directly to the treadmill belt. Interestingly, the treadmill fitted with 10-mm-thick midsole material produced the same improvement in efficiency as the treadmill fitted with 20-mm-thick midsole material. Apparently, just as flexible running tracks providing ¼ inch (7 mm) of deflection allow for the fastest running times (refer back to page 55), ⅘ inch (10 mm) of midsole cushioning provides the ideal amount of energy return with less weight and only a minimal reduction in sensory perception. Remember, the EVA used in the research by Robbins and Waked (10) that resulted in increased impact forces was 1–3 inches (2.5–7.5 cm) thick, which was more likely to dampen sensory input and produce a paradoxical response to cushioning.

Changing the Midsole's Heel-to-Toe Drop

As mentioned, throughout the 1980s, 1990s, and early 2000s all running shoes were made with an additional ⅖ and ⅘ inch (10 and 20 mm) of midsole material, creating what is referred to as the "heel-to-toe drop" (or "heel-to-toe differential") (Fig. 5.7). This degree of heel elevation was considered essential for offloading

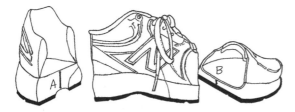

Fig. 5.7. *The heel-to-toe drop is the difference in midsole thickness beneath the heel (A) and the forefoot (B).* This particular sneaker has ⅘ inch (22 mm) of midsole material beneath the heel, and ½ inch (12 mm) of midsole material beneath the forefoot, creating a ⅖ inch (10 mm) heel-to-toe drop.

the Achilles tendon and absorbing impact force when the heel hit the ground. In an attempt to reduce weight and more closely duplicate the way the foot moves when barefoot, different manufacturers began to gradually reduce the amount of midsole material beneath the heel.

Zero-drop running shoes were eventually introduced with the same amount of cushioning in the forefoot and rearfoot and are often considered "more natural" because they allow your foot to function as if you were barefoot. Proponents of zero-drop shoes claim the excessive cushioning associated with the high heel-to-toe drop running sneakers cause you to strike the ground with a more pronounced heel strike, which also results in smaller knee flexion angles at touchdown, as well as less ankle dorsiflexion during midstance (15). Advocates of running shoes with a ½ inch (12 mm) heel-to-toe drop claim that the added cushioning in the heel provides comfort and protects the wearer from injuries.

To resolve the controversy regarding heel-to-toe drop, researchers from France had 553 runners wear running shoes manufactured with 0, ¼, ⅖ inch (0, 6, 10 mm) of heel-to-toe drop (16). The sneakers, which were identical except for the degree of heel elevation, were randomly prescribed and the runners were followed for six months. The fact that the shoes were identical except for heel elevation is what makes this paper significant: Because there are so many differences between different models of running shoe, it's impossible to evaluate the effect of one factor without controlling all other factors. Prior studies evaluating the effect of heel height can't guarantee that their outcomes were actually the result of the heel-to-toe drop or some other attribute of the shoe.

At the end of the six-month French study, while there was no overall difference in injury rates, a lower risk of injury in occasional runners was linked to the 0 and ¼ inch (6 mm) heel-to-toe drop running shoes, while experienced runners wearing the 10 mm heel-to-toe drop shoes were less likely to be injured. Although this was just one study, it tallies with what I've observed in practice in that faster high-mileage runners prefer sneakers with ⅖–⅘ inch (10–12 mm) of heel-to-toe drop, while slower recreational runners do well with 0 and ¼ inch (6 mm) heel-to-toe drop models. As with midsole stiffness and weight, the heel-to-toe drop is an important factor associated with improved comfort, and you should experiment with different models until you find the midsole height that feels best for you.

RUNNING SHOES FROM 2010 TO CURRENT MINIMALIST RUNNING SHOES

Inspired in part by the popular book *Born to Run* by Christopher McDougall, minimalist running shoes were initially designed to mimic barefoot running (Fig. 5.8). According to the paleoanthropologist Daniel Lieberman,

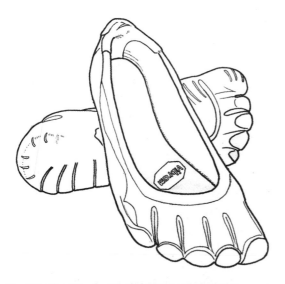

Fig. 5.8. *The Vibram FiveFingers running shoe is designed to mimic barefoot activity.*

to protect their heels from injury, barefoot runners naturally switch to a more forward contact point, which theoretically improves the storage and return of energy and more effectively dampens impact forces (17).

While the possibility of improved energy return and dampened impact forces sounds appealing, it is necessary that runners wearing minimalist shoes actually switch to the more forward contact point in order to obtain these benefits. Unfortunately, this is not always the case. In a study of runners transitioning to minimalist shoe wear, 35% of the runners continued to make ground contact with their heels in spite of wearing the minimalist shoes for more than two years (18). Although runners with midfoot strike patterns may benefit from minimalist shoes, slow runners who continue to strike the ground with their heels are more likely to be injured, since vertical loading rates beneath the heel are nearly 40% higher with a minimalist shoe when rearfoot striking (19). Furthermore, research showing that a 10-mm-thick midsole does not reduce efficiency, since it improves the storage and return of energy, suggests that even fast runners can afford the protection provided by conventional midsoles (14).

Another problem with minimalist shoe wear is that you are more likely to be injured while breaking them in. In a frequently cited study published in *Medicine and Science in Sports and Exercise*, researchers from Brigham Young University noted that 10 out of 19 runners transitioning into minimalist shoes became injured, compared to only one out of 17 runners in the control group wearing conventional running shoes (20). I feel that the high injury rate linked to minimalist shoes has everything to do with the fact that modern foot architecture is significantly different than that of our barefoot ancestors. Remember, the early hominids had robust toes and forefeet that were 16% wider than ours, so they could easily manage the forces associated with the push-off phase of running. In addition to having stronger, wider forefeet, our ancestors were also tiny. *Homo erectus*, the first hominid to routinely run, was only 5 feet 2 inches (1.57 m) tall and weighed about 110 pounds. Given the tiny stature and wide forefeet of these hominids, it's not surprising that heavier male runners are much more likely to be injured while wearing minimalist shoes (21).

In the most detailed studies of minimalist shoes to date, researchers from Australia (22) evaluated the short- and long-term effects of wearing minimalist shoes as runners gradually transitioned from 0–100% minimalist shoe use for their daily runs. For the first six weeks of the study, the authors had 50 recreationally competitive male runners gradually transition into wearing minimalist shoes for 35% of their total weekly running mileages. All runners were habitual rearfoot strikers and had been accustomed to conventional running shoes. After the 6-week break-in, runners were instructed to continue transitioning into the minimalist shoes by increasing their allocated use by 5% each week for an additional 20 weeks. At the 6- and 20-week marks, researchers measured running performance, running economy, calf strength, lower limb bone mineral density, stride length, and cadence.

By week six of the study, runners transitioning into minimalist shoes showed slight improvements in running economy and performance, which the authors attributed to the reduced weight of the minimalist shoes. Two of the 50 runners switched from a heel to a forefoot contact point during the first six weeks. When the study finally concluded after 20 weeks, regular use of minimalist running shoes was shown to have absolutely no effect on performance, running economy, stride length, cadence, bone mineral density, or even point of initial contact (the two runners who transitioned to a forefoot contact reverted to their typical rearfoot strike by week 20). Significantly, the minimalist shoes did slightly increase ankle plantar flexor strength, which was consistent with prior research demonstrating that eight weeks of running in minimalist shoes increased intrinsic foot muscle cross-sectional area (23). The authors state that because of the limited benefits linked to using minimalist shoes for 100% of their training, runners "may need to consider limiting minimalist shoe use to lower percentages of total training volume because greater minimalist shoe volume has been previously associated with increased injury risk."

My takeaway from this study is that when worn throughout the day while walking and/or for brief periods of slow running, minimalist shoes favorably stimulate the muscles of the arches and calves without overloading them, often resulting in significant increases in strength and volume of the muscles of the arches and legs (23). Over time, this may result in not just strength gains, but also an improved ability to store energy in the muscles and tendons of the arches and legs, and return energy to them. This statement is supported by the fact that compared to runners wearing conventional running shoes, experienced minimalist runners have larger and more resilient Achilles tendons (24). Increases in muscle strength and tendon resiliency can have long-term benefits, especially in master's runners, who slow down as they age, not because of decreased force output in their hips or knees but because their calves weaken as they get older (25).

MAXIMALIST RUNNING SHOES

At about the time the popularity of minimalist shoes began to fade (in part due to the high injury rates), an obscure French company named Hoka One One came out with the first maximalist running shoe: the Mafate (Fig. 5.9).

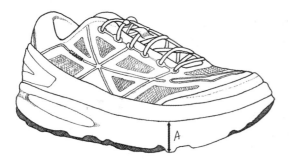

Fig. 5.9. *The Hoka One One Mafate can have as much as 1½ inches (37 mm) of midsole cushioning (A).*

The company name originates from the Maori language, meaning "to fly over earth," and the One One portion of the name is pronounced Oh-nay On-nay. The earliest Hoka models were specifically designed to help runners manage the extreme impact forces associated with fast downhill running, by stacking huge amounts of midsole material into the shoe. Because these shoes are so thick, the term "stack height" was developed to refer to the total amount of shoe material between the foot and the ground. It's usually expressed by two numbers: The first stack height number is the thickness beneath the heel, and the second is the thickness beneath the forefoot. Compared to zero-drop minimalist shoes with a stack height of ½/½ inch (12/12 mm), it is not uncommon for maximalist shoes to have stack heights of well over 1⅕ inches (30 mm). The Hoka One One Bondi, for example, has a stack height of 1½/1¼ inches (37/33 mm).

Immediately popular with the ultra-running community, maximalist shoes have been catching on with recreational runners. Other running shoe manufacturers have noticed the success of the maximalist shoes, and companies such as Altra, Vasque, New Balance, Brooks, and Adidas have developed their own models, each with its own unique shape, stack height, and heel-to-toe drop.

Because of the excessive midsole material, you would think that maximalist shoes would increase impact forces, according to the original research published by Robbins and Waked as previously discussed. In fact, initial research suggested that wearing maximalist shoes did indeed increase impact force. In 2018, researchers from Oregon State University compared vertical ground reaction forces between the Hoka One One and a traditional New Balance running shoe (26). Consistent with prior research on the relationship paradox between midsole thickness and impact force, the subjects wearing Hoka One Ones had significantly higher impact forces and loading rates than those wearing conventional running shoes. The results of this study were in agreement with one study (27) but in conflict with another (28). The problem with all of these studies is that the researchers compared completely different running shoes, which have too many different features to make a judgment possible about stack height alone.

In 2020, to determine the effect of stack height in isolation, researchers from San Jose State University performed a detailed study comparing ground reaction forces and three-dimensional motion as 20 recreational runners ran in three different types of running shoe: maximalist, traditional, and minimalist (29). Unlike prior studies, these researchers used the same running shoe in each category (New Balance Boracay) and they just varied the stack height for each shoe: The maximalist shoe had 1¼ inches (33 mm) rearfoot and 1⅕ inches (29 mm) forefoot cushioning, the traditional had ⅘ inch (22 mm) rearfoot and ⁷⁄₁₀ inch (18 mm) forefoot cushioning, and the minimalist had ⅖ inch (10 mm) rearfoot and ¼ inch (6 mm) forefoot cushioning. Other than the thickness of the midsoles, the shoes were all identical.

After analyzing the three-dimensional motion and impact forces associated with the different shoes, the authors determined that runners wearing the maximalist shoes pronated much farther than runners wearing the traditional and minimalist shoes. The excessive rolling-in was especially apparent as the runners were pushing off. The authors state that "the eversion mechanics in the maximal shoe may place runners at a greater risk of injury." Previous research has linked a wide range of lower limb and leg injuries to excessive pronation (30, 31). Despite the potential for increasing pronation, many of the maximalist models are gaining popularity, not just in the running community but also in professions such as nursing, where foot pain is the number one cause of occupational injury. After a brief break-in period, the altered movement patterns identified with wearing maximalist shoes would more than likely self-correct.

NEW CATEGORIES: FAST, SOFT, OR STABLE

Given the new changes in structure and function of the latest running shoes, the old categories of cushioning, stability, and motion control are no longer adequate for classifying all the new models. To that end, many experts now categorize running shoes as fast, soft, or stable. In keeping with the 1% rule, the fast models are lighter and typically possess slightly lower heel drops than the other models. The stable shoes tend to weigh just slightly more than soft models, but often possess reinforcement struts and/or plates embedded in their midsoles to provide support.

What makes all of these models different from their clunky predecessors is that almost every manufacturer now uses its own high-tech midsole foams, which provide stability and cushioning at a fraction of the weight of the early PU/EVA midsoles used in the 1980s and 1990s. Most of the new midsoles incorporate proprietary mixes of TPU (thermoplastic polyurethane) beads, lightweight EVA, various bags containing gel or air, and/or Pebax, the amazingly lightweight thermoplastic polymer made from polyamide blocks for strength and polyether for flexibility.

In the soft models, Salomon worked with Dow Chemicals to create the Sonic 3 Balance, which contains one layer of a memory-like foam to absorb shock, and another layer that is light and responsive. Another popular soft model is the Asics Nimbus. In addition to its special gel lining that wraps its heel, the Gel-Nimbus 22 has a layer of lightweight FlyteFoam Lyte placed on top of a full layer of FlyteFoam Propel, a high-rebound elastomer to provide extra spring during push-off. The New Balance Fresh Foam X 1080 was voted Editors' Choice among soft running shoes by Runner's World in 2020. What I like about this model is that the Fresh Foam midsole has a molded heel made with a deep pocket that wraps around the back of the foot to eliminate unwanted movement. In my opinion, a well-fitting heel counter is one of the most important things to look for when choosing a running shoe. Another popular soft running shoe is the Adidas Adizero Boost range. The midsole of this shoe is made with Adiprene, a proprietary blend of urethane polymers cured with special chemicals to enhance strength and resilience. This unique foam retains the ability to absorb shock even at subfreezing temperatures. Adiprene is highly effective at storing and returning energy, which is why these shoes are so frequently worn by the world's fastest runners.

Unlike the heavy motion control shoes of the past, several of the new stability models come in weighing less than 10 ounces (284 g). The Nike React Infinity Run Flyknit weighs only 9.6 ounces and is designed with a wide forefoot, a flared midsole, and a slight ramp beneath the midfoot, which is designed to "give your foot proprioceptive cues." Whether this is true or not is open for debate, but I've been working with different people in the running shoe industry for decades and most of them didn't know what proprioception was 30 years ago so I look at this statement as a sign they're moving in the right direction. Another stability shoe, the Mizuno Wave Inspire Waveknit, has special reinforcement plates embedded in the midsole near the inside of the medial arch. These plates provide additional support should your foot roll in too much. The New Balance 860 stability shoe has kept its varus posts to control motion, but the ramp angle has been reduced to make it feel smoother. In contrast, in the Brooks Adrenaline the rearfoot post has been scrapped all together in favor of more subtle changes to the shape of the midsole.

When it comes to fast running shoes, the hands-down winner is the Nike Air Zoom Alphafly NEXT% (who names these things?). Eliud Kipchoge made history wearing these shoes by being the first person to run 26.2 miles in under two hours. Nike boasts that regardless of skill level, the Alphaflys and their predecessor, the Vaporflys, can improve economy by as much as 4%, which translates into a 3.4% increase in speed for the world's fastest marathon runners, and a 4% improvement in speed for three-hour marathon runners (32). While shoe companies can be like politicians in that they have a tendency to tell you what you want to hear, the claims of 4% improvements in performance and economy may actually be true. In addition to weighing less than 7 ounces (200 g), the Alphaflys have special air chambers located beneath the forefoot (called "air pods"), and a graphite plate has been embedded in the midsole that can store and return energy during propulsion (Fig. 5.10). (Think of the graphite poles used in pole vaulting: They bend as the athlete is starting to ascend and then snap back again to propel them over the high bar.)

What really makes the Alphafly and Vaporfly shoes so fast is the new Pebax midsole, which is uncommonly compliant and resilient. In a 2017 study published in *Sports Medicine*, Wouter Hoogkamer and his colleagues (32) had 18 high-caliber runners complete a series of five-minute running trials wearing one of three shoes: the Nike Zoom Streak 6 (midsole lightweight EVA with a rearfoot airbag and a 23/15 stack height), the Adidas Adizero Adios Boost 2 (TPU midsole with a 23/13 stack), and the Nike Vaporfly ZoomX (Pebax midsole with an embedded carbon plate and a 31/21 stack height). After equalizing the weights by adding lead pellets to the lighter shoes, the examiners measured oxygen consumption and CO_2 production as the elite runners ran at different speeds on different days. At the end of the study, the subjects wearing the Vaporflys lowered their metabolic cost of running by a shocking 4%. Even more impressive, this 4% improvement occurred at every running speed on every day of the study. The only drawback was that athletes wearing the Nike Vaporflys had slight increases in their stride

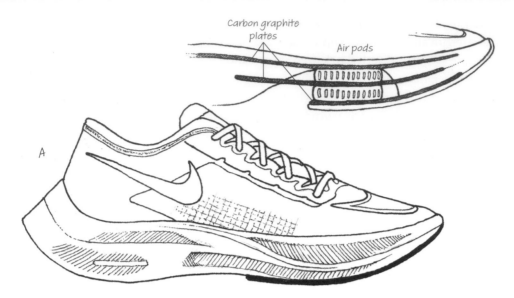

Fig. 5.10. ***The Nike Vaporfly (A) has a graphite plate embedded in the forefoot between two layers of Pebax foam.*** *The Nike Air Zoom Alphafly NEXT% (top) has three carbon graphite plates (arrows) with four separate air pods located beneath the forefoot (two on each side).*

lengths and impact forces, which could translate into a greater prevalence of hamstring and/or knee injuries.

While the carbon plate may have played a slight role in the improved economy, it more than likely was the Pebax midsole, which has just the right blend of stiffness and energy return. The authors claim that to improve performance, a midsole must have high compliance (the ability to deform) and high resilience (the ability to return energy). They use the example of running on a sandy beach: The sand is compliant, so you sink into it, but it's not resilient, so you have to work hard to push forward. Like a springy indoor track, Pebax midsoles come close to that perfect blend of compliance and resilience. The high compliance makes it so you don't have to flex your knees and hips to absorb shock, while the resilience offloads your arch muscles by returning free energy.

Dr. Hoogkamer and his colleagues didn't measure joint motion so it's not possible to determine exactly why the runners became so efficient.

Whatever the mechanism, these shoes represent the most innovative changes in shoe production since Goodyear discovered rubber. Critics of the new technologies claim that the shoes provide an unfair advantage, and as of February 2020, World Athletics decided to ban shoes containing more than one rigid embedded plate or blade and/or any shoe that had a sole height greater than 1⅗ inches (40 mm). The actions of World Athletics reminded me of the 2008 Olympics in Beijing, where Speedo introduced a full-body swimsuit that reduced the drag from water resistance. After athletes wearing the suits shattered dozens of world records, the International Swimming Federation took only a few months to ban all full-body swimsuits from competition.

An important point about these running shoes that no one has discussed is that all of the tests to date have been done on elite athletes. The ability of a midsole to store and return energy is dependent upon the ability of the midsole material (or air pods) to compress just the right amount so that the stored energy can be returned.

The midsole compliance and resilience that works for a 130-pound (60 kg) elite male running at a 4:30 minute/mile pace would probably not work that well for a heavier and slower recreational runner. Think of the springs on a pogo stick. If a 200-pound (90 kg) male got on a pogo stick designed for a 70-pound (30 kg) child, he would quickly stretch the spring to its maximum length, have a lag period, and then have to use his own legs to jump up. Conversely, if a 70-pound child got on a pogo stick designed for a 200-pound male, he or she wouldn't be able to stretch the springs enough for the pogo stick to work. Midsole materials are comparable to pogo stick springs in that they have to be adjusted to match the weight of the person using them.

In regard to running, the midsole/air pods would also have to be adjusted depending upon running speed, which affects the forces beneath the foot. Nike claims that the pressure and size of the air pods will someday be adjustable in order to maximize individual performance, although the cost of customization may be prohibitive. In my opinion, rather than looking to footwear to improve your ability to store and return energy, you'd be better off doing specific exercises and drills to enhance your tendon resiliency. In the 2017 paper evaluating the Vaporflys, Dr. Hoogkamer and his colleagues state that "regardless of the shoes worn, in human running, the vast majority of the mechanical energy storage and return occurs within our natural biological structures." To me, that sentence speaks volumes.

SELECTING THE RUNNING SHOE THAT'S RIGHT FOR YOU

Assuming you don't have a company like Nike bending over backward to design the perfect running shoe for your particular mechanics, given all the different companies and models out there, it can be a bit overwhelming trying to find the running shoe that's right for you. Some experts continue to claim that you should pick a shoe on the basis of your arch height, while others recommend that you should pick a shoe on the basis of how much pronation you may or may not have. To resolve the controversy, Dr. Nigg looked at the relationship between running shoe prescription and running injuries and determined that when runners self-select running shoes on the basis of comfort alone, they are much less likely to be injured (33). Dr. Nigg also proved that self-selected comfortable running shoes improve efficiency by reducing oxygen consumption. Apparently, you may not have to spend $250 on a pair of Vaporflys to get slight improvements in efficiency.

The only problem with Dr. Nigg's research is that it only included studies up to 2014. According to the latest research, high-mileage recreational runners should avoid zero-drop shoes and stick to running shoes with a minimum of ⅓ inch (8 mm) heel elevation, while low-mileage runners would probably do better with a 0 to ¼ inch (6 mm) heel drop sneaker (16). Because they increase rearfoot pronation during contact (29), maximalist shoes should be avoided by beginner runners unless the fit is perfect and they feel really comfortable. That being the case, then by all means buy them but take your time breaking them in. You could also consider doing some preemptive tibialis posterior exercises to reduce the rate of rearfoot pronation associated with using maximalist shoes. I've also noticed that unlike the motion control models from the 1980s and 1990s, runners who pronated excessively prefer stability shoes, while high-arched runners prefer soft shoes. Early motion control models, such as the Brooks Beast, have been replaced with more comfortable, flexible models that can decelerate the velocity of pronation and provide support without bulk. Softer models have been proven to decrease impact forces, which is why high-arched runners find them so comfortable.

If you're a serious runner and looking to get that extra 4% associated with the Nike Vaporflys, consider reducing your stride length for the first few weeks of breaking them in. Remember, Hoogkamer and his colleagues (32) showed that Vaporflys produced slight increases in impact forces and stride lengths, which could increase the risk of a hamstring injury. Because hamstring strains have over a 70% annual reinjury rate, the slight improvement in performance would be meaningless if you're unable to run. As when wearing rearfoot eversion and maximalist shoes, your hamstrings should quickly adapt to the slight increase in stride length that can occur with wearing the Vaporflys. You could also do preemptive eccentric hamstring exercises to prevent injury.

Because the most important predictor of comfort is that the shoe fits your foot perfectly, you should know how to check length, width, and fit of the heel counter. To check length, make sure you're fitting the running shoe to your larger foot (everyone has slight differences between right and left shoe size) and when standing, the tip of your longest toe should be about the width of your thumbnail from the end of the shoe. Selecting the proper shoe width, in both the forefoot and the rearfoot, is essential. The widest part of the forefoot of the shoe should match the location of your metatarsal head. As mentioned previously, you should always look for a running shoe that cradles your heel firmly (Fig. 5.11).

In a paper published more than 30 years ago, Jorgenson (34) proved that a snug heel counter

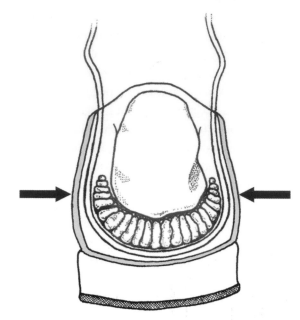

Fig. 5.11. *A firm heel counter (arrows) compresses the sides of the rearfoot, preventing the calcaneal fat pad from displacing from beneath the bottom of the foot.* No synthetic material comes close to matching the shock-absorbing capabilities of the human fat pad.

has the ability to reduce impact forces at foot strike, decrease activity in the quadriceps and calf musculature during stance, and improve overall efficiency (33). The impressive outcomes in this study can be traced directly to the fact that a snug heel counter prevents displacement of the calcaneal fat pad, which has been proven to absorb shock better than any synthetic material. Although Pebax didn't exist at the time, I'm sure that if a head-to-head comparison between the calcaneal fat pad and Pebax were performed today, your fat pad would win hands down. The bottom line when it comes to purchasing a running shoe—rather than listening to an expert on running shoes tell you what shoe is right for you, trust your own judgment. For just as runners intuitively know how to self-select their ideal stride length while running, so too they apparently know how to self-select the ideal running shoe.

REFERENCES

1. D'Aout K, Pataky T, DeClerq D, Aerts P. The effects of habitual footwear use: foot shape and function in native barefoot walkers. *Footwear Sci.* 2009;1(2):81–94.
2. Zipfel B, Berger L. Shod versus unshod: the emergence of forefoot pathology in modern humans? *Foot.* 2007;17:205–213.
3. Changizi M, Weber R, Kotecha R, et al. Are wet-induced wrinkled fingers primate rain treads? *Brain Behav Evol.* 2011;77:286–290.
4. Trinkaus E, Shang H. Anatomical evidence for the antiquity of human footwear: Tianyuan and Sunghir. *J Archeol Sci.* 2008;35:1928–1933.
5. Crisp Sayings. *The New York Times.* September 2, 1887.
6. Nigg B, Morlock M. The influence of lateral heel flare of running shoes on pronation and impact forces. *Med Sci Sports Exerc.* 1987;19:294.
7. Frederick EC. The running shoe: dilemmas and dichotomies in design. In: Segesser B, Pforringer W (eds). *The Shoe in Sport.* Chicago: Yearbook Medical Publishers, 1989:31.
8. Knapik J, Trone D, Swedler D, et al. Injury reduction effectiveness of assigning running shoes based on plantar shaped in Marine Corps basic training. *Am J Sports Med.* 2010;38:1759–1767.
9. Ryan M, Valiant G, McDonald K, Taunton J. The effect of three different levels of footwear stability on pain outcomes in women runners: a randomized control trial. *Br J Sports Med.* 2011;45(9):715–721.
10. Robbins S, Waked E. Balance and vertical impact in sport: role of shoe sole materials. *Arch Phys Med Rehabil.* 1997;78(5):463–467.
11. Robbins S, Hanna A. Running-related injury prevention through barefoot adaptation. *Med Sci Sports Exerc.* 1987;19:148–156.
12. Mennit-Gray J, Yokoi T. The influence of surface characteristics on the impulse characteristics of drop landings. *Proc Am Soc Biomech Ann Meet.* 1989, Burlington, VT:92–93.
13. DeClercq D, Aerts P, Kunnen M. The mechanical behavior characteristics of the human heel pad during foot strike in running: an in vivo cineradiographic study. *J Biomech.* 1994;27:1213–1222.
14. Tung K, Franz J, Kram R. A test of the metabolic cost of cushioning hypothesis in barefoot and shod running. *Proc Am Soc Biomech Ann Meet.* 2012, Gainesville, FL.
15. Chambon N, Delattre N, Gueguen N, et al. Shoe drop has opposite influence on running pattern when running overground or on a treadmill. *Eur J Appl Physiol.* 2015;115(5):911–918.
16. Malisoux L, et al. Influence of the heel-to-toe drop of standard cushion running shoes on injury risk in leisure-time runners: a randomized controlled trial with 6-month follow-up. *Am J Sports Med.* 2016;44:2933.
17. Lieberman D, Venkadesan M, Werbel W, et al. Foot strike patterns and collision forces in habitually barefoot versus shod runners. *Nature.* 2010;463(7280):531–535.
18. McCarthy C, et al. Like barefoot, only better. ACE Certified News; September 2011:8–12.
19. Goss D, Lewek M, Yu B, Gross M. Accuracy of self-reported foot strike patterns and loading rates associated with traditional and minimalist running shoes. *Proc Am Soc Biomech Ann Meet.* 2012, Gainesville, FL.
20. Ridge S, Johnson A, Mitchell U, et al. Foot bone marrow edema after 10-week transition to minimalist running shoes. *Med Sci Sports Exerc.* 2013;45(7):1363–1368.
21. Fuller G, Thewlis J, Buckley D, et al. Body mass and weekly training distance influence the pain and injuries experienced by runners

using minimalist shoes: a randomized controlled trial. *Am J Sports Med.* 2017;45:1162–1170.

22. Fuller J, Thewlis D, Tsiris M, et al. Longer-term effects of minimalist shoes on running performance, stride in bone density: a 20-week follow-up study. *Eur J Sport Sci.* 2019;19:402–412.

23. Ridge S, Olsen M, Bruening D, et al. Walking in minimalist shoes is effective for strengthening foot muscles. *Med Sci Exerc.* 2019;51(1):104–113.

24. Histen K, Arntsen J, L'Hereux L, et al. Achilles tendon properties of minimalist and traditionally shod runners. *J Sport Rehab.* 2017;26:159–164.

25. Paquette M, DeVita P, Williams D. Biomechanical implications of training volume and intensity in aging runners. *Med Sci Sports Exerc.* 2018;50(3): 510–515.

26. Pollard C, Ter Har J, Hannigan J, et al. Influence of maximal running shoes on biomechanics before and after a 5K run. *Orthop J Sports Med.* 2018;6:1–5.

27. Kulmala J-P, Kosonen J, Nurminen J, et al. Running in highly cushioned shoes increases leg stiffness and amplifies impact loading. *Sci Rep.* 2018;8(1):1–7.

28. Hannigan JJ, Pollard CD. A 6-week transition to maximal running shoes does not change running biomechanics. *Am J Sports Med.* 2019;47(4):968–973.

29. Hannigan J, Pollard C. Differences in running biomechanics between a maximal, traditional, and minimal running shoe. *J Sci Med Sport.* 2019;23:15–19.

30. Kuhman DJ, Paquette MR, Peel SA, et al. Comparison of ankle kinematics and ground reaction forces between prospectively injured and uninjured collegiate cross-country runners. *Hum Mov Sci.* 2016;47:9–15.

31. Becker J, Nakajima M, Wu WFW. Factors contributing to medial tibial stress syndrome in runners: a prospective study. *Med Sci Sports Exerc.* 2018;50(10):2092–2100.

32. Hoogkamer W, Kipp S, Farina E, et al. A comparison of the energetic cost of running in marathon racing shoes. *Sports Med.* 2018;48(4):1009–1019.

33. Nigg B, Baltich J, Enders H, et al. Running shoes and running injuries: myth busting and a proposal for 2 new paradigms: "preferred movement path" and "comfort filter." *Br J Sports Med.* 2015;49:1290–1294.

34. Jorgenson J. Body in heel-strike running: the effect of a firm heel counter. *Am J Sports Med.* 1990;18:177.

CHAPTER 6

TREATMENT PROTOCOLS

In spite of the fact that our bodies are remarkably well designed to handle the forces associated with recreational running, nearly 50% of runners are injured each year. Even worse, 90% of first-time marathon runners are injured while training for their big race (1). After reviewing the literature to determine the factors responsible for running injuries, van Mechelen et al. (2) conclude that up to 75% of all running injuries are the result of overtraining. This finding is consistent with several studies showing that the potential for injury dramatically increases when you run more than 35–40 miles (55–65 km) per week (1, 2). This number makes perfect sense when you consider that for the past two million years, our ancestors had foraging distances of about eight miles (13 km) per day (3), and almost all of that distance was covered while walking.

If you're a recreational runner and your goal is to finish a marathon, the easiest way to do that is to develop a running form that places the least strain on your body. Ground running and slow hybrid running won't allow you to set a world record, but they'll greatly increase the likelihood that you'll cross the finish line. It is also important that less experienced marathon runners follow the right training protocols when ramping up their mileage. To that end, experts at Furman University (4) have developed a training approach that allows you to train for full and/or half marathons without having to run too many miles. By utilizing cross-training techniques,

such as swimming and biking, these authors have developed specific training schedules based on an individual's running goals and overall fitness.

While injury rates for recreational runners can be reduced with low-mileage training protocols and/or converting to ground or hybrid running, elite and sub-elite distance runners don't have that option. In order to be competitive, these athletes have to average 80–120 miles (130–200 km) per week, which almost always includes grueling speed workouts. To tolerate the stresses connected with aggressive training, competitive runners have to work hard to address specific strength, flexibility, coordination, and/or bony alignment problems that can increase the likelihood of injury. As discussed in Chapter 3, asymmetry in any of a variety of functional tests correlates strongly with future injury, and these risk factors have to be addressed in order to remain injury free. Competitive runners also need to develop the specific running form that allows them to store and return energy and reduce the forces associated with the braking phase. Performing the at-home gait analysis described in Chapter 4 can help with that.

Because the best predictor of future injury has always been prior injury (5, 6), whether you run a marathon in six hours or in two hours, you have to rehab each and every injury to the fullest extent. Remember, annual reinjury rates among runners with hamstring strains can be as high as 70%, but when rehabbed properly, the reinjury rates drop to 7% (7). To help you recover and get you back to running, the following section reviews home treatment protocols for some of the more common running-related injuries. Just to be safe, prior to initiating any home program, consider setting up an appointment with a sports chiropractor or physical therapist who is familiar with treating running injuries to make sure you have the correct diagnosis. You should also consider scheduling a few sessions with an experienced trainer to have your form evaluated while you're performing your stretches and/or exercises.

ACHILLES TENDINITIS

Despite its broad width and significant length, the Achilles tendon of runners is injured with surprising regularity. In a 2006 study of 69 military cadets participating in a six-week basic training program (which included distance running), 10 of the 69 trainees suffered an Achilles tendon overuse injury (8). The prevalence of this injury is easy to understand when you consider the tremendous strain runners place on this tendon; e.g., during the push-off phase of running, the Achilles tendon is exposed to a force of up to eight times the body weight. This is close to the maximum strain the tendon can tolerate without rupturing. Also, when you couple the high strain forces with the fact that the Achilles tendon significantly weakens as we get older, it is easy to see why this tendon is injured so frequently.

Anatomically, the Achilles tendon represents the conjoined tendons of the gastrocnemius and soleus muscles. Approximately 5 inches above the Achilles attachment to the back of the heel, the tendons from these two muscles unite to form a single thick Achilles tendon (Fig. 6.1).

These conjoined tendons are wrapped by a single layer of cells called the "paratenon." This sheath-like envelope is rich in blood vessels necessary to nourish the tendon. The tendon itself is composed primarily of two types of connective tissue known as "type 1 collagen" and "type 3 collagen." In a healthy Achilles tendon, 95% of the collagen is type 1, which is stronger and more flexible than type 3. It is the strong cross-links and parallel arrangement of the type 1 collagen fibers that give the Achilles tendon its strength.

Unlike the vast majority of tendons in the body, the Achilles tendon is unique in that at about the point where the gastrocnemius and soleus muscles unite, the tendon suddenly begins to

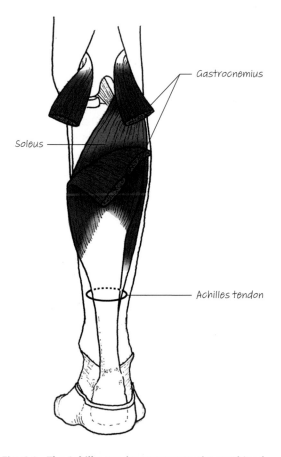

Fig. 6.1. *The Achilles tendon represents the combined tendons from the gastrocnemius and soleus muscles.*

twist, rotating a full 90° before it attaches to the back of the heel. As mentioned in Chapter 3, this extreme twisting significantly improves efficiency while running because it allows the tendon to function like a spring, absorbing energy during the early phases of the gait cycle and returning it in the form of elastic recoil during the propulsive period.

Despite the clever design and significant strength of the Achilles tendon, the extreme forces it is exposed to cause it to break down all too frequently. Depending on the location of the damage, Achilles tendon overuse injuries are divided into several categories: insertional tendinitis, paratenonitis, and non-insertional tendinosis.

As the name implies, "insertional tendinitis" refers to inflammation at the attachment point of the Achilles on the heel. This type of Achilles injury typically occurs in high-arched, inflexible individuals, particularly if they possess what is known as a "Haglund's deformity," a bony prominence near the Achilles attachment on the heel. Because a bursa is present near the Achilles attachment (bursae are small sacs that contain lubricants that lessen shearing of the tendon against the bone), it is very common to have an insertional tendinitis with a bursitis (Fig. 6.2).

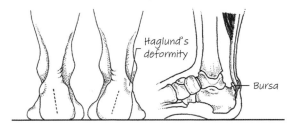

Fig. 6.2. *Insertional Achilles tendinitis injuries are frequently associated with a bony prominence called a "Haglund's deformity."* Because of chronic stress at the Achilles attachment point, an inflamed bursa often forms between the Achilles tendon and the heel.

Until recently, the perceived mechanism for the development of insertional tendinitis was pretty straightforward: Excessive running causes the Achilles tendon to break down on the back portion of the Achilles attachment, where pulling forces are the greatest. While this makes perfect sense, research has shown that just the opposite is true: The Achilles tendon almost always breaks down in the *forward* section of the tendon, where pulling forces are the lowest (9) (Fig. 6.3).

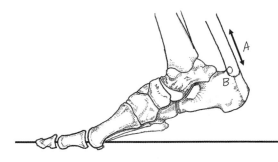

Fig. 6.3. *Location of Achilles insertional injuries.* Tension in the Achilles tendon during push-off places greater strain on the back of the Achilles tendon (**A**). Paradoxically, almost all insertional Achilles tendon injuries occur in the forward section of the Achilles tendon (**B**).

By placing strain gauges inside different sections of the Achilles tendons and then loading the tendons with the ankle positioned in a variety of angles, researchers from the University of North Carolina discovered that the back portion of the Achilles tendon is exposed to far greater amounts of strain (particularly when the ankle was moved upward), while the forward section of the tendon, which is the section most frequently damaged with insertional tendinitis, was exposed to very low loads. The authors suggest that the lack of stress on the forward aspect of the Achilles tendon (which they referred to as a "tension shielding effect") may cause that section to weaken and eventually fail. As a result, the treatment of Achilles insertional tendinitis should be to strengthen the forward-most aspect of the tendon. This can be accomplished by performing

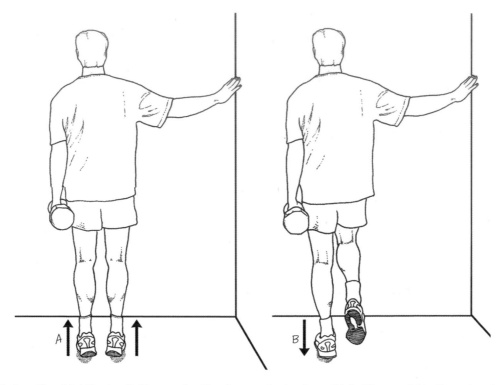

Fig. 6.4. *Insertional Achilles tendinitis exercise.* Standing on a level surface while holding a weight with one hand and balancing against the wall with the other, raise both heels as high as you can (**A**) and then slowly lower yourself on just the injured leg (**B**). Perform 3 sets of 15 repetitions daily on both the injured side and the uninjured side. Use enough weight to produce fatigue.

a series of eccentric load exercises through a partial range of motion (Fig. 6.4). It is particularly important to exercise the Achilles tendon with the ankle maximally plantar flexed (i.e., standing way up on tiptoes) because this position places greater amounts of strain on the more frequently damaged forward portion of the tendon.

Runners with high arches are especially prone to insertional Achilles injuries and they often respond very well to lateral heel wedges. These wedges, which are pasted to the outer portion of an insole, are used to distribute pressure away from the outer aspect of the tendon. Conventional heel lifts are always a consideration, but be careful: They may feel good at first but the calf muscles quickly adapt to their shortened positions, and the beneficial effect of

the heel lift is lost. Heel lifts also increase stress on the sesamoid bones and the plantar fascia, and should therefore be used for no more than a few weeks.

Rather than accommodating tight calves with heel lifts, a better approach is to lengthen the calves with gentle stretches. As mentioned, the most effective calf stretch is the neutral position stretch, which can be done with the knee straight and bent to target the gastrocnemius and soleus, respectively (refer back to Fig. 3.22). Because aggressive stretching can damage the insertion, the stretches should be performed with mild tension. You should perform this stretch routine for about a minute, and repeat the process every three or four hours daily. If calf inflexibility is extreme and does not respond to stretching, a night brace should be considered. These braces, which are typically used to treat plantar fasciitis, are a very effective way to lengthen the gastrocnemius and soleus muscles. My favorite night brace is called the "Cub," which tends to be more comfortable than any of the other commercially available night braces (Fig. 6.5).

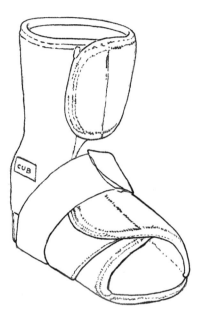

Fig. 6.5. *Night brace.*

The next type of Achilles tendon overuse injury is paratenonitis. This injury, which is very common in runners, manifests as an inflammatory reaction in the outer sheath of the cells surrounding the tendon. Overpronators are particularly prone to this injury because rapid pronation creates a whip-like action that can damage the tendon sheath (particularly the inner side). The first sign of the injury is a palpable lump that forms about 2 inches (5 cm) above the Achilles attachment. This mass represents localized thickening in response to microtrauma. If running is continued, the size of the lump increases and it eventually becomes so painful that running is no longer possible. Treatment for Achilles paratenonitis is to immediately reduce

the swelling with frequent ice packs. If you're flat-footed, you might want to consider trying orthotics (start with over-the-counter models), as excessive foot pronation was proven in 2017 to cause twisting of the Achilles tendon (10), depriving it of blood in a way comparable to wringing a wet towel. The impaired circulation associated with this twisting action increases the risk of chronicity. Night braces are also effective with paratenonitis because tendons immobilized in lengthened positions heal more quickly (11).

If caught in time and the problem is corrected, Achilles paratenonitis is no big deal. However, if untreated, this injury can turn into a classic Achilles non-insertional tendinosis, which involves degeneration of the tendon approximately 1–2 inches (2.5 cm–5 cm) above the attachment on the heel. Because this section of the tendon has such a poor blood supply, it is prone to injury and tends to heal very slowly.

Unlike insertional tendinitis and paratenonitis, non-insertional tendinosis is a degenerative noninflammatory condition (i.e., the suffix *osis* refers to "wear and tear," while *itis* refers to "inflammation"). In response to the repeated trauma caused by running through the injury, specialized repair cells called "fibroblasts" infiltrate the tendon, where, in an attempt to heal the injured regions, they begin to synthesize collagen. In the early stages of tendon healing, the fibroblasts manufacture almost exclusively type 3 collagen, which is relatively weak and inflexible compared to the type 1 collagen found in healthy tendons. If everything goes right, as healing progresses, greater numbers of fibroblasts appear and collagen production shifts from type 3 to type 1. Unfortunately, many runners don't give the tendon adequate time to remodel (which can take up to six months), and a series of small partial ruptures begin to occur that can paradoxically act to lengthen the tendon, resulting in an increased range of upward motion at the ankle. At this point, the pain is significant and the runner is usually forced to stop running altogether.

Various factors may predispose to the development of non-insertional tendinosis. In the previously mentioned study of military recruits, the subjects developing Achilles injuries were overly flexible and had weak calves (8). It is likely that these two factors create a whipping action that strains the Achilles tendons. More recently, in 2019, researchers from the United Kingdom (12) proved that weakness of the soleus plays an important role in the development of Achilles injuries. These authors compared gastrocnemius and soleus muscle strength in 38 runners with Achilles injuries, and 39 asymptomatic control runners,

and determined that the injured runners had isolated strength deficits in the soleus. Importantly, the authors state that "the soleus weakness more than likely predated the injury." This research is consistent with prior studies showing that the tendon fibers originating from the soleus are exposed to more stress and undergo greater elongation than tendon fibers originating from the gastrocnemius (13, 14). As a result, in order to successfully manage any type of Achilles injury, strength and endurance deficits in the soleus should always be addressed.

The good news about non-insertional tendinosis is that there is an exercise intervention you can do at home that's been proven to be effective. Referred to as "heavy load eccentric exercises" (15), this treatment involves wearing a weighted backpack while standing on the edge of a stair with your heels hanging off the stair (Fig. 6.6).

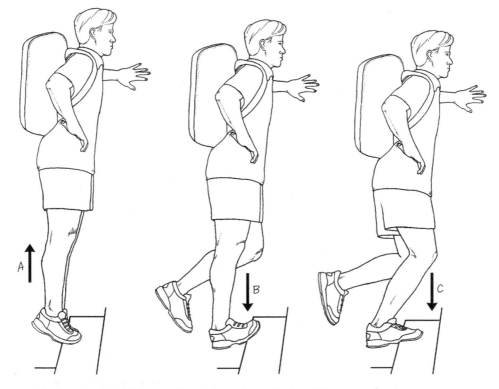

Fig. 6.6. *Heavy load eccentric Achilles exercise.* *(Redrawn from Alfredson [15].)*

Using both legs, you raise your heels as high as possible and then remove the uninjured leg from the stair. The injured leg is then gradually lowered through a full range of motion. The uninjured leg is then placed back on the stairway and both legs are again used to raise the heels as high as possible. This process is repeated with the knee straight and flexed, and runners should perform 3 sets of 15 repetitions daily for 12 weeks. The orthopedic surgeon who first published the eccentric protocols, Hakan Alfredson, recommends the eccentric protocol be continued unless your Achilles pain becomes "disabling." I find Alfredson's approach a little extreme, so I tell athletes to reduce the weight while exercising if the pain exceeds more than 4 on a scale from 0 to 10 (0 being no pain, 10 being unbearable pain).

While the 3 sets of 15 protocol works well for recreational athletes, competitive runners have to work harder to heal a non-insertional Achilles injury. In a 2014 study evaluating tendon resiliency with different strengthening protocols, researchers from Taiwan discovered that high-level athletes undergo no change in tendon resiliency unless they perform 4 sets of 80 repetitions (16). This research explains why elite athletes do not do as well with conventional eccentric protocols as recreational athletes. (Almost all studies on eccentric exercise use the 3 sets of 15 protocol.) I recommend the 4 sets of 80 repetitions protocol for runners averaging more than 50 miles (80 km) per week.

Non-insertional Achilles injuries also respond very well to the tibialis posterior strengthening exercise illustrated in Fig. 6.7. In a 2008 study comparing three-dimensional motion between runners with and without Achilles tendinopathy, researchers from East Carolina University determined that compared to controls, runners

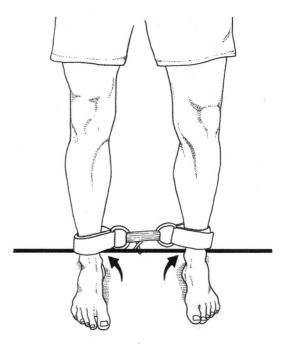

Fig. 6.7. *Closed-chain tibialis posterior exercise.*
By wrapping a TheraBand between two ankle straps (which can be purchased at www.performbetter.com), this exercise is performed by alternately raising and lowering your arches against resistance provided by the TheraBand. Performing 3 sets of 25 repetitions daily is usually enough to strengthen the tibialis posterior.

with Achilles tendinopathy failed to rotate their legs outward during the push-off phase (17).

The authors theorized that tibialis posterior weakness forces the leg to twist in excessively, which in turn increases strain on the Achilles tendon. After reading this article, I began adding tibialis posterior exercises to the standard protocols for managing Achilles tendinitis and noticed reduced recovery times and better long-term outcomes.

In addition to strengthening exercises, an alternate method for improving Achilles function is deep tissue massage. The theory is that aggressive massage breaks down the weaker type 3 collagen fibers and increases circulation so healing can occur. To test this theory, researchers from the Biomechanics Lab at Ball State University (18) surgically damaged the Achilles tendons in a group of rats. In one group, an aggressive deep tissue massage was performed for three minutes on the 21st, 25th, 29th, and 33rd day post injury. Another group served as a control. One week later, both groups of rats had their tendons evaluated with electron microscopy. Not surprisingly, the tendons receiving deep tissue massage showed increased fibroblast proliferation, which would create an environment favoring tendon repair.

A more high-tech method of breaking down scar tissue is extracorporeal shock wave therapy. This technique involves the use of costly machinery that blasts the Achilles with high-frequency sonic vibrations. Recent research has shown comparable outcomes between shock wave therapy and heavy load eccentric exercises in the treatment of non-insertional Achilles tendinosis. As a result, shock wave therapy is typically used only after conventional methods have failed.

Regardless of whether the Achilles injury is insertional or non-insertional, a great method for lessening stress on the Achilles tendon is to strengthen the toe muscles, especially the flexor digitorum brevis and flexor hallucis longus. These muscles, which originate along the back of the leg and attach to the toes, lie deep to the Achilles and work synergistically with the soleus to raise the heel during propulsion. Contraction of the flexor hallucis and digitorum longus while running significantly lessens strain on the Achilles tendon because they decelerate elongation of the tendon. The easiest way to strengthen the long toe muscles is with the ToePro exercise platform (see Fig. 3.27). An alternate way to strengthen these muscles is to get on an AIREX balance pad and lean forward into a wall while pushing down with your toes.

I typically recommend 3 sets of 25 repetitions performed daily.

To make sure the toe muscles are working properly, an injured runner should forcefully curl the toes downward into the insole during the push-off phase of the running cycle. This naturally strengthens the toe muscles and reduces strain on the Achilles tendon. It's easy to see if you have weakness in these muscles by looking at the insole of your running shoe. Normally, when the flexor digitorum muscles are strong, you will see well-defined indents beneath the tips of the toes, whereas in runners with weak digital flexors there will be no marks beneath the toes and signs of excessive wear will be visible in the center of the forefoot only.

It's important to emphasize that runners with Achilles injuries should almost always avoid cortisone injections because they weaken the tendon by shifting the production of collagen from type 1 to type 3. In a study published in the *Journal of Bone and Joint Surgery* (19), cortisone was shown to lower the stress necessary to rupture the Achilles tendon and was particularly dangerous when done on both sides because it produced a systemic effect that further weakened the tendon.

An overview of the management of Achilles tendon disorders can be summarized as follows: Warm up slowly by running at least one minute per mile slower than your usual pace for the first mile and try to remain on flat surfaces. If you are a midfoot or a forefoot striker, consider switching to a rearfoot strike, since this reduces strain in the Achilles tendon during initial contact. Because excessive pronation has been shown to decrease blood flow to the Achilles tendon (10), runners who are excessive pronators should consider wearing stability running shoes, specifically ones with duodensity midsoles and toe springs (see Fig. 5.5).

Overpronators should also consider wearing orthotics. Because they encourage a forward contact point, minimalist shoes and racing flats should be avoided. Lastly, if you have a tendency to be stiff, spend extra time performing the neutral position stretch illustrated in Fig. 3.22, and if you're overly flexible, you should consider performing eccentric load exercises preventively. To evaluate strength, try doing 25 heel raises on each leg to see if you fatigue quicker on one side. If one leg is weaker, fix the strength asymmetry with the exercise illustrated in Fig. 6.6.

SESAMOIDITIS

The sesamoids are the two sesame-seed-shaped bones located beneath the first metatarsal head. Situated inside the tendons of the flexor hallucis brevis, the sesamoids are extremely important while running because they increase the mechanical advantage afforded to the flexor hallucis brevis, greatly improving this muscle's ability to generate force. Because generating force beneath the big toe has been proven to lessen pressure beneath the central forefoot by as much as 30%, properly functioning sesamoids are necessary to prevent a wide range of forefoot injuries, including metatarsal stress fractures and interdigital neuromas.

Runners frequently injure their sesamoids because the bones are situated in a primary weight-bearing area and are subjected to tremendous forces during the push-off phase while running. Runners with high arches are especially prone to sesamoiditis because high arches cause an excessive amount of force to be centered beneath their inner forefeet (Fig. 6.8).

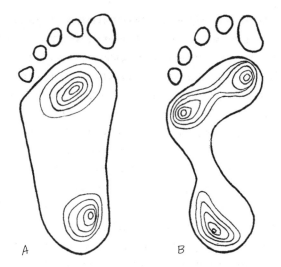

A   B

Fig. 6.8. *Center of pressure distribution in runners with low arches (A), and high arches (B).*

The initial symptom associated with sesamoiditis is a "throbbing pain" located directly beneath the ball of the foot. Treatment for sesamoid injuries is to reduce pressure by incorporating a sub-one balance beneath the first metatarsal head (Fig. 6.9). This balance can be made at home by cutting a ⅛-inch-thick (3 mm) piece of felt

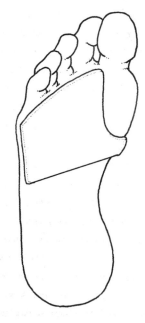

Fig. 6.9. *The sub-one balance.*

into a J-shaped balance and attaching it directly beneath the insole of the running shoe. If you don't feel like making one, pre-made sub-one balances can be purchased online.

Less often, runners with low arches injure their sesamoids. The most common mechanism for injury is that excessive pronation drives the inner forefoot into the ground with greater force, contusing the inner sesamoid (Fig. 6.10). Custom or over-the-counter orthotics are often effective when treating sesamoid injuries in low-arched runners because they distribute pressure away from the sesamoid onto the medial arch.

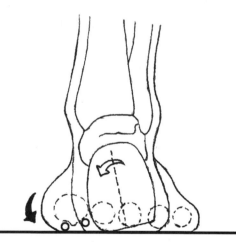

Fig. 6.10. *Excessive pronation (white arrow), drives the inner sesamoid into the ground (black arrow).*

Regardless of the cause, the flexor hallucis brevis almost always responds to chronic sesamoid injury by reflexively tightening. Increased tension in this muscle often worsens the sesamoid injury because it causes the sesamoid to be pulled into the bony groove located beneath the first metatarsal head when the big toe moves upward during push-off. A similar injury occurs in the knee, when chronic injury to the patella causes the quadriceps to tighten, which in turn causes the patella to jam against its bony groove. Tightness in the quadriceps is a proven

perpetuator of chronic patellar injury, and every sports medicine specialist knows the importance of stretching the quads when treating kneecap injuries. In contrast, the same sports experts rarely recommend lengthening the flexor hallucis brevis to treat sesamoiditis. This is too bad because lengthening this muscle is a simple and effective way to treat the condition.

To determine if you have a contracture of the flexor hallucis brevis, gently bend your big toes back and compare the range between both feet. If the side with the painful sesamoid has a reduced range, you need to lengthen the muscle. To do this, start by massaging the flexor hallucis brevis for a minute or so, and then gently pull the big toe back until you feel mild resistance (Fig. 6.11). At that point, hold the stretch for 35 seconds while simultaneously massaging the muscle.

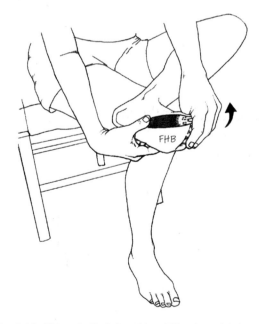

Fig. 6.11. *Flexor hallucis brevis mobilization.* *Lightly massage the flexor hallucis brevis (FHB) and follow with a gentle stretch by lightly pulling the big toe back (**arrow**). You can find the flexor hallucis brevis by starting at the base of the big toe and angling down and back, making sure to massage the entire muscle. With practice, you can find tight points in the muscle.*

The flexor hallucis brevis stretch should always be comfortable and if it produces anything more than mild discomfort, you'll need an x-ray or an MRI to rule out a stress fracture/tendon injury. On occasion, a severely injured sesamoid needs to be immobilized with a walking boot.

METATARSALGIA AND METATARSAL STRESS FRACTURES

Not surprisingly, given the central forefoot supports up to seven times body weight during push-off, metatarsal injuries are extremely common in the running community. "Metatarsalgia" refers to a bruising of one of the metatarsals, while metatarsal stress fractures occur when the metatarsals can no longer tolerate the strain and they begin to break. The second and third metatarsal heads are the most likely to produce metatarsalgia, while the third and fourth metatarsal shafts are the most likely to fracture. Metatarsalgia can easily be diagnosed by pressing firmly on the suspected metatarsal head. Conversely, metatarsal stress fractures can be diagnosed by feeling for a localized region of swelling along the shaft of the suspected metatarsal. Because x-rays miss about 40% of metatarsal stress fractures in the early stages, they are relatively useless for identifying stress fractures within the first few days following injury. After about a week, the repair line can be seen forming in the fractured bone.

A frequently overlooked cause of metatarsalgia and metatarsal stress fractures is tightness in the gastrocnemius. A tight gastrocnemius is dangerous while running because it forces the heel to leave the ground prematurely, driving the forefoot into the ground with excessive force. In a study evaluating the prevalence of tight ankles and metatarsal injuries, it was determined that individuals with tight calves were 4.6 times more likely to fracture their metatarsals than a more flexible control group (20). As a result, it is essential that runners keep their gastrocnemius muscles flexible. On occasion, runners with chronically tight calves should consider sleeping with night braces and/or perform prolonged stretches on slant boards.

The metatarsals are also prone to injury if the muscles to the toes are weak. As mentioned, strong toe muscles distribute pressure away from the metatarsal heads to the tips of the toes, while also lessening the bending strains in the metatarsal shafts (see Fig. 2.34). These muscles can be strengthened with the exercises illustrated in Fig. 3.27. To evaluate if toe weakness is perpetuating a metatarsal injury, pull the insole out of your running shoe and look at the wear pattern: There should be clear indents beneath the toes. If you have more wear and tear beneath the center of the forefoot with little to no evidence of indentations beneath the toes, you need to perform toe strengthening exercises.

In addition to distributing pressure by strengthening the toes, another effective method for treating metatarsalgia is to try wearing metatarsal pads and/or toe crests (Fig. 6.12).

In chronic cases of metatarsalgia, you can attach a Morton's platform beneath the first metatarsal head (Fig. 6.13). Because the first metatarsal is twice as wide and four times as strong as the neighboring metatarsals, it is better able to tolerate the redistribution of pressure away from the painful neighboring metatarsal heads. This addition is especially helpful when pain is centered directly beneath the second metatarsal head.

Regardless of the cause, all metatarsal injuries should be treated by reducing your stride length

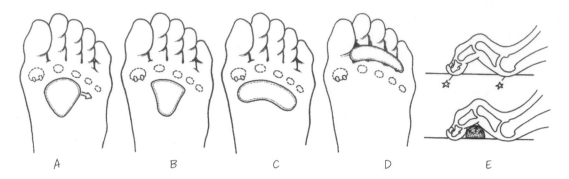

Fig. 6.12. *(A) Heart-, (B) stomach-, and (C) kidney-shaped metatarsal pads distribute pressure away from the metatarsal heads.* These pads should be placed as close to the metatarsal heads as possible. Toe crests **(D)** are attached with an elastic strap that loops around the third toe. By distributing pressure over the entire toe **(E)**, toe crests reduce pressure beneath the metatarsal heads in the tips of the toes **(stars)**.

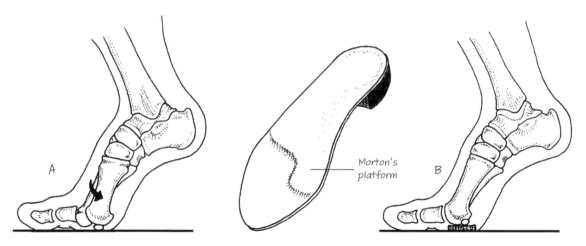

Fig. 6.13. *Morton's platform.* Placing a 1/8-inch-thick (3 mm) piece of felt beneath the first metatarsal head distributes pressure away from the neighboring second metatarsal. This can be added to an over-the-counter orthotic or placed beneath the bottom of your insole. A sports podiatrist can build a Morton's platform into a custom orthotic.

and avoiding forefoot contact points. Runners with a history of metatarsal injury should also avoid minimalist shoes, since they may cause a switch to a forefoot strike pattern, greatly increasing the weight borne by the metatarsals. Minimalist shoes are especially troublesome in runners with narrow forefeet and tight calves. As with all stress fractures, runners should avoid taking anti-inflammatory medications because they can interfere with bone healing. To improve bone health, runners should pay close attention to their diet, particularly their intake of vitamin D3, protein, and trace minerals. Dietary factors associated with recovering from stress fractures are discussed later in this chapter.

INTERDIGITAL NEURITIS/NEUROMA

Interdigital injury results from entrapment of one or more of the interdigital nerves located in the forefoot (Fig. 6.14). While this condition may involve any of the interdigital nerves, the nerve located between the third and fourth toe is the most frequently injured.

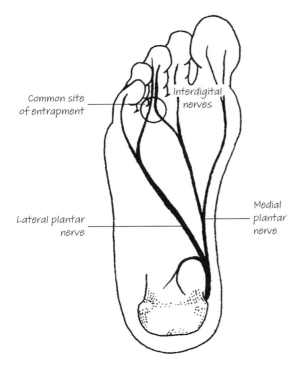

Fig. 6.14. *The interdigital nerves are branches of the medial and lateral plantar nerves.*

A common early symptom of this condition is a slight tingling between the toes. Affected runners often complain that their socks are "bunched" in the forefoot, and say that the discomfort is reduced when they take off their shoes. Initially, the nerve injury is mild and is referred to as an "interdigital neuritis," because the nerve is inflamed but not seriously damaged. Over time, repeated irritation of the nerve results in the formation of a thickened ball of scar tissue inside the nerve called a "Morton's neuroma." The formation of a Morton's neuroma is troublesome because it increases the likelihood of chronicity, since the thickened nerve is more readily pinched. Clinically, it is often possible to identify a neuroma by squeezing the forefoot and feeling for the presence of a Mulder's click: a clunk-like sound that occurs when a swollen bursa located between the metatarsal heads is displaced.

Until recently, the most popular theory regarding the origin of interdigital neuritis was that upward motion of the toes during propulsion tethered the interdigital nerves against the transverse ligament (Fig. 6.15). This theory was disproved in 2007, when researchers from Korea performed detailed dissections of 17 interdigital neuromas in order to identify the exact location of nerve entrapment (21). To everyone's surprise, in each case the nerve was shown to be compressed beneath the tip of the metatarsal head and the base of the toe, not beneath the transverse ligament.

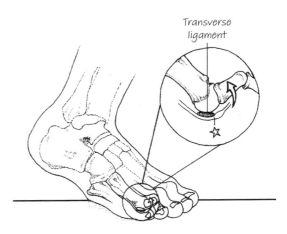

Fig. 6.15. *Until recently, it was believed that the interdigital nerve was tethered when it pulled against the transverse ligament.*

After reading this paper, I changed the way I treated interdigital nerve injuries. Prior to this study, like most sports doctors, I treated interdigital neuritis/neuroma by placing metatarsal pads behind the involved metatarsal heads in order to lift the transverse ligament off the inflamed interdigital nerve. After discovering the nerve is actually pinched downstream from this location, I began treating interdigital neuritis by placing a U-shaped felt support beneath the forefoot (Fig. 6.16).

The felt support treatment protocol turned out to be way more effective than conventional

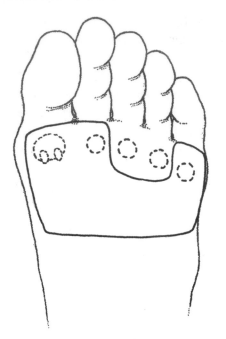

Fig. 6.16. *A U-shaped felt balance distributes pressure away from the third and fourth metatarsal heads during push-off.*

metatarsal pads because these pads do not support the metatarsal heads during the propulsive period (they are positioned too far back). In contrast, a U-shaped pad placed beneath the forefoot distributes pressure away from the involved metatarsals during the propulsive period, when the interdigital nerves are being compressed. The thickness of the pad is dependent upon the severity of the symptoms. I like to initially start with a 1/8-inch-thick (3 mm) piece of felt with the U-shaped cutout placed directly beneath the third and fourth metatarsal heads. If symptoms persist, consider adding another ¹⁄₁₆ inch (1.6 mm) of felt to distribute a greater amount of pressure toward the neighboring metatarsals. Rarely, the nerve injury is so severe that the thickened neuroma needs to be surgically removed.

As with metatarsalgia, an often-overlooked perpetuating factor for interdigital neuritis is

tightness in the gastrocnemius. As previously mentioned, tightness in this muscle results in a premature lifting of the heel that can amplify forces centered beneath the metatarsal heads during propulsion. Additionally, because the big toe can distribute pressure away from the central metatarsal heads, runners suffering from interdigital neuritis should strengthen the muscles that stabilize the big toe. I tend to avoid strengthening the little toes because movement of the toes while performing the exercise sometimes irritates the interdigital nerve.

Finally, to reduce pressure centered beneath the metatarsal heads during daily activities, women should avoid wearing high heels, and runners with midfoot and forefoot strike patterns should consider switching to a rearfoot strike pattern. To lessen the pressure on the nerve during propulsion, you should develop a shorter stride length with an increased cadence. Once the nerve injury resolves, you can begin running with your more natural stride but make sure you keep your calves flexible by performing straight leg stretches routinely. Interdigital neuromas can be frustrating to treat because once the nerve thickens, it never reduces in size and you will be prone to this injury in the future. As a result, it is important to treat interdigital neuritis very aggressively in the early stages of the injury.

BUNIONS

The medical term for a bunion is "hallux abducto valgus," from the Latin *hallux* for "big toe" and *abducto valgus* for "pulled out and rotated" (Fig. 6.17).

While no one is sure exactly why bunions form, an inherited tendency for loose ligaments seems to be a factor. In a series of interesting papers

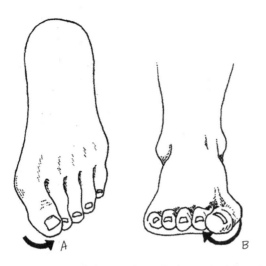

Fig. 6.17. *Hallux abducto valgus.* *The big toe is abducted (**A**) and in valgus (**B**).*

evaluating potential factors associated with the development of bunions, researchers found that laxity of the thumb (a marker for whole body laxity) was one of the best predictors of bunion formation (22) (see Fig. 3.19). In fact, thumb laxity turned out to be a better predictor for the development of future bunions than x-ray measurements.

Runners with painful bunions are often difficult to treat because the inward angled big toe is ineffective at generating force. As a result, the pressure normally centered beneath the big toe is transferred to the central forefoot. Over time, a painful callus develops beneath the central forefoot that increases the potential for developing metatarsal stress fractures.

One of the key factors present in almost all runners with bunions is weakness of the abductor hallucis (Fig. 6.18). Once weakened, this muscle is no longer able to stabilize the big toe, allowing the bunion to worsen.

Another important muscle in managing bunion pain is the peroneus longus. Because

this muscle attaches to the base of the first metatarsal, it has the ability to stabilize the inner forefoot, protecting the bunion from excessive force. While the ToePro exercise platform is an effective way to strengthen both the abductor hallucis and the peroneus longus, it can sometimes aggravate bunion pain if the runner raises his or her heel too high. I typically recommend avoiding raising the heel more than 1 inch (2.5 cm) off the ground while performing ToePro exercises, and runners with large bunions should consider wearing toe separators to improve the alignment of the big toe while exercising.

Despite a lack of clinical evidence supporting their use, custom and prefabricated orthotics are the most common treatment for bunions. Although there's no research suggesting they alter the long-term development of bunions, runners with painful bunions often respond very well to orthotics, possibly because they effectively distribute pressure over a broader area (24) and/or increase peroneus longus activity when worn by flat-footed individuals (25). These combined factors may help distribute pressure away from the overloaded central forefoot and improve stability of the first metatarsal. In my

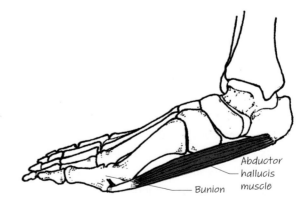

Fig. 6.18. *Rolling onto the big toe forces you to use the abductor hallucis (AH), which is weak in people with bunions (23).*

experience, runners tend to prefer graphite or thin plastic orthotics because these orthotics are less bulky and do not elevate the heel (even a slight heel lift increases pressure centered beneath the first metatarsal head). When large bunions are present, toe separators are often necessary to stop the toes from butting against one another.

As with all forefoot injuries, maintaining a flexible gastrocnemius is important in order to reduce pressure on the forefoot during propulsion. Shoe gear must accommodate the widened forefoot, and minimalist shoes should be avoided because they may cause initial ground contact to switch from the heel to the forefoot. To reduce pressure on the forefoot, runners with bunions should consider reducing their stride length and increasing their cadence. Despite the fact that bunion surgery is performed over 200,000 times a year in the US, surgical correction should always be a last resort because the failure rate is so high (26). In my experience, runners are especially prone to poor outcomes following bunion surgery because of the extreme forces placed on the foot during push-off.

HALLUX LIMITUS AND RIGIDUS

From the Latin for "limited big toe motion," *hallux limitus* is a degenerative condition in which the big toe becomes progressively stiffer and more painful. Hallux rigidus is an extreme version of this condition in which the big toe joint is completely fused and rigid. While hallux rigidus is relatively rare, hallux limitus is surprisingly common in the running community because even a slight reduction in the range of motion in the big toe joint can cause trouble while running.

Occasionally the result of trauma, hallux limitus is more likely to develop in runners with Egyptian toes, since a long big toe is exposed to greater force during propulsion (Fig. 6.19). Despite its prevalence, many doctors are unaware of this condition and frequently misdiagnose hallux limitus as a bunion. This is unfortunate because these two conditions are treated differently.

The easiest way to diagnose hallux limitus is by evaluating the range of motion in the big toe joints. When hallux limitus is present, there is asymmetric motion between the right and left big toe joints. Another way to differentiate hallux limitus from a bunion is by noting the location of the bone spur on the metatarsal head. When a bunion is present, the spur forms on the side of the metatarsal head. In contrast, when hallux limitus is present, the bone spur forms directly on top of the metatarsal head (Fig. 6.20).

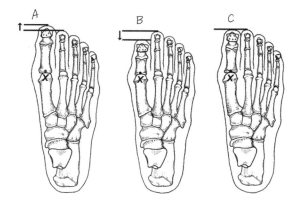

Fig. 6.19. *Variation in toe length.* An Egyptian toe is present when the big toe is longer than the second toe (**A**). Conversely, a Greek toe occurs when the big toe is significantly shorter than the second toe (**B**). Square toes are present when the first and second toes are of equal length (**C**). The next time you go to the Museum of Natural History, take a look at the Egyptian and Greek statues: Egyptian sculptures almost always have long big toes, while Greek statues possess short big toes.

A

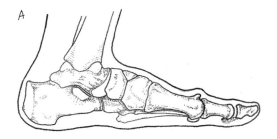

B

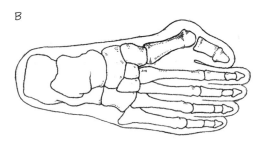

Fig. 6.20. *Bone spur formation in hallux limitus (A) and bunions (B).*

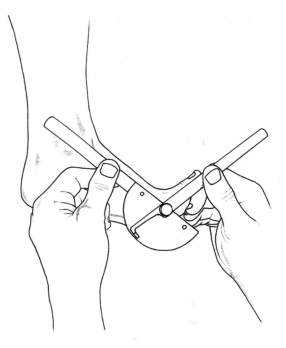

Fig. 6.21. *Measuring the range of motion in the big toe joint. This measuring device can be purchased at any hardware store.*

The severity of hallux limitus is determined by measuring the range of motion in the big toe joint (Fig. 6.21). Because this joint normally moves about 45° during propulsion, hallux limitus tends to produce pain when the range of big toe motion drops below 40°. Runners with low arches are especially prone to developing painful hallux limitus because they have more force centered beneath their big toes during propulsion, and their big toe joints need to move through larger ranges of motion (19, 20).

The goal when treating hallux limitus is to restore as much range of motion as possible. As long as the spur on the top of the metatarsal head is not too large, it is possible to restore as much as 30° of range of motion by performing the massage and stretch illustrated in Fig. 6.11. In addition to increasing the range of motion available to the big toe joint with home stretches, it is also important to increase the range of motion available in the ankle. In my experience, runners with even severe hallux limitus rarely complain of pain as long as their ankles are flexible. In many cases, it is necessary to perform slant board exercises for up to five minutes per day in order to obtain the ankle motion necessary for preventing hallux limitus from becoming painful.

Another popular treatment for hallux limitus is to prescribe custom or over-the-counter orthotics. While it was originally believed that orthotics allowed the big toe to move through a larger range of motion during propulsion, three-dimensional research has proven that this is not the case. Almost a decade ago, Dr. Deb Nowaczenski and I performed a pilot study in which we measured three-dimensional motion in the big toe joint while subjects wore different types of orthotic (27) (Fig. 6.22).

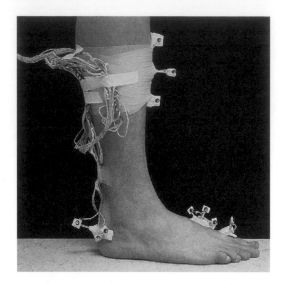

Fig. 6.22. *Measuring three-dimensional motion in the first metatarsal.*

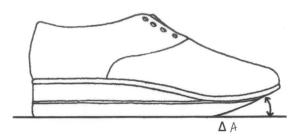

Fig. 6.23. *Rocker bottom. By tapering just past the metatarsals (**A**), a rocker bottom provides a pivot point that allows you to shift into your propulsive period with limited motion of the big toe.*

the Achilles tendon, this treatment approach is surprisingly well tolerated by most runners.

If these treatment protocols fail, a surgical intervention known as a "cheilectomy" may

While preliminary results suggested that it was possible to improve motion, follow-up studies showed that no matter what type of orthotic the subjects wore, their big toe joints continued to move through the same range of motion. Nonetheless, orthotics have been proven to lessen pain in subjects with hallux limitus and should therefore be considered as a viable treatment option (28).

In situations where it is not possible to restore range of motion (e.g., a large dorsal spur has already formed), the goal of treatment is to accommodate the stiffened joint. The easiest way to do this is to wear running shoes with stiff midsoles and large toe springs that prevent the big toe joints from bending. In difficult cases, it is possible to accommodate hallux limitus by having a cobbler install a rocker bottom into the midsole of the running shoe (Fig. 6.23).

Another option is to consider wearing an orthotic with a Morton's extension in the shell (Fig. 6.24). Despite slightly increasing strain on

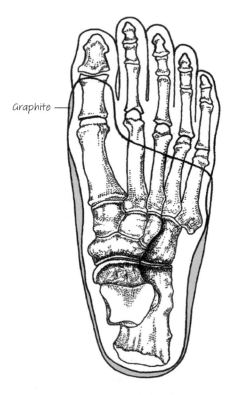

Graphite

Fig. 6.24. *A "Morton's extension in the shell" is usually made from a graphite material that is extended beneath the big toe. The graphite extension reduces movement of the big toe during push-off.*

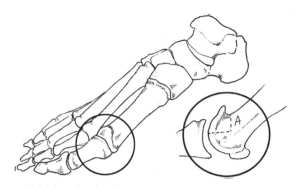

Fig. 6.25. *A cheilectomy is a surgical procedure in which the spur on top of the first metatarsal is removed (A).*

be necessary (Fig. 6.25). While the long-term outcomes of this approach are pretty good, surgery should always be a last option.

PLANTAR FASCIITIS

By far, the most common cause of heel pain in runners is plantar fasciitis. The word *fascia* is Latin for "band," and the inner portion of the plantar fascia, which runs from the heel to the base of the big toe, represents the strongest and most frequently injured section of the band. Until recently, it was assumed that excessive lowering of the medial arch in flat-footed individuals increased tension in the plantar fascia and overloaded the insertion of the plantar fascia on the heel bone. In fact, the increased tension on the heel was believed to be so great that it was thought to eventually result in the formation of a heel spur.

Although the connection between increased plantar fascial tension and the development of heel spurs is generally accepted in the medical community, research in 2003 proved that it is not the plantar fascia that causes the spur to form. A detailed study of 22 heel bones with spurs revealed that bone spurs form at the origin of the flexor digitorum brevis, not the plantar fascia (29). This research emphasizes the important interactions occurring between the plantar fascia and the intrinsic muscles of the arch: The plantar fascia functions passively to store and return energy, while the arch muscles play a more dynamic role in "variable load sharing." Apparently, the intrinsic muscles work with the plantar fascia to prevent lowering of the arch during early stance, while also assisting with arch elevation during propulsion. This explains why the development of plantar fasciitis is not correlated with arch height, and the best predictor of the development of plantar fasciitis is the speed in which the toes move upward during the propulsive period (30).

When the flexor digitorum brevis is strong, it effectively decelerates upward movement of the toes during propulsion while equally distributing pressure between the tips of the toes and the metatarsal heads. Weakness of this small but important muscle allows the digits to move rapidly through larger ranges of motion, pulling on the plantar fascia with more force. As a result, successful treatment requires decelerating the speed in which the toes move up by strengthening the arch muscles. The speed in which the toes move may also be lessened by wearing a running shoe with a high toe spring.

In the most thorough study of plantar fasciitis to date, Sullivan et al. (31) took 202 people with heel pain and compared them to 70 asymptomatic control participants. They determined that in addition to toe weakness and calf tightness, people with chronic heel pain had significant weakness of the peroneals. This finding was significant, as prior to their research, no one had even considered that the peroneals played even the slightest role in the development of plantar fasciitis. It was after reading this paper that I decided to manufacture the ToePro exercise platform, as it effectively strengthens the toes and peroneals while simultaneously stretching the calf. After completing 3 sets of 25 repetitions on the ToePro, I have runners just stand and stretch the backs of their calves by letting their heels touch the ground while their forefeet are resting on the ToePro. Runners with extreme calf tightness should consider sleeping with a night brace, especially if they wake up with pain.

Because the plantar fascia attaches to the base of the big toe, a group of researchers from Ithaca College of Physical Therapy (32) came up with a clever treatment for plantar fasciitis in which the big toe is stretched for 10 seconds, 30 times per day (Fig. 6.26). Compared to conventional treatments for plantar fasciitis,

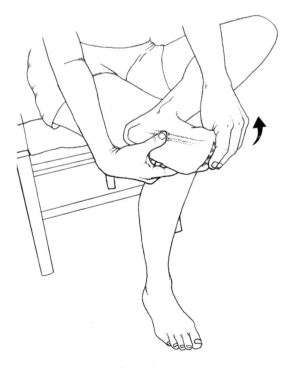

Fig. 6.26. *The plantar fascia home stretch.* *The stretch is held for 10 seconds and repeated 30 times per day. The plantar fascia should be lightly massaged while performing this stretch.*

this stretch routine produced significantly better outcomes.

In addition to stretching the calves and strengthening the toe and peroneus muscles, chronic plantar fasciitis often responds well to low-dye taping and to custom and prefabricated orthotics, which are equally effective in the short-term treatment of the condition (33). As demonstrated by researchers from the Orthopedic Bioengineering Research Lab in Illinois (34, 35), buttressing the arch and/or placing a varus wedge beneath the rearfoot significantly reduces plantar fascial strain.

Whenever possible, runners with plantar fasciitis should avoid making initial ground contact with their midfoot or forefoot, since these strike patterns significantly increase tension in the plantar fascia. Because surgery often results in a gradual destruction of the medial arch (the plantar fascia is an important stabilizer of the arch, and when it is surgically cut, the arch eventually collapses), this type of intervention should always be a last resort. An effective alternative to surgery is shock wave therapy, which is theorized to stimulate repair and accelerate healing. Many chiropractors, PTs, and sports podiatrists perform this procedure in their offices.

HEEL SPURS AND CALCANEAL STRESS FRACTURES

The second most common cause of heel pain is calcaneal spur syndrome. These bony spurs are more likely to be a problem in slightly overweight older runners. The easiest way to differentiate heel spur pain from plantar fasciitis is to take a few steps while walking on your heels and while walking on your tiptoes. Because the plantar fascia is injured during push-off and heel spurs hurt when your foot hits the ground, runners with plantar fasciitis complain of discomfort while walking on their toes, whereas runners with heel spur syndrome find it painful to walk on their heels. In fact, heel spur patients often make initial ground contact with the outer forefoot in an attempt to lessen the pressure beneath the heel during the contact period.

It is important to diagnose plantar fasciitis and heel spur syndrome correctly because the treatment protocols for the two are different: Plantar fasciitis is treated with orthotics, stretches, and exercises, while heel spur syndrome is treated with heel cups and well-fitting heel counters. For both of these conditions, cortisone injections should be a last resort, especially in individuals with heel spur syndrome, because they may result in further degeneration of the calcaneal fat pad. In every situation, runners with heel spur syndrome should avoid minimalist shoes and should consider wearing running shoes with extra midsole material placed beneath the heel.

It is also possible that chronic heel pain is the result of an undiagnosed calcaneal stress fracture. A simple test to rule out a calcaneal fracture is the squeeze test. Because the outer layer of bone in the heel is so thin, compressing the sides of the calcaneus between the thumb and the index finger produces significant discomfort when a stress fracture is present. This test should be performed on both sides of the body. If you feel more pain on one side while applying the same pressure, set up a time to get an x-ray or MRI to make sure the bone isn't fractured. If a calcaneal stress fracture is present, it is important to identify what caused the stress fracture, such as underlying osteoporosis and/or vitamin D deficiency.

BAXTER'S NEUROPATHY

Baxter's neuropathy occurs when the nerve that supplies the little toe (also known as "Baxter's nerve") becomes trapped beneath the plantar fascia. Although rare, high-mileage runners occasionally get this injury. Because most sports docs aren't familiar with Baxter's neuropathy, the proper diagnosis is delayed and the injured runner spends a lot of time and effort receiving ineffective treatments.

To see if you might have Baxter's neuropathy, actively separate your toes: When Baxter's neuropathy is present, you are unable to separate the fourth and fifth toes on the involved side (Fig. 6.27). If Baxter's neuropathy is present, custom and prefabricated orthotics are often helpful, since they may lessen the "scissoring" of the nerve against the plantar fascia. I tend to prescribe soft over-the-counter orthotics because rigid custom orthotics occasionally dig into Baxter's nerve where it passes beneath the arch.

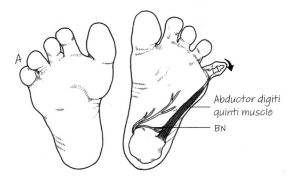

Fig. 6.27. **Baxter's neuropathy test.** *When the nerve to the abductor digiti minimi is compressed, you are unable to abduct the fifth toe (**A**). (**BN** = Baxter's nerve.)*

An alternate method for treating Baxter's neuropathy is to perform the nerve glides illustrated in Fig. 6.28. This technique has

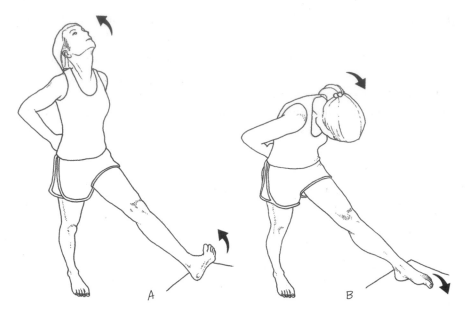

Fig. 6.28. *Nerve glide technique.* *To mobilize Baxter's nerve, place your heel on an elevated platform and then alternately tilt your neck back while moving your ankle and toes in the same direction (**A**). This position is held for five seconds and followed by bending your head and torso forward while pointing your ankle and toes (**B**).*

been proven to mobilize nerves in the arms and hands (36), and is believed to loosen the adhesions responsible for maintaining the nerve in a fixed position.

If conservative management of Baxter's neuropathy does not produce a rapid reduction in symptoms, consider setting up an appointment with a foot surgeon experienced in treating this condition. Surgical release of the scar tissue responsible for pinching Baxter's nerve has pretty good outcomes. Unfortunately, the longer you delay treatment, the less favorably this condition responds to surgical intervention.

TIBIALIS POSTERIOR TENDINITIS

The tibialis posterior is the deepest and most central muscle of the leg. The tendon of the tibialis posterior forms in the lower third of the leg and angles sharply forward as it passes behind the inner ankle bone (Fig. 6.29). The tibialis posterior tendon is similar to the Achilles tendon in that it rotates before it attaches, allowing it to store and return energy like a spring.

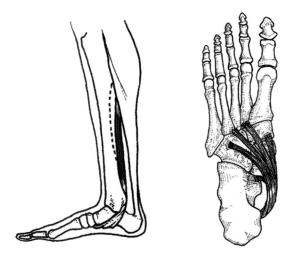

Fig. 6.29. *The tibialis posterior tendon.* *Notice the multiple attachment points to the bottom of the foot.*

The tibialis posterior is a powerful muscle possessing extensive attachments throughout the midfoot making it the most important stabilizer of the arch. When your foot hits the ground while running, this muscle stores energy as the arch begins to flatten and returns this energy to elevate the arch during propulsion. In my experience, high-mileage runners with low arches are especially prone to tibialis posterior tendinitis, especially if they are weak and/or hypermobile (check your thumb laxity with the test on page 88). The excessive force associated with repeatedly lowering the arch eventually overloads the tendon. Early symptoms associated with tibialis posterior tendinitis include pain beneath the inner ankle bone, especially while running on uneven surfaces.

Clinically, an early sign of tibialis posterior tendinitis is the inability to perform an equal number of heel raises on both sides. In the early stages of tibialis posterior tendon injuries, the tendon is inflamed but not lengthened and the arches are the same height. As the tendon injury progresses, the arch on the side of the damaged tendon begins to collapse and the runner is unable to lift his or her heel without significant discomfort.

Treatment for early-stage tibialis posterior tendon injuries consists of either over-the-counter or custom-made orthotics possessing large varus posts. Almost always, soft orthotics are preferred over hard orthotics. In addition to orthotics, runners with mild tibialis posterior tendon injuries usually respond favorably to strengthening exercises. The alternate ToePro exercise is especially helpful, and I typically have runners perform four 30-second isometric contractions after performing this exercise, with the knee bent and the heel down

(see Fig. 3.30, D). The same exercise can also be performed on an AIREX balance pad by leaning sideward against the wall and keeping your knee flexed. Because aggressive exercises can injure the tendon, you should consult a sports specialist familiar with treating tibialis posterior injuries prior to performing strengthening exercises.

Although mild to moderate tibialis posterior tendon injuries typically respond well to orthotics and exercises, severe tibialis posterior tendon injuries can be dangerous, and early diagnosis is the key to keeping you running. Because of their potential to progress, it is very important to diagnose tibialis posterior tendon injuries early, and while I'm not an advocate of expensive tests, runners with chronic tibialis posterior tendon injuries should consider getting an MRI to evaluate the degree of tendon damage.

ANKLE SPRAINS

In the United States alone, 23,000 people sprain their ankle each day (Fig. 6.30), resulting

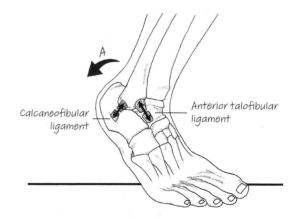

Fig. 6.30. *Inversion ankle sprain. Although an ankle can be sprained in any direction, the most common ankle sprain occurs when the rearfoot inverts (**arrow A**). The sudden movement can damage the anterior talofibular ligament and/or the calcaneofibular ligament.*

in 1.6 million doctor office visits yearly (37). The direct and indirect costs (e.g., lost days from work) associated with treating ankle sprains exceeds $1.1 billion annually (38). To make matters worse, these numbers do not take into account the long-term disability often associated with ankle sprains. In a ten-year follow-up of patients suffering ankle sprains, 72% showed signs of arthritis in the ankle joint (39).

Given the serious long-term consequences associated with ankle sprains, it is important to identify which runners are prone to spraining their ankles. Although numerous factors have been proven to correlate with the development of ankle sprains (such as high arches, impaired balance, tight calves, and decreased cardiovascular fitness), by far the best predictors of future ankle sprains are prior ankle sprains and being overweight. In fact, overweight athletes with a prior history of ankle sprain are 19 times more likely to suffer another ankle sprain (40). Because force centered on the ankle can exceed seven times body weight while running, even a few extra pounds will greatly increase the potential for ankle sprain.

A previous ankle sprain can result in impaired coordination and calf tightness that can increase your potential for reinjury. In a three-dimensional study of motion in the foot and ankle while walking, individuals with a prior history of ankle sprain had reduced ground clearance during swing phase, and the foot was tilted in excessively when it hit the ground (41).

Despite the strong connection between prior sprain and future sprain, there is a counterintuitive inverse relationship between the severity of ligament damage and the potential for reinjury. In a two-year follow-up study of 202 elite runners presenting with inversion ankle sprains, researchers determined that runners with the worst ligament tears rarely suffered reinjury (reinjury rates in this group were between 0 and 5%), while runners with less severe ankle sprains suffered significantly higher rates of re-sprain (18% of runners with moderate sprains were reinjured during this two-year period) (42). Previous research, however, confirmed that patients with completely torn ankle ligaments treated with surgical reconstruction had worse short- and long-term outcomes than individuals who refused surgical intervention (43). Clearly, runners with severe ankle ligament injuries should try to avoid surgery.

Regardless of the degree of ligament damage, the goal of treating an ankle sprain is to restore strength, flexibility, balance, and endurance as quickly as possible during the first few days following injury. Adding an elastic bandage to a standard air cast has been proven to reduce the length of time to full recovery by 50% (44). Table 6.1 outlines a popular treatment protocol for managing ankle sprains, and Fig. 6.31 illustrates an effective tubing exercise that can be performed once symptoms of the acute sprain are reduced.

Besides the standard exercise routines, it is also important that problems with balance be addressed. The simple addition of an inexpensive foam balance pad can significantly reduce the risk of injury. In one study, there was a 77% decrease in the rate of reinjury when overweight athletes with a prior history of ankle sprain performed balance training on a foam stability pad for five minutes on each leg for four

Table 6.1. *Ankle rehabilitation program (42).*

Phase 1. You are unable to bear weight.
A) Use a compressive wrap with U-shaped felt pad placed around fibula. Change every four hours.
B) Actively abduct/adduct toes for five seconds, repeat 10 times.
C) Write out alphabet with toes, five times per day.
D) Ride a stationary bike, 15 minutes per day.
E) Perform ankle rock board while seated (non-weight-bearing), 30 circles, clockwise and counter-clockwise, twice per day. Perform for three minutes on uninjured ankle while standing (exercising your uninjured ankle on the rock board has been shown to increase stability in the injured limb).

Phase 2. You can walk with minimal discomfort and the sprained ankle has 90% full range of motion.
A) Stretch all stiff joints in legs and hips.
B) Perform TheraBand exercises (Fig. 6.31) in all directions, 3 sets of 25 in each direction.
C) Perform double-leg and then single-leg heel raises on the involved side, 3 sets of 10 reps, twice per day.
D) Perform standing closed-eye balance for 30 seconds, five times per day.
E) Perform standing single-leg ankle rock board for one minute, five times per day.

Phase 3. You can hop on the involved ankle without pain.
A) Run at 80% full speed, avoiding forefoot touchdown.
B) Exercise on a mini-trampoline, 3 sets of 30 jumps forward, backward, and side to side. Begin on both legs, then progress to single leg.
C) Perform plyometrics on a 20-inch (50 cm) and a 10-inch (25 cm) box, positioned 3 feet (90 cm) apart. Jump from one box to the ground and then onto the other box, landing as softly as possible. Perform 3 sets of 5 reps. This is an advanced drill and should be performed with care.

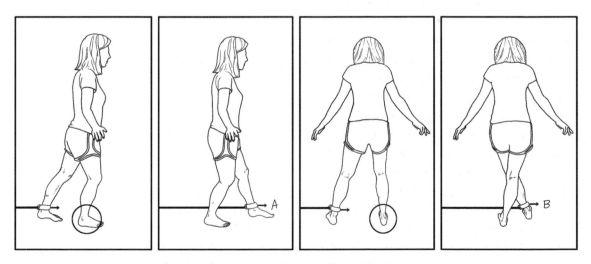

Fig. 6.31. *Ankle exercise. The sprained ankle (circled) is placed on the ground and a resistance band with an ankle cuff is wrapped around the opposite ankle. While maintaining balance on the injured ankle, the uninjured leg pulls the TheraBand forward (**A**), and to the side (**B**). You then rotate 180° and repeat the exercise by pulling the uninjured leg back and then out. While I typically don't like resistance bands, this exercise creates a twisting force in the involved ankle that duplicates the forces while walking and running on unstable surfaces.*

weeks (45). Another study from the Netherlands (46) found that individuals treated with balance board exercises reduced their subsequent reinjury rates by 47%.

Because foam pads and balance boards do not put your foot through a full range of motion, I prefer the Two-to-One Ankle Rockboard. Unlike conventional rock boards that move your foot equally in both directions, the Two-to-One Ankle Rockboard forces your foot to tilt in twice as much as it tilts out (which is how your ankle is designed to move). By standing with your hip and knee straight, you move your ankle so the periphery of the board touches the ground. The rock board places your foot in the position of a future sprain and then forces you to use your muscles to pull yourself out of the risky position. At first, you may need to do this exercise while seated, but after a few days, you can perform it while standing.

Lastly, runners with sprained ankles occasionally develop a condition known as "lateral gutter syndrome." In this syndrome, scar tissue forms inside the ankle joint, which can get pinched when the ankle moves upward. Lateral gutter syndrome is particularly troublesome when the person affected runs uphill. Even though this condition does not show up on an x-ray or MRI, a simple test you can do to confirm this diagnosis is to stand with both feet straight and slowly squat down while keeping your heels on the ground. If lateral gutter syndrome is present, you will feel pin-point pain localized slightly in front of the outer ankle. Unfortunately, lateral gutter syndrome does not respond well to conventional treatments, and it is often necessary to have the scar tissue removed with arthroscopic surgery. The long-term outcomes for this procedure are excellent.

COMPARTMENT SYNDROMES

The muscles of the leg are located in five separate compartments, each of which is separated by specialized walls made of fascia (Fig. 6.32).

Exercise can increase muscular volume by as much as 20%, so the fascial envelopes surrounding each compartment must be capable of stretching to accommodate the expanding muscle compartments. If the fascial envelopes are stiff and unable to expand sufficiently, pressure inside the affected compartment increases, causing the capillaries and veins to collapse. Without adequate venous drainage, the compartment's pressure continues to increase, eventually resulting in muscle and/or nerve damage.

Compartment syndromes are divided into two types: acute and chronic. Although rare, the acute form of compartment syndrome is a surgical emergency because pressure inside the muscle quickly becomes so high that the muscle may be badly damaged. Although sports specialists and runners need to be aware of the potential for acute compartment syndromes, this type of injury is uncommon. More often, runners develop chronic compartment syndromes in which the increased pressure causes discomfort but does not result in long-term muscle damage.

Teenage runners are especially prone to compartment syndromes. The anterior and deep posterior compartments are most likely to be affected, and at first, the runner usually complains of a throbbing pain in the middle of the leg. If the condition worsens, runners with compartment syndromes may present with signs of nerve damage: tingling in the leg

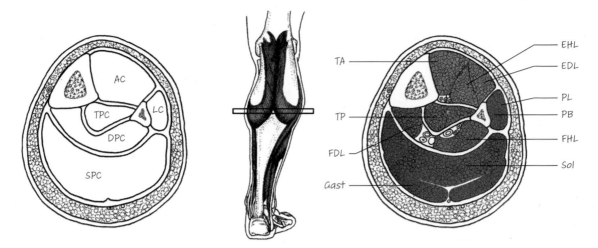

Fig. 6.32. *Cross-section through the middle of the leg revealing the five compartments: AC* = anterior compartment; ***TPC*** = *tibialis posterior compartment;* ***LC*** = *lateral compartment;* ***DPC*** = *deep posterior compartment;* ***SPC*** = *superficial posterior compartment. (Muscle abbreviations:* ***TA*** = *tibialis anterior;* ***EHL*** = *extensor hallucis longus;* ***EDL*** = *extensor digitorum longus;* ***FL*** = *peroneus longus;* ***FB*** = *peroneus brevis;* ***FHL*** = *flexor hallucis longus;* ***Sol*** = *soleus;* ***Gast*** = *gastrocnemius;* ***FDL*** = *flexor digitorum longus;* ***TP*** = *tibialis posterior.)*

and/or extreme muscle weakness. Approximately 45% of individuals with chronic compartment syndromes also have fascial hernias, a condition in which a small portion of the muscle protrudes from its compartment. The herniated muscle looks like a small marble caught beneath the skin. Fortunately, muscle hernias are often asymptomatic and may even be protective, since they allow for reductions in internal muscle pressures.

The treatment of chronic compartment syndrome is dependent upon the specific compartment involved and the shape of the runner's foot: Flat-footed runners presenting with a posterior compartment syndrome should be treated with over-the-counter or custom orthotics incorporating varus posts, while runners with high arches presenting with lateral compartment syndromes should be treated with valgus posts attached beneath the insoles. Regardless of arch height, runners with anterior compartment syndromes should be told to make

initial ground contact with a midfoot strike pattern, while runners with superficial and deep posterior compartment syndromes should be encouraged to run with a heel-first strike pattern. In every situation, runners with chronic compartment syndrome should reduce their stride lengths and find a running shoe that works best for them.

Because compartment syndrome tends to be chronic, it is often necessary to incorporate cross-training techniques, such as stationary bike riding and/or wet vest running in a pool. I tend to discourage runners with this injury from swimming because flutter kicks tighten the deep posterior compartment, which may prolong the length of time to full recovery. To improve flexibility of the fascial envelopes, a home program of stretches and self-massage is invaluable (Fig. 6.33).

Because the compartment muscles are difficult to stretch, runners with compartment

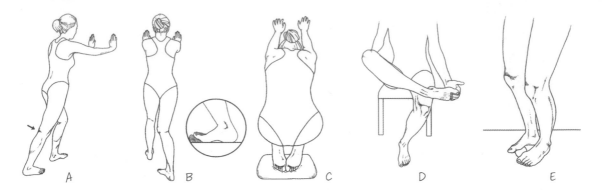

Fig. 6.33. *Compartment stretches.* *The gastrocnemius is stretched with the knee straight (arrow in **A**), while the soleus and tibialis posterior are stretched with the knee bent and the foot pointing (**B**). The flexor digitorum longus is isolated by placing a rolled-up towel beneath the toes while performing stretch **B** (inset). The anterior compartment is stretched by placing a towel beneath the toes and leaning back (**C**), or by sitting with your leg in a figure 4 position (i.e., with the foot of the involved side touching the opposite knee) while pulling the toes back (**D**). The peroneus longus is stretched by placing a tennis ball beneath your forefeet while bending your knees (**E**).*

syndromes should routinely incorporate massage sticks and/or foam rollers to more effectively lengthen the fascia (the Black & Decker car polisher works great as well). Heating the involved compartment prior to using massage sticks and/or rollers increases the speed in which the fascia is lengthened. Care must be taken when massaging the lateral compartment because the superficial fibular nerve can easily be irritated (Fig. 6.34). If you feel tingling along the top of the foot or the outside of the leg while working on the lateral compartment, immediately stop massaging that area.

If compartment symptoms persist, surgeons often recommend a "fascial release" in which an incision is made along the length of one or more fascial envelopes. Although this type of surgery relieves pain in approximately 60% of cases (47), as many as 13% of patients may experience postoperative complications, and for unknown reasons, women respond less favorably than men.

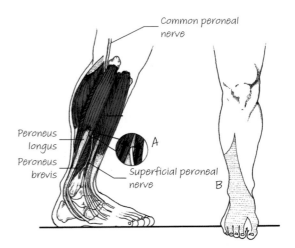

Fig. 6.34. *Location of the superficial fibular nerve (A).* *When using massage sticks or foam rollers, avoid massaging the middle portion of the outside of the leg with too much force, since this may irritate the superficial fibular nerve. You can tell if you're compressing the nerve because you'll feel a tingling along the outer leg and the top of the foot (**B**).*

MEDIAL TIBIAL STRESS SYNDROME

"Medial tibial stress syndrome" refers to a condition of localized pain along the inner aspect of the lower tibia. The classic sign of this injury is palpable tenderness over a 2–3 inch

(5–7.5 cm) area just above the inner ankle bone. Originally believed to be caused by the soleus and/or flexor digitorum longus muscles pulling on the periosteum (a sensitive membrane surrounding the outer surface of bone), medial tibial stress syndrome has been verified by research to involve the bone itself. In a detailed study comparing bone geometry in injured and uninjured athletes, Franklin et al. (48) confirmed that runners with medial tibial stress syndrome have narrower tibias compared to an uninjured exercising control group, proving that medial tibial stress syndrome is also a bony injury, and not just a soft tissue injury. This is supported by other studies showing that the tibia in medial tibial stress syndrome subjects is more porous than in control subjects (43).

This injury is surprisingly common in the running community. In an online survey of 748 high school track and field athletes, 41% of females and 34% of males reported suffering a medial tibial stress injury. Injury to the medial tibia occurs four to six times more often than Achilles tendinitis and plantar fascial injuries, and the best predictor of the development of medial tibial stress injury is higher weekly mileages and faster running. While no single cause has been identified, numerous theories for the development of this injury have been suggested, including muscle weakness/tightness, decreased bone density, hormonal imbalances, and excessive pronation. Extrinsic factors, such as running on asphalt and/ or canted roads, have also been implicated in the development of this condition.

To evaluate potential causes for the development of medial tibial pain, a prospective clinical study was performed in which 122 male and 36 female cadets were followed after measuring a variety of biomechanical risk factors, such as ankle flexibility, limb length discrepancy, and foot type (49). At the end of a 12-month training program, 23 cadets developed medial tibial pain, and even though no factors predicted injury in females, the injured males were more likely to present with greater ranges of hip rotation and smaller diameter calves. This research suggests that hip and calf strengthening exercises should be recommended for male runners presenting with this injury. In my experience, both male and female runners with medial tibial stress syndrome benefit from flexor digitorum longus exercises.

Although orthotics are almost always recommended in the treatment of medial tibial stress syndrome, research regarding their effectiveness has produced mixed results. In 2011, a large, well-designed study confirmed that orthotics may prevent the development of medial tibial stress injury (50). In a randomized controlled trial of 400 military trainees performing a seven-week basic training program, researchers prescribed customized foam orthotics modified with posts, arch supports, and heel cups. These additions were added on a case-by-case basis depending upon the amount of pressure centered beneath each foot. A control group of military trainees was treated with standard insoles. After seven weeks of basic training, 22 cadets from the control group developed medial tibial stress syndrome, compared to only two in the orthotic group. Given the outcomes of this study alone, orthotics should be considered by all runners with a history of medial tibial stress syndrome.

The most popular home treatment for the management of medial tibial stress syndrome continues to be stretching. Despite its popularity, several studies have shown that stretching does not protect against the development of medial tibial injury (51). Nonetheless, once the injury has occurred, it is important to restore the soleus and flexor digitorum longus muscles to their degree of flexibility present prior to the injury. The stretches illustrated in Fig. 6.33, B (and inset), isolate these two muscles. Night braces are also helpful when treating this condition and a wedge can be placed beneath the toes to stretch the long toe muscles.

The development of medial tibial stress syndrome has been associated with higher weekly mileages and faster running, so those with this injury should reduce their training volume and intensity until symptoms subside. Neoprene calf wraps are helpful when returning to sport, and taping the inner side of the leg is also useful, since it may enhance proprioception. To reduce strain on the medial compartment muscles, injured runners should run on soft trails. Because medial tibial stress syndrome is associated with reduced bone strength, it is important to evaluate dietary factors, such as daily intake of vitamin D, calcium, magnesium, and protein (you need a minimum of 50 grams (1.75 oz.) of protein each day). Finally, while anti-inflammatory medications are routinely prescribed for the management of this condition, an award-winning study by Cohen et al. (52) confirms that many nonsteroidal anti-inflammatory drugs can negatively affect tendon-to-bone healing in laboratory animals, and regular use of these drugs should therefore be discouraged.

STRESS FRACTURES

In any given year, more than one in five runners will sustain a stress fracture (53). In the US alone, this translates into nearly two million stress fractures annually (54). In one of the largest studies to date, Matheson and colleagues (55) evaluated 320 athletes with stress fractures and noted that 4% of stress fractures occurred when playing basketball, 5% when playing tennis, and 8% when taking aerobics classes, while a surprising 69% of these athletes developed stress fractures when running. While it is generally believed that runners get stress fractures because the high impact forces associated with running cause the bones to break down, this is not always the case. In Matheson's classic study of 320 athletes with stress fractures, only 20% of the stress fractures could be related to an increase in running mileage and/or the transition to training on a hard surface (55).

In most situations, stress fractures are not the result of weak bones cracking when exposed to excessive stress; they are more likely to be the result of various biomechanical factors in which healthy bones break down when exposed to otherwise manageable impact forces. Though rarely a consideration, muscle strength plays an important role in the prevention of stress fractures. In an interesting study of muscle volume and the development of stress fractures, researchers from Australia (49) determined that a ⅖ inch (10 mm) reduction in calf circumference was associated with a fourfold increase in the incidence of tibial stress fracture. This is consistent with studies demonstrating that certain muscles prevent tibial fractures by adjusting to bony vibrations by pre-tensing prior to heel strike (56, 57).

In addition to dampening the potentially dangerous bony oscillations following heel strike, key muscles play an important role in creating compressive forces that allow various bones to resist the bending strains present while running. For example, the piriformis muscle of the hip has been shown to reinforce the femoral neck, thereby preventing it from bending with the application of vertical forces (Fig. 6.35).

Without adequate support from the piriformis and the neighboring hip abductor, the femoral neck might crack when exposed to the normal bending forces present during midstance while running. The best ways to strengthen the muscles responsible for protecting the femoral neck are illustrated in Fig. 6.36.

While the piriformis has been proven to protect the femoral neck, the iliotibial band has recently been shown to create a stabilizing force that protects the shaft of the femur from stress fractures while running (Fig. 6.37).

During the midstance phase, the tensor fasciae latae and gluteus maximus muscles create a compressive force in the iliotibial band that prevents the femur from bending. As a result, weakness of certain hip muscles may increase the likelihood of suffering a femoral shaft stress

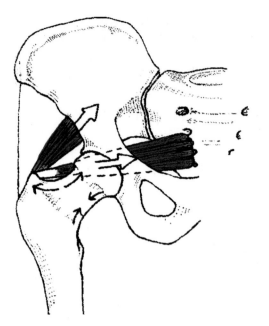

Fig. 6.35. *The piriformis and gluteus medius muscles (white arrows) create a compressive force that protects the femoral neck from stress fractures while running (black arrows).*

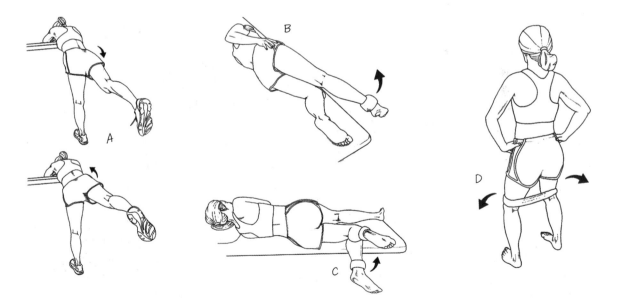

Fig. 6.36. *Piriformis and gluteus medius strengthening exercises. A)* Standing piriformis exercise: While standing on the involved leg, raise and lower the opposite pelvis (*arrows*). *B)* Sidelying gluteus medius exercise: While lying on the edge of a bed or a bench, raise and lower the upper leg (*arrow*). To increase resistance, this exercise can be performed with an ankle weight. *C)* Piriformis exercise: This muscle can be exercised by lying on your side and raising and lowering the ankle with the knee flexed 90° (*arrow*). *D)* Standing piriformis exercise: With a TheraBand positioned above your knees, separate your knees against resistance provided by the band (*arrows*).

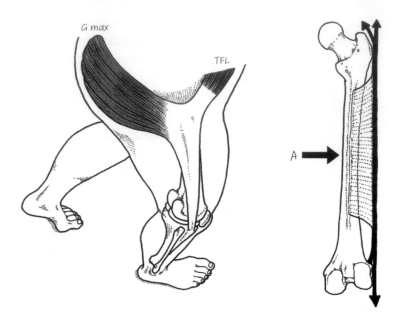

Fig. 6.37. *Because the iliotibial band has a fibrous slip that covers the back of the femur (A), the glute max and the tensor fasciae latae create a compressive force that protects the femur from stress fractures while running.*

fracture. The exercises illustrated in Fig. 6.36 will help protect your femur from this injury.

As previously mentioned, the toe muscles play an important role in protecting the metatarsal shafts from stress fractures, and runners with a prior history of metatarsal stress fracture should work hard to strengthen all of the toe muscles. To determine if your toes are working properly, inspect the insoles of your running shoes. Ideally, you'll notice visible indents beneath the tips of all of the toes.

Tightness in the gastrocnemius is also an underappreciated cause of certain stress fractures. In addition to increasing the risk of metatarsal stress fracture by more than 400% (20), a tight calf also increases the potential of suffering a navicular stress fracture (58). Navicular stress fractures are extremely dangerous in runners, since they tend to heal poorly because of the bone's naturally limited blood supply. In some cases, the navicular can

only heal after surgeons reinforce the midportion of the bone with a metal screw. Because 45% of athletes suffering navicular stress fractures do not return to sport (59), tight runners should try to prevent this injury by routinely stretching their calves.

While strengthening exercises and stretches are helpful when treating a variety of stress fractures, figuring out ways to prevent tibial fractures, especially in young women, has been difficult. This is unfortunate because tibial stress fractures are very common. In their 12-month study of 111 track and field athletes, researchers from the University of Melbourne (53) noted that almost 50% of all stress fractures occurred in the tibia.

To determine why runners get so many tibial stress fractures, researchers from the University of Tennessee (60) performed three-dimensional motion analysis on female runners with and without a history of tibial stress fracture. To their surprise, runners with prior tibial stress fractures consistently attempted to absorb shock by excessively lowering their opposite hip rather than flexing their knee.

In my opinion, the number one cause of tibial stress fractures is a crossover gait pattern. As described in Chapter 4, this gait pattern causes the leg to make ground contact at an angle, altering the transfer of force through the tibia. This altered force can result in chronic reinjury. I had one athlete present with six tibial stress fractures (two on one side and four on the other) over a two-year period, and despite going to numerous facilities for treatment, no one ever evaluated her gait. Needless to say, a gait analysis revealed a crossover gait that was so bad that she'd worn down the insides of her heel counters as a result of her feet hitting one another during swing phase. I had her put a chalk line in the center of a treadmill and told her to make sure the inner portion of her running shoe never crossed the chalk line. I saw her years later for a different injury and she was able to return to high-mileage running without ever suffering a tibial stress fracture again. As with all injuries, runners dealing with stress fractures should receive a detailed gait analysis to identify possible causes.

In order to allow runners to return to sport following a stress fracture, many practitioners continue to recommend the "10% rule," in which the injured runner is told to increase his/her running distance by 10% per week. Even though the 10% rule continues to be used by most sports experts, a study published in the *American Journal of Sports Medicine* in 2007 showed that this approach does not alter reinjury rates (61). To complicate things even more, because runners heal at different rates, the conventional formulas used to predict recovery time for specific stress fractures are extremely inaccurate.

For example, some experts incorrectly claim that metatarsal stress fractures heal in six weeks, while femoral stress fractures heal in 12 weeks. No two runners heal at the same rate so these formulas are useless.

Fortunately, three of the best running doctors in the world have developed what I think is the best return-to-running protocol ever published (62). The program consists of a pre-entry stage and three running stages. The pre-entry stage requires the runner be pain free for five consecutive days while performing normal daily activities. After that, they begin the five-week program described in Table 6.2. I like this paper so much that I recommend injured runners get the original article, as it's full of detailed information and great illustrations outlining the different causes and treatments for stress fractures.

As mentioned, runners with stress fractures should always receive detailed biomechanical and gait evaluations to identify the risk factors that could perpetuate injury. Nutritional factors should also be considered, and all runners should have a vitamin D blood level of 30–40 ng/dL. While some runners would rather get their vitamin D from sun exposure, this is not an option for runners in cities like Boston, New York, Chicago, and Seattle, as sunlight lacks the necessary UVB rays to produce a safe level of vitamin D from November through April in most northern states of the US (63). Vitamin D levels in cold climates are lowest during the month of March, which some experts claim is the cause of the high rates of colds and flus during that month (vitamin D is also important for immune function).

Some nutritionists recommend that runners consume large doses of vitamin D, but recent

Table 6.2. *A graduated running program to return a runner to 30 minutes of pain-free running.*

Stage	Day	Description
0		*Pre-entry to graduated running program* *Pain during walking in normal activities of daily living*
1		INITIAL LOADING AND JOGGING (50% NORMAL PACE) WITH INCREASING DURATION
	1	Walk 30 minutes
	2	*Rest*
	3	Walk 9 minutes and jog 1 minute (3 repetitions)
	4	*Rest*
	5	Walk 8 minutes and jog 2 minutes (3 repetitions)
	6	*Rest*
	7	Walk 7 minutes and jog 3 minutes (3 repetitions)
	8	*Rest*
	9	Walk 6 minutes and jog 4 minutes (3 repetitions)
	10	*Rest*
	11	Walk 4 minutes and jog 6 minutes (3 repetitions)
	12	*Rest*
	13	Walk 2 minutes and jog 8 minutes (3 repetitions)
	14	*Rest*
2		RUNNING WITH INCREASING INTENSITY
	1	Jog 30 minutes
	2	*Rest*
	3	Run 30 minutes at 60% normal pace
	4	*Rest*
	5	Run 30 minutes at 60% normal pace
	6	*Rest*
	7	Run 30 minutes at 70% normal pace
	8	*Rest*
	9	Run 30 minutes at 80% normal pace
	10	*Rest*
	11	Run 30 minutes at 90% normal pace
	12	*Rest*
	13	Run 30 minutes at full pace
	14	*Rest*
3		RUNNING ON CONSECUTIVE DAYS
	1	Run 30 minutes at full pace
	2	Run 30 minutes at full pace
	3	*Rest*
	4	Run 30 minutes at full pace
	5	Run 30 minutes at full pace
	6	*Rest*
	7	Run 30 minutes at full pace
4		RETURN TO RUNNING

Modified from Warden et al. [62].

research shows that this can actually reduce bone density. In a 2019 study of 311 participants receiving either 400, 4,000, or 10,000 IU of vitamin D daily for three years, researchers from Canada (64) found that subjects taking the highest doses had the greatest reductions in bone mineral density. Because vitamin D deficiency correlates with accelerated muscle loss and an increased likelihood of falling (65), runners should have their vitamin D levels tested in the winter months, especially in the colder northern climates. Although it tastes horrible, cod liver oil is one of the best natural sources of vitamin D.

In addition to large doses of vitamin D being problematic for bone health, the latest research also suggests that ketogenic diets are also terrible for bone strength (66). These diets, which are low in carbohydrates and high in fat, are popular with ultra-distance runners because they allow these athletes to more effectively utilize their fat stores for energy, which comes in handy when you are trying to run 100 miles. Unfortunately, even short-term use of ketogenic diets can be harmful to bones. In a 2020 study of 30 world-class racewalkers forced to consume either a high-carbohydrate diet or a low-carbohydrate/high-fat diet (the typical ketogenic diet), in less than four weeks, athletes on the ketogenic diet had accelerated bone breakdown and impaired remodeling. The authors of the study state that the detrimental effects of ketogenic diets could have "major consequences to health and performance."

While the best way to maintain proper bone health is with a balanced diet, my favorite supplement for athletes recovering from stress fractures is a product called "Bone Up." Manufactured by Jarrows Formulation, this supplement contains microcrystalline hydroxyapatite compound, magnesium, boron, molybdenum, zinc, and a range of micronutrients important for bone repair. Keep in mind that bone is much more than calcium, and in order to heal properly, it needs a wide range of nutrients.

The single biggest concern when managing stress fractures in runners is the presence of an untreated eating disorder, which is an epidemic in the collegiate running community. These complex disorders are beyond the scope of this book, and coaches and friends are encouraged to openly discuss the possibility of this diagnosis and refer out to appropriate specialists. Compared to the 1980s and 1990s, when coaches would routinely tell runners that they would "run a little faster if only they were thinner," the heightened awareness of these disorders and the availability of experts have improved the rates of recovery from these extremely difficult to treat disorders.

PATELLOFEMORAL PAIN SYNDROME

Also referred to as "retropatellar pain" (or pain behind the kneecap), patellofemoral pain syndrome affects 25% of the running population. A classic sign that you have this injury is that your kneecap aches when you sit for long periods, and the pain goes away when you straighten your leg. Despite the fact that researchers have spent decades studying patellofemoral pain, identifying the cause of this condition has been difficult. Early research suggested that the most likely cause of patellofemoral pain syndrome was a sideward shifting of the kneecap into the lower femur. The most frequently cited factors responsible for abnormal movement of the kneecap included an increased Q angle and/or weakness of the inner quadriceps muscle, the vastus medialis obliquus (also known as the "VMO") (Fig. 6.38).

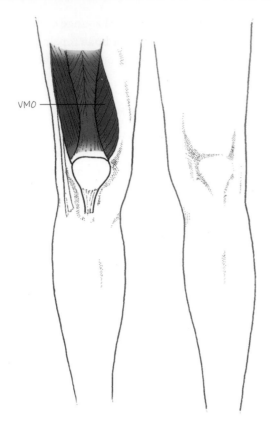

VMO

Fig. 6.38. *The vastus medialis obliquus (VMO).*

To correct the abnormal sideward movement of the patella, sports specialists prescribe a variety of VMO strengthening exercises, such as toe-out leg extensions and wall presses while squeezing a ball. Unfortunately, dozens of studies have shown that these exercises do not target the VMO. Rather, these exercises more effectively strengthen the *outer* quadriceps muscle, potentially worsening patellofemoral pain when the stronger outer quadriceps muscle pulls the patella sideward with more force. In spite of their proven ineffectiveness, VMO exercises continue to be a first-line intervention for the management of this common condition.

To get a better understanding of what really happens with patellofemoral injuries, a group of researchers placed people in specialized

MRI scanners to evaluate patellofemoral movement while they flexed their knees (67). Surprisingly, the MRIs revealed that the primary cause of patellofemoral problems was not a shifting of the patella into the stable femur, but a shifting of the outer aspect of the femur into the stable patella. CT and functional MRI evaluations in 2008 and 2010 support this observation, confirming that the most likely cause of patellofemoral pain while running is abnormal motion of the femur, not altered motion of the patella (68, 69).

Hip weakness has been cited as the most likely cause of the exaggerated rotation of the femur. In a three-dimensional evaluation of runners with and without patellofemoral pain syndrome, researchers from Indiana University (70) proved that runners with weak hip abductors allow their femurs to turn in excessively, and the degree of rotation increases when the runners are fatigued. Runners with anteverted hips, external tibial torsion, and/or weakness of the hip rotators (as measured with the testing device illustrated in Fig. 3.26) are especially prone to retropatellar injuries.

As previously mentioned, in addition to the strengthening exercises listed in Fig. 3.36, runners with excessive inward rotation of the hips should perform gait retraining, in which they consciously focus on improving the faulty movement pattern. The forward step-down test (see Fig. 3.35) is a simple means of determining if hip weakness predisposes you to patellofemoral injury. This test is also useful to monitor progress, and you should consider cross training until you are able to perform the forward step-down test while keeping the hip and knee straight.

A frequently cited cause of retropatellar pain is low arches. The belief is that because runners with low arches pronate more, their lower legs are forced to twist inward excessively, dragging the kneecap against the femur. While this seems logical, the connection between excessive and increased inward rotation of the leg is based on the mitered hinge analogy (refer back to Fig. 3.5), which has been proven to be incorrect. As discussed in Chapter 5, three-dimensional research in 2001 confirmed that although runners with low arches do pronate more, their lower legs rotate the same amount as people with high arches (71). As a result, runners with low and high arches have the same potential for developing patellofemoral pain syndrome. The equal ranges of tibial rotation in runners with high and low arches explains why so many recent studies have shown a limited connection between pronation and patellofemoral pain.

Despite the limited connection between pronation and retropatellar pain, runners with painful kneecaps frequently report that orthotics lessen their discomfort. The easiest way to determine if an orthotic will reduce your patellofemoral pain is to do a simple trial in which you wear an over-the-counter orthotic while performing a few single-leg squats. According to researchers from Australia (72), if you feel more comfortable performing the squats while wearing the orthotics, the potential for orthotics to produce a marked reduction in knee pain increases from 25% to 45%. New research confirms that the best outcomes for managing retropatellar pain occur when over-the-counter orthotics are prescribed along with a few simple foot exercises (73). This study is consistent with prior research showing that you're more likely to get good results when prescribing orthotics if you simultaneously prescribe foot exercises.

The final aspect to consider when treating chronic patellofemoral pain is flexibility of the quadriceps. Researchers from Belgium (74) evaluated multiple factors associated with the development of patellofemoral pain and determined that tightness in the quadriceps is a clear risk factor. In fact, quadriceps inflexibility was a better predictor of patellofemoral pain than an increased Q angle, which doctors often correct by surgically reconstructing the knee.

You can evaluate quadriceps flexibility by lying face down and measuring the distance from the back of your heel to your hip (Fig. 6.39). The measurement should be repeated on both sides, and in most situations, you should be able to get your heels within 4 inches (10 cm) of each hip.

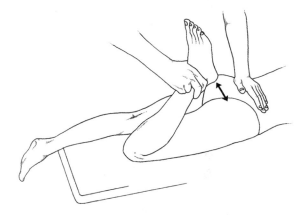

Fig. 6.39. *Measuring quadriceps flexibility.*

If either quadriceps is inflexible, roll the tight muscle with a foam roller or a massage stick and then perform the stretch illustrated in Fig. 6.40. The stretch should be held for 30 seconds and repeated five times per day.

A common mistake is to only massage the lower portion of the quadriceps. Because the outer quadriceps muscle (vastus lateralis) runs up to the outside of the hip (Fig. 6.41), it is important to work the entire muscle, not just the lower portion. Because the vastus lateralis plays an

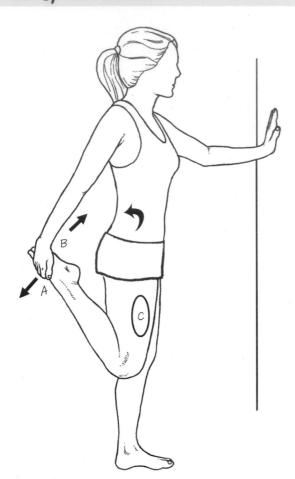

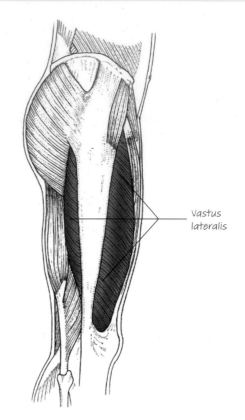

Fig. 6.41. *The vastus lateralis is a large muscle, running from the hip to the outer knee.*

Fig. 6.40. *The central quadriceps muscle (rectus femoris) is stretched while maintaining a pelvic tuck (arrow), while the vastus lateralis is stretched by pulling your heel toward your opposite hip.* Prior to stretching the vastus lateralis, you should warm the central portion of this muscle up (**C**) with a Black & Decker car polisher. The muscle energy stretch can be performed by lightly pushing your foot down into your hand (**arrow A**), then relaxing and gently pulling your heel closer to the opposite hip (**arrow B**). Repeat this process by moving back to the starting position and performing the stretch three times.

important role in shock absorption, loosening up the central portion of the muscle is especially important.

To lessen patellofemoral pressure while running, consider shortening your stride and switching to a more forward strike pattern.

Increasing your cadence by just 5% has been proven to reduce knee pressure (38). Finally, because running amplifies impact forces fivefold, overweight runners should consider losing a few pounds, as even small reductions in body weight can significantly lessen the pressure behind the kneecap. When returning to sport following a retropatellar injury, you may want to try wearing a neoprene knee brace or consider using Kinesiotape over the top of the patella. The Triple Stick Strap is a compressive brace that is easy to use and helps stabilize the kneecap while you are recovering (Fig. 6.42). As with almost all injuries, an active dynamic warm-up (see Fig. 4.5) should be performed prior to running, and you should make the first mile of your typical run at least one minute per mile slower than usual.

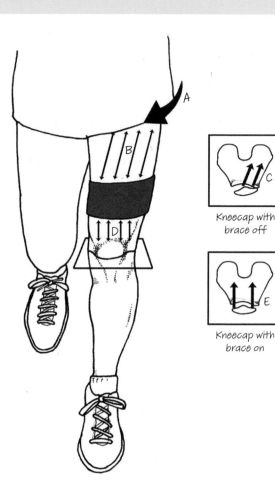

Fig. 6.42. *Managing patellofemoral pain with the Triple Stick Strap.* *Excessive inward rotation of the thigh while running (**A**) causes the quadriceps to pull the kneecap sideward (**B** and **C**). Placing the Triple Stick Strap securely above the kneecap compresses the quadriceps, allowing for improved alignment of the kneecap (**D** and **E**).*

Kneecap with brace off

Kneecap with brace on

PATELLAR TENDINOPATHY

Patellar tendinopathy is a degenerative condition characterized by local tenderness of the patellar tendon at its attachment to the patella. Because stress in the tendon is greatest when the knee is flexed excessively, this injury is more prevalent in sprinters and high-mileage endurance runners than in recreational runners. In an attempt to identify potential risk factors for the development of patellar tendinopathy, van der Worp (75)

performed an extensive review of the literature and found *some* evidence suggesting that reducing body weight, increasing thigh flexibility, and using orthotics to control excessive pronation can be effective methods for reducing the risk of injury. However, the evidence correlating a lessened potential for injury with a specific treatment intervention was weak. As in the case of patellofemoral pain syndrome, the ability of an orthotic to favorably modify symptoms associated with patellar tendinopathy is unpredictable. For these reasons, an orthotic device should only be prescribed if while wearing an arch support you respond favorably to specific functional tests; e.g., performing repeat step-downs off a 4-inch (10 cm) platform with and without over-the-counter orthotics.

Vigorous deep tissue massage followed by frequent stretching of the quadriceps is almost always helpful, since a flexible quadriceps absorbs force that would otherwise be absorbed by the patellar tendon. In one of the best papers ever published on patellar tendon injuries, researchers from Hong Kong (76) demonstrated that tightness in the outer quadriceps muscle plays a huge role in the development of this injury. Using a high-tech ultrasound device to measure elasticity in different sections of the quadriceps, these researchers showed that the outer quadriceps muscle, the vastus lateralis, lengthened significantly more than the other quadriceps muscles as the knee flexes to absorb forces during ground contact. The clinical significance of this is that tightness in the vastus lateralis would generate more force in the patellar tendon, greatly increasing the likelihood of injury. These researchers examined over 65 athletes and determined that athletes suffering patellar tendinopathy had 26.5% greater tension in the vastus lateralis, which was associated with the development of patellar tendinopathy.

The authors state that "traditional stretching of the whole quadriceps muscle might not be targeted to the tight muscle heads."

A very effective way to lengthen the vastus lateralis is by massaging the central portion of the muscle with a Black & Decker car polisher for five minutes, followed by a series of gentle hold-relax stretches. The best way to do the stretches is to stand in the position shown in Fig. 6.40.

In addition to improving vastus lateralis flexibility, another way to reduce tendon strain while running is to wear a compressive strap around the knee (see Fig. 6.42). Several studies have shown that compressive straps reduce tendon strain by distributing the forces generated by muscle contraction over a broader area (77, 78).

Of all the proposed treatment protocols, the most effective way to fix patellar tendinopathy is to increase the strength of the patellar tendon itself. In an in-depth study of the effects of heavy weight training on patellar tendinopathy in athletes, researchers from Denmark (79) used electron microscopes to evaluate tendon fragments removed from individuals with and without patellar tendinopathy, before and after completing a 12-week exercise protocol. The training sessions consisted of three weekly sessions of squats, leg presses, and hack squats. The subjects completed 4 sets of each exercise with a two- to three-minute rest between sets. Before and after completing this rigorous training program, biopsies of tendons in the patients with patellar tendinopathy were compared to biopsies of tendons taken from a healthy control group. As demonstrated with electron microscopes, the exercise group developed an increase in the number of small tendon fibers, which improved the overall flexibility of the patellar tendon (Fig. 6.43).

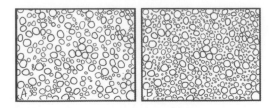

Fig. 6.43. *Electron microscopy of tendon biopsies taken before (A) and after (B) a 12-week strength training program.* Note the significant increase in small-sized fibrils following strength training.

The changes to the patellar tendon made it significantly more resilient, allowing the athletes to exercise with considerable reductions in tendon pain and swelling. The authors speculate that overuse may cause small tears to form inside the patellar tendon, resulting in a reduced formation of new fibrils (hence the older, fatter, less populated fibril population). It is theorized that slow, heavy resistance training leads to an increase in tendon production, which in turn produces a greater number of tendon fibers with the formation of numerous small-sized fibrils. The changes in tendon fiber density occurred rapidly, and by week 12, there was no difference between the patellar tendinopathy group and the control group. The Danish researchers (79) related the reduced tendon stiffness to the increased production of new fibrils: Because the smaller fibrils have fewer cross-links between them, the tendon itself becomes more resilient, since fewer cross-fibrils allow for greater flexibility.

While heavy load resistance training increases tendon flexibility and decreases pain, the heavy weights used in this protocol could potentially cause injury when performed by recreational runners. An alternate protocol for strengthening the patellar tendon is to perform the long-step lunges without strides illustrated in Fig. 6.44.

The long-step forward lunge has been proven to reduce strain on the patella, and I recommend

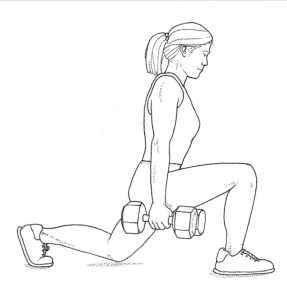

Fig. 6.44. *The long-step forward lunge. While maintaining your feet in a fixed position, raise and lower your body by straightening your legs. (Redrawn from Escamilla et al. [80].)*

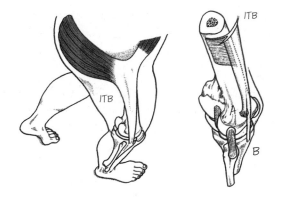

Fig. 6.45. *The iliotibial band (ITB) has two separate attachment points along the outer knee (A and B).*

that runners with patellar tendinopathy perform this exercise 50 times per day, with each repetition lasting six seconds (a three-second eccentric phase followed by a three-second concentric phase). In my experience, this exercise protocol is just as effective as the heavy resistance protocol described by the Danish researchers, but because only light weights are used, the risk of injuring the kneecap is greatly reduced.

As with patellofemoral pain, runners with patellar tendinopathy should consider switching to a forefoot strike pattern, reduce stride length, and/or increase self-selected cadence by 5%. Over-the-counter knee braces and/or placing Kinesiotape over the patellar tendon can make it a little less painful when returning to running.

ILIOTIBIAL BAND COMPRESSION SYNDROME

The iliotibial band is an interesting fibrous structure that originates from the gluteus maximus, gluteus medius, and tensor fasciae latae muscles and attaches to two separate points on the outside of the knee (Fig. 6.45).

Runners with iliotibial band compression syndrome often describe the pain as a burning sensation along the outside of the knee. While most sports textbooks will tell you that runners develop this injury when the band snaps back and forth over a small bony prominence located on the outside of the knee (traumatizing a bursa trapped beneath), more recent research confirms that the band does not snap back and forth and that a trapped bursa is not the cause of the pain.

In their thorough analysis of iliotibial band anatomy and function, researchers from the University of Wales (81) proved that what appears to be a forward/backward displacement of the band during knee flexion is actually an illusion created by alternating tensions generated by the tensor fasciae latae and gluteus maximus muscles (Fig. 6.46). Using MRI, the authors conclusively proved the band does not snap back and forth, but is compressed into the outer side of the femur when the knee is flexed, with peak compression occurring at 30° flexion.

To identify the biomechanical factors potentially responsible for the development of this common

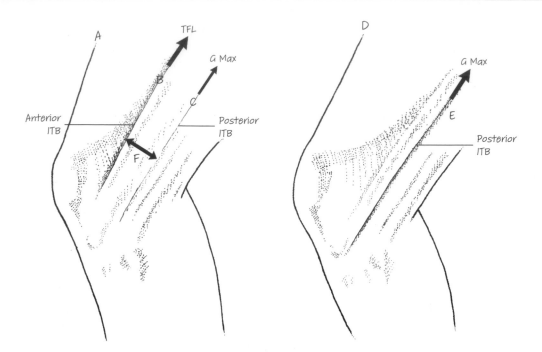

Fig. 6.46. *The iliotibial band (ITB). When the knee is slightly bent (**A**), the tensor fasciae latae (**TFL**) pulls with more force than the gluteus maximus (**G Max**), causing the front of the ITB to become more prominent (compare **B** and **C**). When the knee bends more (**D**), greater tension is created in the gluteus maximus, and the back of the iliotibial band becomes more prominent (**E**). The shifting of tension from the front to the back of the ITB (**F**) creates the illusion that the band is snapping forward and backward.*

injury, William Ferber and colleagues (82) performed three-dimensional motion analysis of 35 runners with iliotibial band syndrome and compared rearfoot, knee, and hip movements to 35 age-matched controls. Compared to the control group, the iliotibial band syndrome group exhibited significantly greater collapse of the opposite hip with increased inward rotation of the involved knee. Importantly, there was no appreciable difference in rearfoot pronation between the two groups. In fact, runners with iliotibial band syndrome had slightly reduced ranges of pronation compared to the control group, which is consistent with research suggesting that this injury is more likely to happen in people with high arches (83). The authors state that the excessive dropping of the opposite hip and twisting of the involved knee causes an amplified compression of the

band against the outer side of the knee. To treat this condition, runners with this injury should strengthen their hips and perform the gait retraining techniques described on page 137.

While strengthening exercises and gait retraining play an important role in the management of iliotibial band compression syndrome, it is also important to evaluate hip abductor flexibility, since tightness in the tensor fasciae latae, gluteus medius, and gluteus maximus muscles can increase tensile strain on the band. In an extremely detailed study of the effect of stretching on the iliotibial band and proximal muscles, researchers surgically implanted strain gauges into the iliotibial bands of 20 cadavers and evaluated the effect of three different stretches on lengthening the band (84). These same researchers also evaluated elasticity of the iliotibial band in live athletes by using special ultrasound machines. Their detailed analysis confirmed that the iliotibial band itself is extremely rigid and resistant to stretch, since it lengthened less than 0.2% when pulled by the hip muscles with maximum force. Because of the extreme inflexibility of the iliotibial band, the authors stress that treatments aimed at reducing tension in the band are a waste of time, since massage will not loosen the band.

Other experts confirm that it is physically impossible to loosen the iliotibial band itself because the connective tissue that makes up the band is as strong as Kevlar, the material used in bullet-proof vests (85). Rather than needlessly massaging the band, a more effective approach is to reduce tension in the muscular component of the band by massaging trigger points in the gluteus maximus, gluteus medius, and tensor fasciae latae muscles. After a few minutes of massage, it is recommended to lengthen these muscles with the stretches illustrated in Fig. 6.47.

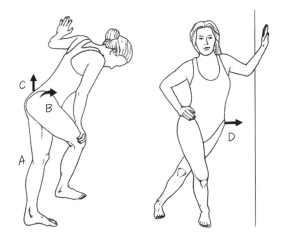

Fig. 6.47. *Iliotibial band stretches. The involved leg is kept in a straight position (**A**), while you bend forward at the hip (**B**). To stretch the back portion of the band, the involved hip is moved toward the wall (**C**). To stretch the TFL component of the band, move the involved hip toward the wall while keeping your spine upright (**D**).*

HAMSTRING STRAINS

Of all the gait-related muscle injuries, hamstring strains have the highest rate of recurrence, with as many as one-third of injured runners suffering reinjury within the first few weeks following a return to sport. With stride lengths exceeding 15 feet, sprinters are especially vulnerable to this injury, and it can take up to four months of aggressive rehabilitative exercises before a return to sport is possible.

Even though the hamstrings consist of four different muscles, runners almost exclusively injure the outer hamstring muscle, the long head of the biceps femoris. The reason for the higher injury rate in the outer hamstring muscle was a mystery until 2005, when researchers from the University of Wisconsin determined that because the biceps femoris attaches lower down the leg, it is under greater strain when the swinging leg is moving forward (86) (Fig. 6.48).

In a 2008 MRI study evaluating the location of hamstring strains in different athletes, the only runner to injure a hamstring muscle other than the biceps femoris was an older man who severely strained his inner hamstring while performing stretches prior to running, not while running (87). This is consistent with research showing that dancers almost always injure their inner hamstring muscles, which are very sensitive to stretch injuries.

Runners typically strain the biceps femoris just before the lead foot hits the ground, when tension in the outer hamstring muscle is greatest. As with most injuries, the single best predictor of future injury is prior injury, possibly because the injured muscle heals with less flexibility and/or impaired coordination. Because of the extremely high recurrence rate associated with

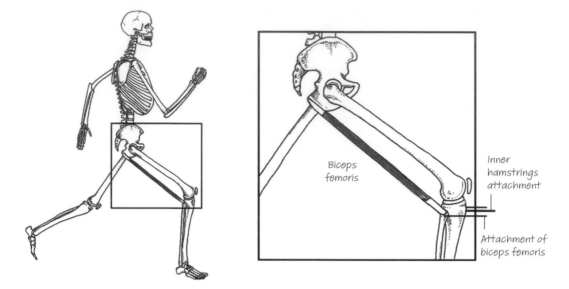

Fig. 6.48. *Because the biceps femoris attaches lower down the leg, runners tend to strain this hamstring muscle almost exclusively.*

biceps femoris strains, rehabilitation of this injury must be comprehensive and address all possible factors associated with chronicity. While hamstring inflexibility is often cited as a potential cause, there is little evidence to support this theory. Recent research confirms that strength, not muscle stiffness, plays the most important role in preventing hamstring injury.

In an impressive study comparing the success of different treatment regimens used in the management of acute hamstring strains, Sherry and Best (7) proved that compared to a conventional protocol of static stretching and hamstring resistance exercises, an exercise regimen including agility and trunk stabilization exercises produces significantly better short- and long-term outcomes (see Table 6.3 for a summary of these exercises). Compared to conventional rehabilitation, the agility and stabilization group returned to sport sooner (22 days vs. 37 days), and suffered fewer reinjuries during the first two weeks after returning to sport (55% of the conventional rehab group were reinjured,

compared to no reinjuries in the progressive agility and trunk stabilization group).

The beneficial effects of the agility and stabilization exercises were even present one year following the return to sport, as 70% of the athletes treated with conventional stretches and exercises were reinjured, compared to only 7.7% of the athletes completing the progressive agility and trunk stabilization program. The alternate hamstring exercises illustrated in Fig. 6.49 are also helpful when treating hamstring injuries.

The fact that hamstring inflexibility does not cause hamstring strains does not suggest that an injured hamstring should never be stretched. On the contrary, since a flexible muscle is able to tolerate higher eccentric forces with less muscle damage (88), and individuals with flexible hamstrings are less prone to a variety of injuries (89), lengthening the hamstrings with gentle stretches is almost always appropriate. The stretch illustrated in Fig. 6.50 isolates the long head of the biceps femoris. To reduce stiffness in

Table 6.3. *Hamstring exercise protocol as described by Sherry and Best (7).*

Phase 1
1. Low- to moderate-intensity sidestepping, 3 × 1 minute.
2. Low- to moderate-intensity grapevine stepping (lateral stepping with the trail leg going over the lead leg and then under the lead leg), both directions, 3 × 1 minute.
3. Low- to moderate-intensity steps forward and backward over a tape line while moving sideward, 2 × 1 minute.
4. Single-leg stand, progressing from eyes open to eyes closed, 4 × 20 seconds.
5. Prone abdominal body bridge (performed by using abdominal and hip muscles to hold the body in a facedown straight-plank position with the elbows and feet as the only point of contact), 4 × 20 seconds.
6. Supine extension bridge (see Fig. 3.30, X). Repeat four times, holding 20 seconds.
7. Side plank (see Fig. 3.30, W). Repeat four times, hold 20 seconds on each side.
8. Ice with hamstrings in a stretched position for 20 minutes.

Phase 2
1. Moderate- to high-intensity sidestepping, 3 × 1 minute.
2. Moderate- to high-intensity grapevine stepping, 3 × 1 minute single-leg windmill touches (see Fig. 6.49, B).
3. Push-up stabilization with trunk rotation (performed by starting at the top of a full push-up, then maintain this position with one hand while rotating the chest toward the side of the hand that is being lifted to point toward the ceiling, pause and return to the starting position), 2 × 15 reps on each side.
4. Fast feet in place (performed by jogging in place with increasing velocity, picking the foot only a few inches off the ground), 4 × 20 seconds.
5. Symptom-free practice without high-speed maneuvers.
6. Ice for 20 minutes if any symptoms of local fatigue or discomfort are present.

Key:
Low intensity: a velocity of movement that is less than or near that of normal walking.
Moderate intensity: a velocity of movement greater than normal walking but not as great as sport.
High intensity: a velocity of movement similar to sport activity.
Progression criteria: subjects progressed from exercises in phase 1 to exercises in phase 2 when they could walk with a normal gait pattern and do a high knee march-in-place without pain.

the upper hamstring muscles, this stretch should be performed with the knee flexed 45° and 90°.

Since fatigue increases the potential for hamstring injury, Verral et al. (90) recommend stretching the hamstrings for 15 seconds with the knee bent at different angles while exercising. Over a two-year period, the authors demonstrated significantly reduced rates of hamstring injuries in Australian Rules football players when the stretches were performed during workouts and competition. As this also applies to runners, the results of the study suggest that occasionally stopping to stretch the outer hamstring muscle during your long runs may lessen the potential for reinjury.

In another study of Australian Rules football players, Hoskins et al. (91) demonstrated that occasional chiropractic care can reduce the rate of hamstring injuries and reinjuries. In a one-year study of nearly 60 Australian Rules football players, the authors demonstrated that players treated with occasional chiropractic care throughout the entire season developed significantly fewer hamstring injuries (one vs. five) and reinjuries (none vs. two) than an age-matched control group.

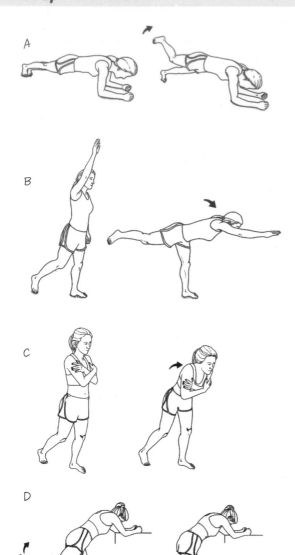

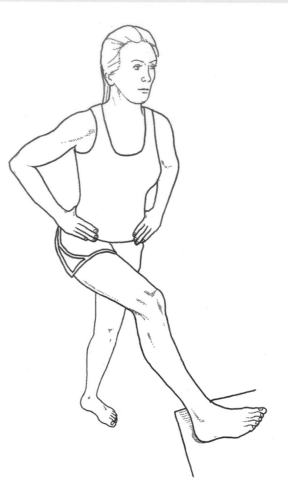

Fig. 6.50. *Stretch for the long head of the biceps femoris.* *While keeping your spine in a neutral position, lean forward by pivoting at the hip while your leg is turned in with your knee slightly bent.*

Fig. 6.49. *Hamstring exercises.* A) *Prone plank march: Hold a plank position and alternately raise one leg at a time for five seconds.* **B)** *Single-leg windmill: While standing on the involved leg, pivot at the hips while maintaining alignment of the opposite arm and leg.* **C)** *Upper hamstring muscle exercise: Stand on the involved leg with the opposite knee slightly bent. While maintaining an arch in your low back, pivot forward at the hips (**arrow**). The opposite leg should barely be contacting the ground during this exercise.* **D)** *Lower hamstring muscle exercise: With arms supported on a stable surface, flex and extend the involved knee while turning the leg in and out.*

While stretches and chiropractic care may be helpful in treating and preventing hamstring injuries, comprehensive strengthening exercises play the most important role in the management of hamstring strains. Because nonsteroidal anti-inflammatories may result in impaired tendon healing (52), the routine use of these drugs should be reconsidered. A safer alternative to improve healing is to perform deep tissue massage directly over the damaged tendon, since this may stimulate repair without adversely affecting tendon strength (18, 92).

PIRIFORMIS SYNDROME

The piriformis muscle takes its name from the word *piriformis* in Latin for "pear-shaped," since the muscle's wide base and tapered attachment resembles a pear. This small but important muscle creates a compressive force that prevents the femoral neck from fracturing while running (see Fig. 2.17). Despite the protection afforded the femoral neck, the piriformis causes a lot of trouble in runners because it sits directly on top of the sciatic nerve, which is the largest nerve in the body (Fig. 6.51).

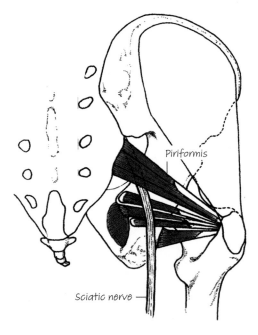

Fig. 6.51. *The sciatic nerve exits the pelvis directly beneath the piriformis.*

In fact, in about 2% of the population, the sciatic nerve exits the pelvis directly through the middle of the piriformis, greatly increasing the potential for developing sciatica. The increased activity present in this muscle while running can produce a chronic pinching of the nerve. Common symptoms associated with piriformis-related sciatica include a toothache type of pain along the outside of the leg and/or a tingling that can travel all the way to the foot.

To differentiate piriformis syndrome from other causes of sciatica (such as a herniated disc in the low back), a simple test you can do on yourself is to pull your knee toward your opposite shoulder while lying on your back. Hold the involved knee toward the opposite shoulder for about 30 seconds and if piriformis syndrome is present, you'll feel a slight tingling along the outside of your leg. In my experience, piriformis syndrome is much more common than herniated discs in runners.

While most researchers refer to piriformis syndrome as an isolated entity in which the sciatic nerve is irritated only by the piriformis, researchers from Austria determined that this muscle fuses with the neighboring obturator internus and/or gluteus medius muscles in more than 40% of the population (93) (Fig. 6.52). In addition to the sciatic nerve getting pinched beneath the piriformis, these researchers proved that the nerve can also be trapped against the obturator internus.

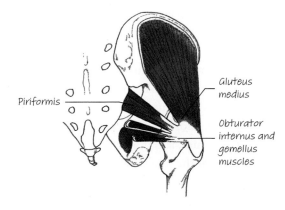

Fig. 6.52. *The tendon of the piriformis frequently merges with the tendons of the obturator internus and gluteus medius muscles.*

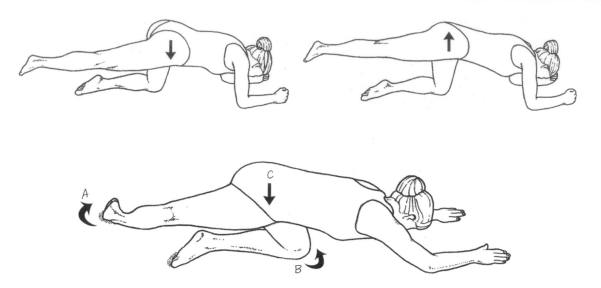

Fig. 6.53. *Hip rotator muscle energy stretch. This is an important stretch because it allows you to access specific fibers of each of the hip external rotators. To stretch the left hip external rotators, get on all fours with your weight supported by the left knee. At first, the right leg is held in a horizontal position. By using the left hip external rotator muscles, raise and lower the right hip up and down (**arrows**). Once the left hip fatigues slightly (after about a minute), touch the right leg to the ground by pulling it back and toward the left (**arrow A**). By varying the degree of hip flexion (**arrow B**) you can isolate specific muscle fibers responsible for limiting motion. The piriformis stretch illustrated in Fig. 3.20, Q, is also an effective way to lengthen the hip external rotators.*

Regardless of which muscles are involved, conventional treatments for piriformis syndrome emphasize stretching the hip rotators to lessen tension on the sciatic nerve. Because the gluteus medius, piriformis, and obturator internus muscles work together to cause this syndrome, it is important to stretch the hip abductors as well as the hip rotators. The most effective method to lengthen the hip external rotators is with the muscle energy stretch illustrated in Fig. 6.53.

Prior to performing the hip rotator stretch, I like to have runners use a softball to massage the piriformis and gluteus medius muscles. Because the piriformis is thickest where it leaves the sacrum, it is important to loosen this specific area of the muscle prior to stretching (Fig. 6.54).

You should be careful while massaging the piriformis to make sure you don't irritate the

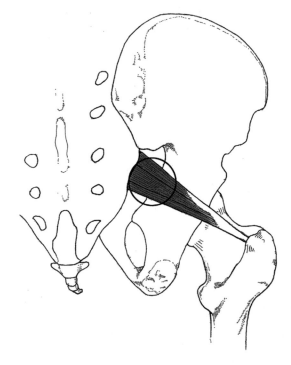

Fig. 6.54. *Prior to stretching, it is important to loosen the section of the piriformis closest to the sacrum (circle).*

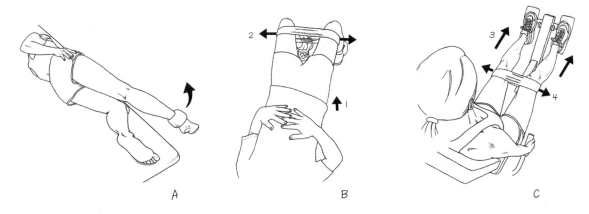

Fig. 6.55. *Gluteus maximus and medius strengthening exercises.* **A**) *While keeping the pelvis stationary with the upper leg hanging off the edge of a workout bench, raise and lower the upper leg through a 45° range of motion.* **B**) *With your shoulders resting flat on the floor, perform a plank by raising your pelvis (**1**) and then actively abduct your hips by pushing your knees outward against resistance provided by a TheraBand (**2**).* **C**) *This exercise requires a leg press, which is available at most gyms. The leg press is performed by moving your knees through the final 30° of extension (i.e., with the knees almost straight). While pushing the press (**3**), you simultaneously abduct your hips against resistance provided by a TheraBand (**4**).*

sciatic nerve: Focus the massage near the sacrum and along the outside of the hip. You can tell if you're accidentally hitting the sciatic nerve because your leg will go slightly numb. To avoid irritating the nerve, it is important to hold stretches for no more than 20 or 30 seconds, since a prolonged stretch can also pinch the nerve. As a rule, the stretches should be done frequently throughout the day for short durations only.

Even though sports doctors suggest that piriformis syndrome can be corrected with stretches alone, it is almost always necessary to strengthen the hip musculature when treating this condition. Some great research shows that compared to conventional stretches alone, hip strengthening exercises hasten recovery and result in improved outcomes when treating piriformis syndrome (94, 95). Fig. 6.55 describes specific exercises that target the gluteus medius and maximus muscles. These exercises are especially important in runners who cannot generate 20% of their body weight in the test illustrated in Fig. 3.26.

To decrease the potential for reinjury, runners with piriformis syndrome often have to change the way they sit and sleep. Because rotating the hip up and out reduces tension in the piriformis, runners with this injury tend to sit and sleep with their legs folded in a figure 4 position (i.e., with the foot of the involved side touching the opposite knee). Even though this position reduces tension on the sciatic nerve and feels comfortable, it is troublesome because it allows the piriformis to tighten even more, potentially worsening the discomfort while running. Most runners are unaware they are rotating the injured side outward, and it can take months to correct the faulty sitting and sleeping positions. To reduce the potential for chronicity, runners with piriformis syndromes should sleep on their side with a pillow folded between their knees, and sit with their knees straight. Because piriformis syndrome tends to produce low-grade discomfort that can go on for months, it is usually possible to continue running with this injury. To reduce strain on the piriformis while running, consider shortening your stride by increasing your cadence 10%.

GREATER TROCHANTERIC PAIN SYNDROME

The greater trochanter is the large bone you feel on the outside of your hip, and greater trochanteric pain syndrome is a condition in which the soft tissues around this bony prominence become chronically painful. Next to arthritis, greater trochanteric pain syndrome is the most frequently encountered hip injury in older runners, especially women. Until recently, it was assumed that this injury resulted from a chronic pinching of the bursa located between the greater trochanter and the iliotibial band. This bursa was thought to be compressed when the upper portion of the band snaps over the greater trochanter while running (Fig. 6.56). The standard medical intervention has been to inject the inflamed bursa with corticosteroids.

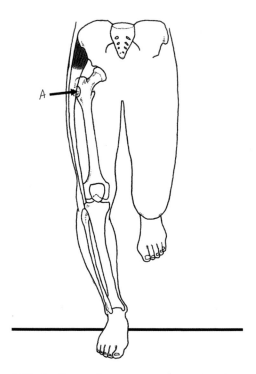

Fig. 6.56. *Until recently, greater trochanteric pain syndrome was thought to result from the iliotibial band compressing a bursa located on the outside of the hip (A).*

Although effective in the short term, corticosteroid injections have been proven to have poor long-term outcomes. More recently, research has shown that it is not the bursa that causes the chronic pain associated with this syndrome, but degeneration of the gluteus medius tendon insertion. By comparing MRI findings between the painful greater trochanter and the opposite symptom-free greater trochanter, researchers from New Zealand proved that inflammation of the bursa has nothing to do with this injury, and that in every situation, the pain could be related to degeneration of the gluteus medius tendon (96). As a result, treatment interventions to correct greater trochanteric pain syndromes should focus on improving tendon function, not reducing inflammation in the bursa.

The most effective way to treat this common condition is with the stretches and exercises described in Table 6.4. In a paper published in 2009 in the *American Journal of Sports Medicine*, strengthening exercises were found to be more effective than corticosteroid injection for the long-term management of greater trochanteric pain syndrome (97). In addition to these exercises, deep tissue massage of the tendon attachment is an effective way to stimulate repair. My favorite way to access the gluteus medius tendon is to have a runner lie face up with the hip pulled slightly outward. I then use my thumb to get right on the attachment point of the gluteus medius tendon and perform cross friction massage. An alternate technique to stimulate repair in this tendon is with the use of shockwave therapy. While strength training has great long-term outcomes, shockwave therapy produces significantly better results during the first four months compared to exercises alone (97).

Table 6.4. *Home training program for greater trochanteric pain syndrome, recommended by Rompe et al. (97).*

Piriformis stretch. Lie on your back with both knees bent and the foot of the uninjured leg flat on the floor. Rest the ankle of your injured leg over the knee of your uninjured leg. Grasp the thigh of the uninjured leg, and pull that knee toward your chest. You will feel a stretch along the buttocks and possibly along the outside of your thigh on the injured side. Hold this stretch for 30 to 60 seconds. Repeat 3 times.

Iliotibial band stretch standing. Cross your uninjured leg in front of your injured leg, and bend down and touch your toes. You can move your hands across the floor toward the uninjured side, and you will feel more stretch on the outside of your thigh on the injured side. Hold this position for 30 seconds. Return to the starting position. Repeat 3 times.

Straight leg raise. Lie on the floor on your back, and tighten up the top of the thigh muscles on your injured leg. Point your toes up toward the ceiling, and lift your leg up off the floor about 10 inches (25 cm). Keep your knee straight. Slowly lower your leg back down to the floor. Repeat 10 times. Do 3 sets of 10.

Wall squat with ball. Stand with your back, shoulders, and head against a wall, and look straight ahead. Keep your shoulders relaxed and your feet 12 inches (30.5 cm) away from the wall, shoulder-width apart. Place a rolled-up pillow or a ball between your thighs. Keeping your head against the wall, slowly squat while squeezing the pillow or ball at the same time. Squat down until your thighs are parallel to the floor. Hold this position for 10 seconds. Slowly stand back up. Make sure you are squeezing the pillow or ball throughout this exercise. Repeat 20 times.

Gluteal strengthening. To strengthen your buttock muscles, lie on your stomach with your legs straight out behind you. Tighten your buttock muscles, and lift your injured leg off the floor 8 inches (20 mm), keeping your knee straight. Hold for 5 seconds, and then relax and return to the starting position. Repeat 10 times. Do 3 sets of 10.

All exercises are performed twice a day, 7 days a week, for 12 weeks.

Reproduced exactly as described by the authors.

Because greater trochanteric pain syndrome is notorious for lasting more than six months, it is often necessary to cross train on a bike or begin swimming while you gradually strengthen the tendon. To avoid reinjury, many runners with this condition report less discomfort by reducing their stride length and increasing cadence by 10%. Greater trochanteric pain syndrome is a surprisingly difficult injury to treat, and it is very important to remain patient while this injury gradually resolves.

ADDUCTOR STRAINS

The adductor muscle group is located in the upper thigh and consists of the adductor longus, brevis, and magnus muscles. Adductor strains are the most common cause of groin pain in runners. Fast runners with long strides are especially prone to developing this injury. Although any of the adductor muscles may be involved, the adductor longus is by far the most frequently injured. While some experts suggest the adductor longus is injured because it has such a poor blood supply, the real reason this muscle is so frequently injured is because its tendon is so small. In a detailed three-dimensional study of the cross-sectional shape of the adductor longus tendon, researchers from NYU (98) observed that within an inch of its attachment to the pelvis, the tendon of the adductor longus thinned rapidly and was less than ⅛ inch (3 mm) in diameter. The rapid narrowing of its upper tendon makes the adductor longus susceptible to strains, particularly when the adductors are assisting with flexing the hip at the initiation of swing phase.

While early research suggested that a lack of flexibility was likely to produce adductor strain, more recent research, in 2010, suggested that prior injury and/or adductor weakness is more likely to produce an adductor injury. In their evaluation of various risk factors responsible for the development of adductor injuries, Engebretsen et al. (99) found that previously injured individuals were more than twice as likely to sustain a new adductor injury, and individuals with weak adductors were four times more likely to be injured. This is consistent with research published in the *American Journal of Sports Medicine*, in which athletes with adductor weakness were 17 times more likely to develop adductor muscle strain, and no correlation between adductor inflexibility and future injury was found (100).

The fact that adductor injuries are the result of adductor weakness, not tightness, is consistent with an evaluation of exercise protocols by Holmich et al. (101). By comparing a conventional treatment program of massage, stretching, and various physical therapy modalities to a 12-week strengthening program, the authors demonstrated that while the conventional treatments of massage and stretching were ineffective, 79% of the strengthened athletes were able to return to their prior level of sport within five months. Table 6.5 lists the exercises used in this study.

Table 6.5. *Adductor strengthening program.*

First 2 weeks

1. Place a soccer ball between your *ankles* while lying face up and squeeze for 30 seconds. Repeat 10 times.
2. Place a soccer ball between your *knees* while lying face up and squeeze for 30 seconds. Repeat 10 times.
3. Sit-ups, both in straight forward direction and in oblique direction; 5 sets of 10 reps.
4. Combined sit-up and hip flexion: Lying on your back with a soccer ball placed between your knees, do a sit-up while flexing your hips and torso (folding knife exercise); 5 sets of 10 reps.
5. Balance training on wobble board for five minutes.
6. One-foot exercises on sliding board, with parallel feet; 5 sets of one-minute continuous work with each leg in both positions. Because most runners don't have access to a sliding board, I recommend doing the grapevine running drills illustrated in the bottom of Fig. 4.5.

Weeks 3 to 12

(Two sets of each exercise, done twice at each training session.)

1. Continue step 2 from above.
2. Perform low back extension exercises while lying facedown over a workout bench or physioball; 5 sets of 10 reps. See Fig. 3.30, R, on page 109.
3. One-leg weight-pulling abduction/adduction standing; 5 reps for each leg (see Fig. 3.30, L and N).
4. Abdominal sit-ups both in straight forward direction and in oblique direction; 5 sets of 10 reps.
5. One-leg coordination exercise flexing and extending knee and swinging arms in same rhythm (cross-country skiing on one leg); 5 sets of 10 reps on each leg.
6. Training in sideward motion on a "Fitter" (a rocking platform that rolls laterally on tracks positioned on top of a curved base) for five minutes. If not available, perform the grapevine exercises illustrated at the bottom of Fig. 4.5 for five minutes.
7. Balance training on wobble board for five minutes.
8. Skating movements on sliding board; 5 sets of one-minute continuous work.

Modified from Holmich et al. [101].

Perpetuating factors such as sleeping on your side with the injured hip adducted and/or sitting in chairs with knees higher than hips should be avoided. Aggressive strengthening exercises should only be prescribed after a full range of hip abduction has been restored. While you're waiting for the adductor injury to heal, compressive thigh wraps made of neoprene reduce stress on the adductor tendon and can allow you to run short distances. Because the adductor tendon is strained at the initiation of swing phase, it is important to run with short strides. Once this condition has healed, you should consider routinely incorporating grapevine drills prior to running. Remember, once this tendon has been injured, it is prone to being chronically reinjured, so you have to warm this tendon up carefully.

OSTEITIS PUBIS

Also referred to as "pubic symphysitis," osteitis pubis occurs when excessive movement of the pelvic bones produces pain in and around the pubic symphysis (Fig. 6.57).

In the early stages of osteitis pubis, the runner complains of vague lower abdominal pain and/or adductor muscle discomfort. As symptoms progress, the pain becomes more localized to the pubic symphysis, and may be amplified by running on uneven surfaces, such as trails. On occasion, the pubic symphysis may make a clicking sound when you stand from a seated position. Because the pubic symphysis is well designed to manage the forces associated with running, osteitis pubis tends to occur only in high-mileage long-distance runners. Elite females returning to sport after having a baby are especially susceptible to developing this injury.

The most common biomechanical causes for osteitis pubis are limb length discrepancy and muscle imbalances. Limb length discrepancies greatly stress the pubic symphysis because the pelvic bones rotate in opposite directions to accommodate the discrepancy (102) (Fig. 6.58).

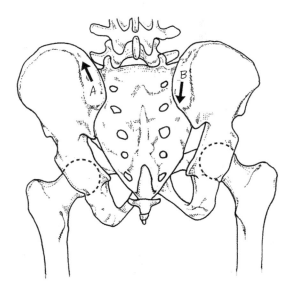

Fig. 6.58. *To accommodate a limb length discrepancy, the pelvis on the side of the short limb tilts forward (A), while the pelvis on the side of the long limb tilts back (B).*

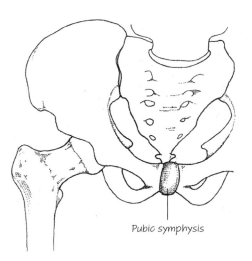

Pubic symphysis

Fig. 6.57. *The pubic symphysis is a fibrocartilaginous disc located in the front of the pelvis.*

While the counter-rotations of the pelvic bones level the pelvis and lessen strain on the lumbar spine, they twist the pubic symphysis and increase the likelihood of developing this injury. As a result, limb lengths should be carefully evaluated, including the evaluation of asymmetrical pronation as a possible cause of limb length discrepancy. When necessary, asymmetrical pronation should be treated with the appropriate lift and/or orthotic.

The typical muscle imbalance responsible for the development of osteitis pubis is weakness of the core muscles coupled with excessive tightness in the hip flexors. This combination allows the pelvis to hyperextend during late midstance, which creates a shearing of the pubic symphysis (Fig. 6.59). Treatment in this situation is to improve

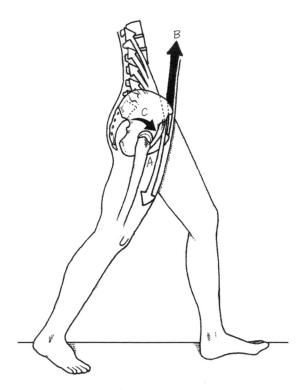

Fig. 6.59. *Tightness in the hip flexors (A), along with weakness of the core (B), stresses the pubic symphysis because the pelvis on that side hyperextends during propulsion (C).*

hip flexibility and strengthen the core muscles. Unfortunately, even when treated properly, osteitis pubis can last six months or more, and the best way to deal with this troublesome condition is to prevent it from occurring in the first place by keeping your hips flexible and your core strong.

LOW BACK DISORDERS

Over the past seven million years, the low back has gradually undergone redesign so it can easily manage the impact forces associated with walking and running. In fact, you're more likely to herniate a disc with prolonged sitting than with high-mileage running. Nonetheless, running-related back injuries do occur and they can usually be related to a variety of mechanical factors, such as muscle weakness/tightness and/or compensation for limb length discrepancy.

A common cause of low back pain in runners is weakness of the core muscles. When your foot hits the ground, weak core muscles allow your lowest lumbar vertebrae to shift forward, potentially damaging the joints of the low back. Weak core muscles are particularly likely to produce low back pain if your hip flexors are tight, because the lumbar spine is forced to hyperextend with each stride. A classic sign of core weakness is that your low back pain is worsened while running downhill and relieved while running uphill.

To test your core strength, try holding a side plank for 60 seconds on each side. If you're unable to maintain the plank for the full 60 seconds, start doing the exercises illustrated in Fig. 6.60. Begin by holding each position for 20 seconds and repeat three times daily. After a few weeks, you should be able to easily hold a side plank for 60 seconds.

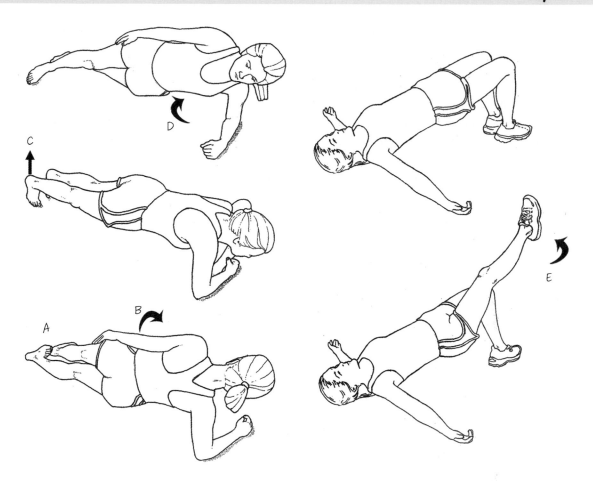

Fig. 6.60. *Core exercises. With the front heel touching the toes of the back foot (**A**), maintain a sidelying plank for 20 seconds. By placing your arms parallel, rotate your torso 90° into a conventional plank (**B**). Try to hold this position for 20 seconds while raising one leg at a time for five seconds (**C**). You finish this exercise by again rotating 90° (**D**), holding the final side plank for 20 seconds. This cycle is usually repeated three times. Another excellent core exercise is to maintain a standard bridge position while raising a straightened lower leg (**E**). The leg is held in an elevated position for five seconds while maintaining the pelvis in a fixed position. Three sets of 5 repetitions while alternating legs is usually sufficient to strengthen the core.*

Another cause of low back pain in runners is tightness of the spinal stabilizer muscles (Fig. 6.61). Because these muscles help absorb impact by decelerating forward motion of the spine, almost all high-mileage runners have tight spinal stabilizers. Tightness in these muscles can produce delayed onset muscle soreness following long runs and can even hurt during the run, since excessive tightness in these muscles can compress the joints of the low back.

To test the flexibility of your spinal stabilizers, stand up and tilt sideward while moving your hand toward the outside of your knee (Fig. 6.62).

Repeat this tilting motion on the opposite side and compare flexibility. If you can reach farther on one side than the other, perform the stretches illustrated in Fig. 6.63. Each stretch is typically held for about 20 seconds and repeated at least three times per day. It usually takes about a

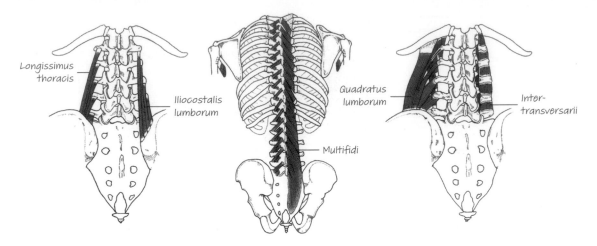

Longissimus thoracis

Iliocostalis lumborum

Quadratus lumborum

Inter-transversarii

Multifidi

Fig. 6.61. *The spinal stabilizers.*

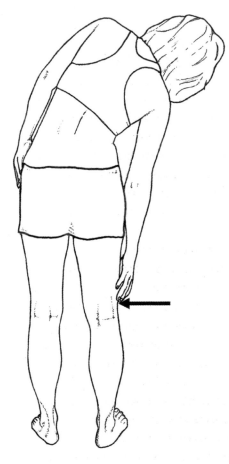

Fig. 6.62. *Testing tension in the spinal stabilizers.*
Compare the distance you can move your hand down your thigh on each side (arrow). Make sure you tilt directly to the side and avoid bending forward or backward.

month of regular stretching to improve flexibility, and after that, you will have to perform the stretches preventively to maintain flexibility.

Despite its strong ligaments, the sacroiliac joint is also an occasional source of pain in runners. Although difficult to diagnose, sacroiliac sprains usually produce a toothache-type pain directly over the joint, and the ligaments covering the back of the joint are frequently painful to touch. The process of transitioning from a sitting to a standing position is surprisingly uncomfortable, and the runner often limps to the opposite side to avoid compressing the inflamed sacroiliac joint. Rare in older runners because the joint is fused by the time you are in your 50s, sacroiliac pain is more likely to occur in young female long-distance runners, especially following childbirth because the hormone relaxin loosens the joints of the pelvis to assist in delivery.

Treating sacroiliac sprains can be difficult because the sacroiliac joint is stabilized almost exclusively by ligaments. One of the only muscles that can provide protection if the sacroiliac joint is unstable is the transversus abdominis, which sends muscle fibers across the front

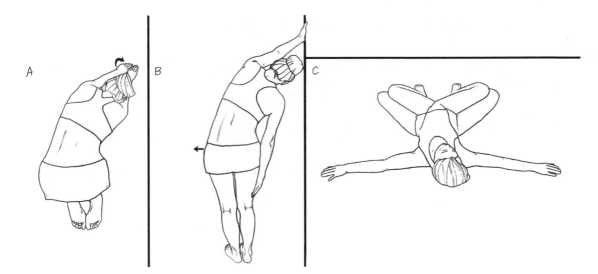

Fig. 6.63. **Low back stretches. A)** *Kneeling quadratus lumborum stretch: Squat down so your hips are directly over your heels and use your hands to pull your torso to the right (arrow). This stretches the left quadratus lumborum.* **B)** *Standing quadratus lumborum stretch: With your feet touching, grab the top of a door jam and shift your pelvis away from the door* (**arrow**). *By grabbing the door jamb at different points and altering the degree of spinal flexion, different spinal stabilizers can be stretched.* **C)** *Lumbar rotational stretch: Lie on your back and gently rock your flexed knees from side to side. This motion stretches the multifidi, and if asymmetrical rotation is present, spend more time moving in the direction of the restriction.*

of the sacrum. To test if you are weak in the transversus abdominis, perform Vleeming's test illustrated in Fig. 3.31. If your pelvis lifts off the table more than a few degrees, do the strengthening exercises illustrated in Fig. 6.60.

An important perpetuator of sacroiliac pain that needs to be corrected is tightness in the piriformis. Because this muscle attaches to the front of the sacrum, a tight piriformis can pull the sacrum to one side, chronically stressing the sacroiliac joints. The muscle energy stretch illustrated at the bottom of Fig. 6.53 is the easiest way to lengthen the piriformis.

To help in the diagnosis and possibly assist in the treatment, runners with painful sacroiliac joints should consider wearing a sacroiliac stabilizing belt. If you feel better while wearing this belt, you probably have a sacroiliac joint injury. Runners with sacroiliac sprains should wear the stabilizing belt until they correct any problem with core

weakness and/or piriformis tightness. In theory, these belts apply a stabilizing compressive force that protects an unstable sacroiliac joint from the excessive shear forces present while running. Even though I see mixed results with these belts, chronic sacroiliac sprains can be difficult to treat so they are always worth trying.

While unlikely to produce low back pain in the general population, small limb length discrepancies can cause chronic low back pain in runners. By embedding metal beads in the sacrum and pelvis while subjects stood on different-sized heel lifts, researchers determined that the pelvis shifts in very specific directions when limb length discrepancies are present (102) (Fig. 6.64).

As a result, in addition to lifts, runners with limb length discrepancies should perform the stretches illustrated in Fig. 6.65. In some situations, chiropractic adjustments may be

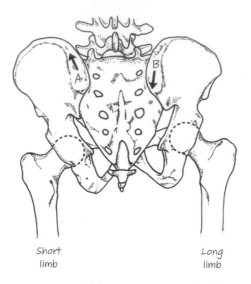

Short   Long
limb   limb

Fig. 6.64. *Pelvic movements to compensate for limb length discrepancy.* *The pelvis on the side of the short limb tilts forward (**A**), while the pelvis on the side of the long limb tilts back (**B**).*

needed to restore motion and reduce tension in the surrounding muscles and ligaments.

Ironically, many runners injure their low backs while performing stretches and exercises

designed to prevent low back pain. For example, many yoga instructors inappropriately recommend spinal unwinds, in which individual vertebra are gradually flexed forward. As pointed out by the spinal researcher Stuart McGill (103), the discs of the lumbar spine were not designed to tolerate forward bending, so to remain injury free, you should avoid flexing your spine excessively. The stretches most likely to injure your back are illustrated in Fig. 6.66.

Another common practice that may inadvertently result in low back injury is the recommendation that runners should run with their spines flat and their belly buttons tucked in. These concepts are taken from tai chi and Pilates, in which drawing in of the bellybutton is believed to recruit the transversus abdominis and stabilize the low back. Unfortunately, this belief is unsubstantiated, since the spine is most stable when held with a slight arch. A mild curve in the low back has been proven to distribute force more evenly between the discs and the joints

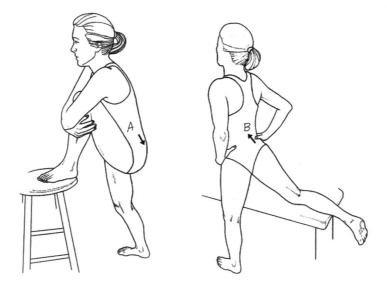

Fig. 6.65. *Home mobilizations for limb length discrepancy.* *On the side of the short limb, pull your knee toward your chest (**A**). This motion flexes the pelvis on that side. On the side of the long limb, place your knee on a chair or workout bench and extend the hip on that side (**B**). The stretches are typically held for 20 seconds and performed five times daily.*

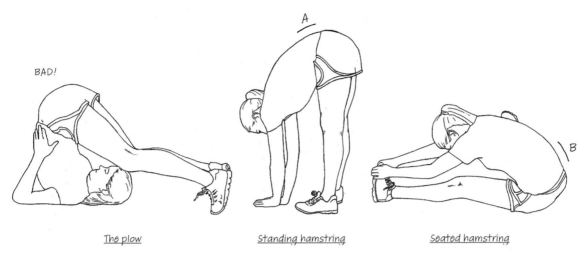

BAD!

The plow

Standing hamstring

Seated hamstring

Fig. 6.66. *Common stretches incorporating excessive forward flexion.* *While the plow stretch is always troublesome, the standing and seated hamstring stretches can be useful as long as you avoid flexing your lumbar spine excessively (**A** and **B**).*

while displacing the gel component of the disc forward (Fig. 6.67).

Maintaining a slight curve while running effectively distributes pressure between the

joints in the discs and allows the muscles of the low back to work in a more efficient manner (Fig. 6.68).

As with all running injuries, the best way to manage low back pain is to identify and correct all potential sources of injury. As pointed out throughout this book, the annual reinjury rates for runners should not be 70%. By quickly treating running injuries with proven treatment

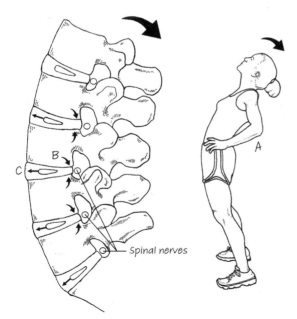

Spinal nerves

Fig. 6.67. *Side view of the lumbar spine.* *Arching your spine into extension (**A**) compresses the back portions of the lumbar discs (**B**), displacing the gel-like nucleus of the discs forward (**C**), away from the spinal nerves.*

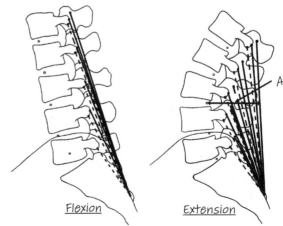

Flexion

Extension

Fig. 6.68. *Extension of the lumbar spine improves muscle efficiency by increasing the length of the lever arm afforded to the spinal stabilizers (A).*

protocols, you can markedly reduce your potential for reinjury. Remember, recreational running is no more stressful on the body than fast walking, and with a little effort, there's no reason you can't continue running into your 80s and 90s.

REFERENCES

1. Fredericson M, Anuruddh M. Epidemiology and etiology of marathon running injuries. *Sports Med*. 2007;37:437–439.

2. van Mechelen W. Running injuries: a review of the epidemiological literature. *Sports Med*. 1992;4:320.

3. Leonard W, Robertson M. Rethinking the energetics of bipedality. *Current Anthropol*. 1997;38:304–309.

4. Pierce B, Murr S, Moss R. *Run Less Run Faster*. New York: Rodale Books, 2007.

5. van Gent R, Siem G, van Middelkoop M, et al. Incidence and determinants of lower extremity running injuries in long distance runners: a systematic review. *Br J Sports Med*. 2007;41:469–480.

6. Reinking M, Austin T, Hayes A. Exercise-related leg pain and collegiate cross-country athletes: extrinsic and intrinsic factors. *J Orthop Sports Phys Ther*. 2007;37:670–678.

7. Sherry M, Best T. A comparison of 2 rehabilitation programs in the treatment of acute hamstring strains. *J Orthop Sports Phys Ther*. 2004;34:116.

8. Mahieu NN, Witvrouw E, Stevens V, et al. Intrinsic risk factors for the development of Achilles tendon overuse injuries. *Am J Sports Med*. 2006;34(2):226–235.

9. Lyman J, Weinhold P, Almekinders LC. Strain behavior of the distal Achilles tendon. *Am J Sports Med*. 2004;32(2):457–461.

10. Wezenbeek E, Willems T, Mahieu N, et al. Is Achilles tendon blood flow related to foot pronation? *Scand J Med Sci Sports*. 2017;27(12):1970–1977.

11. Tabary J, Tabary C, Tardieu C, et al. Physiological and structural changes in the cat's soles muscle due to immobilization at different lengths by plaster casts. *J Physiol*. 1972;224:231–244.

12. O'Neill S, Barry S, Watson P. Plantar flexor strength and endurance deficits associated with the mid-portion Achilles tendinopathy: the role of soleus. *Phys Ther Sport*. 2019;37:69–76.

13. Slane L, Thelen D. Non-uniform displacements within the Achilles tendon observed during passive and eccentric loading. *J Biomech*. 2014;47:2831–2835.

14. Slane L, Thelen D. Achilles tendon displacement patterns during passive stretch and eccentric loading are altered in middle-aged adults. *Med Eng Phys*. 2015;11:1–5.

15. Alfredson H, Pietila T, Jonsson P, et al. Heavy-load eccentric calf muscle training for the treatment of chronic Achilles tendinosis. *Am J Sports Med*. 1998;26(3):360–366.

16. Yin N, Chen W, Wu Y, et al. Increased patellar tendon microcirculation and reduction of tendon stiffness following knee extension eccentric exercises. *J Orthop Sports Phys Ther*. 2014;44:304.

17. Williams D, Zambardino J, Banning V. Transverse-plane mechanics at the knee and tibia in runners with and without a history of Achilles tendinopathy. *J Orthop Sports Phys Ther*. 2008;38:761–767.

18. Davidson CJ, Ganion LR, Gehlsen GM, et al. Rat tendon morphological and functional changes resulting from soft tissue mobilization. *Med Sci Sports Exerc*. 1997;29(3):313–319.

19. Hugate R, Pennypacker J, Saunders M, Juliano P. The effects of intratendinous injections of corticosteroid on the biomechanical properties of rabbit Achilles tendons. *J Bone Joint Surg Am.* 2004;86:794–801.

20. Hughes L. Biomechanical analysis of the foot and ankle for predisposition to developing stress fractures. *J Orthop Sports Phys Ther.* 1985;3:96–101.

21. Kim J, Choi J, Park J, et al. An anatomical study of Morton's interdigital neuroma: the relationship between the occurring site and the transverse metatarsal ligament (DTML). *Foot Ankle Int.* 2007;28:1007–1010.

22. Carl A, Ross S, Evanski P, et al. Hypermobility in hallux valgus. *Foot Ankle Int.* 1988; 8:264–270.

23. Stewart S, Ellis R, Heath M, Rome K. Ultrasonic evaluation of the abductor hallucis muscle in hallux valgus: a cross-sectional observational study. *BMC Musculoskelet Disord.* 2013;14:45.

24. Redmond A, Lumb P, Landorf K. The effect of cast and noncast foot orthoses on plantar pressures and force during gait. *J Am Podiatr Med Assoc.* 2000;90:441–449.

25. Gray E, Basmajian J. Electromyography and cinematography of the leg and foot ("normal" and flat) during walking. *Anat Rec.* 1968;161:1–15.

26. Okuda R, Kinoshita M, Yasuda T, et al. Hallux valgus angle as a predictor of recurrence following proximal metatarsal osteotomy. *J Orthop Sci.* 2011;16:760–764.

27. Michaud T, Nawoczenski D. The influence of two different types of foot orthoses on first metatarsophalangeal joint kinematics during gait in a single subject. *J Manip Phys Ther.* 2006;29:60–65.

28. Welsh B, Redmond A, Chockalingam N, Keenan A. A case-series study to explore the efficacy of foot orthoses in treating first metatarsophalangeal joint pain. *J Foot Ankle Res.* 2010;3:17.

29. Abreu M, Chung C, Mendes L, et al. Plantar calcaneal enthesophytes: new observations regarding sites of origin based on radiographic, MR imaging, anatomic, and paleopathologic analysis. *Skeletal Radiol.* 2003;32:13–21.

30. Wearing S, Smeathers J, Yates B, et al. Sagittal movement of the medial longitudinal arch is unchanged in plantar fasciitis. *Med Sci Sports Exerc.* 2004;36:1761–1767.

31. Sullivan J, et al. Musculoskeletal and activity-related factors associated with plantar heel pain. *Foot Ankle Int.* 2015;36:37–45.

32. DiGiovanni B, Nawoczenski D, Lintal M, et al. Tissue-specific plantar fascia-stretching exercise enhances outcomes in patients with chronic heel pain. A prospective, randomized study. *J Bone Joint Surg Am.* 2003;85(7):1270–1277.

33. Landorf K, Keenan AM, Herbert R. The effectiveness of foot orthoses to treat plantar fasciitis: a randomized trial. *Arch Intern Med.* 2006;166:1305–1310.

34. Kogler G, Solomonidis S, Paul J. Biomechanics of longitudinal arch support mechanisms in foot orthoses and their effect on plantar aponeurosis strain. *Clin Biomech.* 1996;11:243–252.

35. Kogler G, Veer F, Solomonidis S, Paul J. The influence of medial and lateral placement of orthotic wedges on loading of the plantar aponeurosis. *J Bone Joint Surg Am.* 1999;81:1403–1413.

36. Coppieters M, Hough A, Dilley A. Different nerve-gliding exercises induce different magnitudes of median nerve longitudinal excursion: an *in vivo* study using dynamic ultrasound imaging. *J Orthop Sports Phys Ther.* 2009;39:164.

37. McKeon PC, Mattacola CG. Interventions for the prevention of first time and recurrent ankle sprains. *Clin Sports Med.* 2008;27:371–382.

38. Heiderscheit B, Chumanov E, Michalski M, et al. Effects of step rate manipulation on joint mechanics during running. *Med Sci Sports Exerc.* 2011;43:296–302.

39. Verhagen E, van Mechelen W, de Vente W. The effect of preventive measures on the incidence of ankle sprains. *Clin J Sport Med.* 2000;10:291–296.

40. Tyler TF, McHugh MP, Mirabella MR, et al. Risk factors for noncontact ankle sprains in high school football players: the role of previous ankle sprains and body mass index. *Am J Sports Med.* 2006;34:471–475.

41. Delahunt E, Monaghan K, Caulfield B. Altered neuromuscular control and ankle joint kinematics during walking in subjects with functional instability of the ankle joint. *Am J Sports Med.* 2006;34:1970–1976.

42. Malliaropoulos N, Ntessalen M, Papacostsa E, et al. Reinjury after acute lateral ankle sprains in elite track and field athletes. *Am J Sports Med.* 2009;37:1755.

43. Magnusson H, Westlin N, Nyqvist F, et al. Abnormally decreased regional bone density in athletes with medial tibial stress syndrome. *Am J Sports Med.* 2001;29:712–715.

44. Beynnon B, Renstrom P, Haugh L, et al. A prospective, randomized clinical investigation of the treatment of first-time ankle sprains. *Am J Sports Med.* 2006;34:1401.

45. McHugh M, Tyler T, Mirabella M, et al. The effectiveness of a balance training intervention in reducing the incidence of noncontact ankle sprains in high school football players. *Am J Sports Med.* 2007;35:1289.

46. Verhagen E, van der Beek A, Twisk J, et al. The effect of proprioceptive balance board training for the prevention of ankle sprains. *Am J Sports Med.* 2004;32:1385–1393.

47. Styf J. Chronic exercise-induced pain in the anterior aspect of the lower leg: an overview of diagnosis. *Sports Med.* 1989;7:331–339.

48. Franklyn M, Oakes B, Field B, et al. Section modulus is the optimum geometric predictor for stress fractures and medial tibial stress syndrome in both males and female athletes. *Am J Sports Med.* 2008;36:1179.

49. Burne S, Khan K, Boudville P, et al. Risk factors associated with exertional medial tibial pain: a 12-month prospective clinical study. *Br J Sports Med.* 2004;38:441–445.

50. Franklyn-Miller A, Wilson C, Bilzon J, McCrory P. Foot orthoses in the prevention of injury in initial military training: a randomized controlled trial. *Am J Sports Med.* 2011;39:30.

51. Andrish JT, Bergfeld JA, Walheim J. A prospective study on the management of shin splints. *J Bone Joint Surg Am.* 1974;56:1697–1700.

52. Cohen D, Kawamura S, Ehteshami J, Rodeo S. Indomethacin and celecoxib impair rotator cuff tendon-to-bone healing. *Am J Sports Med.* 2006;34:362–369.

53. Bennell K, Malcolm S, Thomas S, et al. The incidence and distribution of stress fractures in competitive track and field athletes. A twelve-month prospective study. *Am J Sports Med.* 1996;24:211–217.

54. Crowell H, Milner C, Hamill J, Davis I. Reducing impact loading during running with the use of real-time visual feedback. *J Orthop Sports Phys Ther.* 2010;40:206.

55. Matheson GO, Clement DB, McKenzie DC. Stress fractures in athletes. A study of 320 cases. *Am J Sports Med.* 1987;15:46–58.

56. Wakeling J, Nigg B. Modifications of soft tissue vibrations in the leg by muscular activity. *J Appl Physiol.* 2001;90:412–420.

57. Wakeling J, Liphardt A, Nigg B. Muscle activity reduces soft-tissue resonance at heel-strike during walking. *J Biomech.* 2003;36:1761–1769.

58. Agosta J, Morarty R. Biomechanical analysis of athletes with stress fracture of the tarsal navicular bone: a pilot study. *Aust J Podiatr Med.* 1999;33(1):13–18.

59. Burne S, Mahoney C, Forster B, et al. Tarsal navicular stress injury: long-term outcome and clinical radiological correlation using both computed tomography and magnetic resonance imaging. *Am J Sports Med.* 2005;33:1875–1881.

60. Milner C, Hamill J, Davis I. Distinct hip and rearfoot kinematics in female runners with a history of tibial stress fracture. *J Orthop Sports Phys Ther.* 2010;40:59–66.

61. Bulst I, Bredeweg S, van Mechelen W, et al. No effect of a graded training program on the number of running-related injuries in novice runners. A randomized controlled trial. *Am J Sports Med.* 2007;16:1–7.

62. Warden S, Davis I, Fredericson M. Management and prevention of bone stress injuries and long-distance runners. *J Orthop Sports Phys Ther.* 2014;44:749–765.

63. Kroll M, Bi C, Garber C, et al. Temporal relationship between vitamin D status and parathyroid hormone in the United States. *PLoS One.* 2015;10:e0118108.

64. Bert L, Billington E, Rose M, et al. Effect of high-dose vitamin D supplementation on volumetric bone density and bone strength: a randomized controlled trial. *JAMA.* 2019;322(8):736–745.

65. Glerup H, Mikkelsen K, Poulsen L, et al. Hypovitaminosis D myopathy without biochemical signs of osteomalacic bone involvement. *Calcif Tissue Int.* 2000;66:419–424.

66. Heikura I, Burke L, Hawley J, et al. A short-term ketogenic diet impairs markers of bone health in response to exercise. *Front Endocrinol.* 2019;10:880.

67. Powers C, Ward S, Fredericson M, et al. Patellofemoral kinematics during weight-bearing and non-weight-bearing knee extension in persons with lateral subluxation of the patella: a preliminary study. *J Orthop Sports Phys Ther.* 2003;33:677–685.

68. Lin YF, Jan MH, Lin DH, Cheng CK. Different effects of femoral and tibial rotation on the different measurements of patella tilting: an axial computed tomography study. *J Orthop Surg Res.* 2008;3:5.

69. Souza R, Draper C, Fredericson M, et al. Femur rotation and patellofemoral joint kinematics: a weight-bearing magnetic resonance imaging analysis. *J Orthop Sports Phys Ther.* 2010;40:277–285.

70. Dierks T, Manal K, Hamill J, Davis I. Proximal and distal influence on the hip and knee kinematics in runners with patellofemoral pain during a prolonged run. *J Orthop Sports Phys Ther.* 2008;38:448.

71. Williams D, McClay I, Hamill J, Buchanan T. Lower extremity kinematic and kinetic differences in runners with high and low arches. *J Appl Biomech.* 2001;17:153–163.

72. Collins N, Crossley K, Beller E, et al. Foot orthoses and physiotherapy in the treatment of patellofemoral pain syndrome: a randomised clinical trial. *BMJ.* 2008;337:a1735.

73. Molgaard C, Rathleff M, Andreasen J, et al. Foot exercises and foot orthoses are more effective than knee focused exercises in individuals with patellofemoral pain. *J Sci Med Sport.* 2018;21:10–15.

74. Witvrouw E, Lysens R, Bellemans J, et al. Intrinsic risk factors for the development of

anterior knee pain in an athletic population: a 2-year prospective study. *Am J Sports Med.* 2000;28:480.

75. van der Worp H, Ark M, Roerink S, et al. Risk factors for patellar tendinopathy: a systematic review of the literature. *Br J Sports Med.* 2011;45(5):446–462.

76. Zhang Z, NG G, Lee W, Fu S. Increase in passive muscle tension of the quadriceps muscle heads in jumping athletes with patellar tendinopathy. *Scand J Med Sci Sports.* 2017;27(10):1099–1104.

77. Takasaki H, Aoki M, Oshiro S, et al. Strain reduction of the extensor carpi radialis brevis tendon proximal origin following the application of a forearm support end. *J Orthop Sports Phys Ther.* 2008;38:257.

78. Wadsworth C, Nielsen D, Burns L, et al. Effect of the counterforce armband on wrist extension and grip strength and pain in subjects with tennis elbow. *J Orthop Sports Phys Ther.* 1989;5:192–197.

79. Kongsgard M, Qvortup K, Larsen J, et al. Fibril morphology and tendon mechanical properties in patellar tendinopathy. Effects of heavy slow resistance training. *Am J Sports Med.* 2010;38:749.

80. Escamilla R, Zheng N, Macleod T, et al. Patellofemoral joint force and stress between a short and long-step forward lunge. *J Orthop Sports Phys Ther.* 2008;38:681–690.

81. Fairclough J, Hayashi K, Toumi H, et al. The functional anatomy of the iliotibial band during flexion and extension of the knee: implications for understanding iliotibial band syndrome. *J Anat.* 2006;208:309–316.

82. Ferber R, Noehren B, Hamill J, et al. Competitive female runners with a history of iliotibial band syndrome demonstrate atypical hip and knee kinematics. *J Orthop Sports Phys Ther.* 2010;40:52.

83. Williams D, McClay I, Hamill J. Arch structure and injury patterns in runners. *Clin Biomech.* 2001;16:341–347.

84. Falvey E, Clark R, Franklyn-Miller A, et al. Iliotibial band syndrome: an examination of the evidence behind a number of treatment options. *Scand J Med Sci Sports.* 2010;20:580–587.

85. Chaudhry H, Schleip R, Ji Z, et al. Three-dimensional mathematical model for deformation of human fasciae in manual therapy. *J Am Osteopath Assoc.* 2008;108:379–390.

86. Thelen D, Chumanov E, Best T, et al. Simulation of biceps femoris musculotendon mechanics during the swing phase of sprinting. *Med Sci Sports Exerc.* 2005;37:1931–1938.

87. Askling C, Tengvar M, Saartok T, Thorstensson A. Proximal hamstring strains of stretching type in different sports: injury situations, clinical and magnetic resonance imaging characteristics, and return to sport. *Am J Sports Med.* 2008;36:1799–1804.

88. McHugh M, Connolly D, Eston R, et al. The role of passive muscle stiffness and symptoms of exercise-induced muscle damage. *Am J Sports Med.* 1999;27:594.

89. Hreljac A, Marshall RN, Hume PA. Evaluation of lower extremity overuse injury potential in runners. *Med Sci Sports Exerc.* 2000;32(9):1635–1641.

90. Verrall GM, Slavotinek JP, Barnes PG. The effect of sport specific training on reducing the incidence of hamstring injuries in professional Australian Rules football players. *Br J Sports Med.* 2005;39:363–368.

91. Hoskins W, Pollard H, Orchard J. The effect of sports chiropractic on the prevention of hamstring injuries: a randomized controlled trial. *Med Sci Sports Exerc.* 2006;38:S27.

92. Loghmani M, Warden S. Instrument-assisted cross-fiber massage accelerates knee ligament healing. *J Orthop Sports Phys Ther*. 2009;39:506–514.

93. Windisch G, Braun E, Anderhuber F. Piriformis muscle: clinical anatomy and consideration of the piriformis syndrome. *Surg Radiol Anat*. 2007;29:37–45.

94. Tonley J, Yun S, Kochevar R, et al. Treatment of an individual with piriformis syndrome focusing on hip muscle strengthening and movement reeducation: a case report. *J Orthop Sports Phys Ther*. 2010;40:103.

95. Hallin RP. Sciatic pain and the piriformis muscle. *Postgrad Med*. 1983;74:69–72.

96. Woodley S, Nicholson H, Livingstone V, et al. Lateral hip pain: findings from magnetic resonance imaging and clinical examination. *J Orthop Sports Phys Ther*. 2008;38:313.

97. Rompe J, Segal N, Cachio A, et al. Home training, local corticosteroid injection, or radio shock wave therapy for greater trochanteric pain syndrome. *Am J Sports Med*. 2009;37:1981.

98. Strauss E, Campbell K, Bosco J. Analysis of the cross-sectional area of the adductor longus tendon: a descriptive anatomic study. *Am J Sports Med*. 2007;35:996.

99. Engebretsen A, Myklebust G, Holme I, et al. Intrinsic risk factors for groin injuries among male soccer players: a prospective cohort study. *Am J Sports Med*. 2010;38:2051.

100. Tyler T, Nicholas S, Campbell R, McHugh M. The association of hip strength and flexibility with the incidence of adductor muscle strains in professional ice hockey players. *Am J Sports Med*. 2001;29:124.

101. Holmich P, Uhrskou P, Ulnits L, et al. Effectiveness of active physical training as treatment for long-standing adductor related groin pain in athletes: a randomized trial. *Lancet*. 1999;353:439.

102. Cummings G, Scholz J, Barnes K. The effect of imposed leg length difference on pelvic bone symmetry. *Spine*. 1993;18:368–373.

103. McGill S. *Low Back Disorders: Evidence-Based Prevention and Rehabilitation*. Champaign, IL: Human Kinetics Publishing, 2002.

INDEX

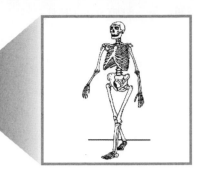

Bold italic numbers denote illustrations, tables and checklists.